Calculating and Reporting Healthcare Statistics

Sixth Edition

Susan White, PhD, RHIA, CHDA

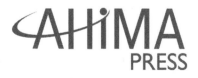

ISBN: **978-1-58426-683-9**
AHIMA Product No.: AB120718

AHIMA Staff:
Jessica Block, MA, Production Development Editor
Chelsea Brotherton, MA, Production Development Editor
Colton Gigot, MA, Production Development Editor
Megan Grennan, Managing Editor
Kimberly Hooker, Production Development Editor
James Pinnick, Senior Director of Publications
Rachel Schratz, MA, Assistant Editor

Cover image: © iStock: jxfzsy

For more information about AHIMA Press publications, including updates, visit http://www.ahima.org/education/press.

American Health Information Management Association
233 North Michigan Avenue, 21st Floor
Chicago, Illinois 60601-5809
ahima.org

Table of Contents

Online Resources
   Student data tables

About the Author

Susan White, PhD, RHIA, CHDA, is the administrator of analytics at the James Cancer Hospital at The Ohio State University Wexner Medical Center. White is an associate professor in the health information management and systems division at The Ohio State University where she teaches data analytics, healthcare finance, and database courses. White served on American Health Information Management Association's National Board of Directors from 2015–2018.

White is the author of AHIMA's *A Practical Approach to Analyzing Healthcare Data,* Third Edition, *Principles of Finance for Health Information and Informatics Professionals,* Second Edition, *Certified Health Data Analytics Exam Preparation,* Second Edition, as well as numerous peer and editor reviewed articles.

White is a regular presenter at the state and national level on healthcare data analytics, alternative payment models and big data. She earned her PhD in statistics from The Ohio State University.

Acknowledgments

Susan White, PhD, RHIA, CHDA, used the prior work compiled by Loretta Horton, Med, RHIA, FAHIMA, to prepare the revisions for this edition of the text. Dr. White offers a special thank you to Lou Ann Wiedemann, MS, RHIA, CDIP, CHDA, FAHIMA, for her technical advice and review of this text.

AHIMA Press and Susan White thank John Barrilleaux, MME, RHIA, and Tracey Pizzino, MSA, RHIT, CHDA, CPhT, for their technical reviews of this edition.

Thank you to each of the following reviewers for their insightful comments, suggestions and guidance throughout the development of this edition.

Gina Augustine, RHIT, COC, CPC
Nora Blankenbecler, MBA, RHIA
Kori Boeckeler, MEd, RHIA
Sonya Braddy, MHSA, RHIA, CCS
Jennifer Briscoe, MBA, RHIA
Nancy Carman, RHIA, CPC
Jane Ellis, MAT, RHIT
Romanza Forsythe, RN, BSN, RHIT
Deborah Gilbert, RHIA
Elisa Gorton, MAHSM, RHIA, CHPS, CHC
Kerry Heinecke, MS, RHIA
Christine Jerson, RHIA
Marissa LaJaunie, MBA, RHIA
Lisa Legere, RHIA
Gloria Madison, MS, RHIA, CHDA, CHTS-IM
Christina Manley, MAEd., RHIT
Maureen Millsom, BA, CHIMA
Tanya Mulder, BBA RHIT
Misty Neal, MBA, RHIA
Olivia Pollard, MA, RHIA, MCP, CLS, CDIP, CHTS-IM, CPHI
Paula Rehfus-Hagstrom, RHIA
Becky Rice, RHIT, CHTS-IS, CHTS-TS
Karen Shuler, MEd
Diana Skarbek, MHA, RHIA, CCS
Sherry Slay, RHIT
Debra Slusarczyk, RHIT
Martin Smith, BA, MAEd
Christopher Wheat, MS, RHIA, CCS, CCS-P

Student and Instructor Resources

For Students

To help students focus and gain more experience with the calculations, **student data tables** are provided for selected exercises in this text. Visit http://www.ahimapress.org/white6839 to register your unique student access code that is provided on the inside front cover of this text to download these files.

For Instructors

AHIMA provides the following supplementary resources to educators who use this text in their courses:

- **Instructor's manual.** Each chapter of the instructor's manual includes suggested student assignments and activities, key points for lecture notes, and a test bank with answers.
- **PowerPoint presentations.** Instructors can enhance their course lectures with these presentation slides that cover the key topics presented in each chapter.
- **Solutions manual.** Answers to all odd-numbered exercises are provided in appendix E at the back of this text. Answers to all exercise are provided to approved educators.
- **Course curriculum map.** Each chapter of this text is mapped to the AHIMA curricula domains for statistics.

Instructor materials for this text are provided only to approved educators. Please visit http://www.ahima.org/publications/educators.aspx for further instructions on how to access instructor resources.

Introduction to Health Statistics

Learning Objectives

At the conclusion of this chapter, you should be able to do the following:

- Recommend healthcare statistics
- Assess sources of data
- Compare and contrast between data and information, validity and reliability, descriptive and inferential statistics, and primary and secondary data sources
- Determine the users of healthcare statistics

Key Terms

Agency for Healthcare Research and
  Quality (AHRQ)
Ambulatory care facility
Census
Centers for Disease Control and
  Prevention (CDC)
Centers for Medicare and Medicaid
  Services (CMS)

Descriptive statistics
Encounter
Home health (HH)
Hospice
Inferential statistics
Inpatient
Inpatient census
Managed care organization (MCO)

Nursing facility
Outpatient
Primary data source
Secondary data source
Visit
Vital statistics
World Health Organization (WHO)

The term *statistics* has two meanings. First, it is a number computed from a larger group of numbers, which collectively constitute a sample of data—for instance, the average number of days that patients stay in the hospital overnight. Second, statistics is more broadly defined as a branch of mathematics concerned with collecting, organizing, summarizing, and analyzing data.

Statistics

Originally, the term *statistics* referred to the collection of data about and for the "state." The word comes from the Italian word *stato*, meaning "state." One need only think of our own government and its statistics-collecting organizations, such as the Bureau of Labor Statistics, the Centers for Disease Control and Prevention (CDC), and the Centers for Medicare and Medicaid Services (CMS), for example.

Health statistics provide information about the health of people and their use of healthcare services. Examples of healthcare statistics include average longevity; birth rates; death rates; number of people with a disease in a county, state, the US as a whole, or the world; and the frequency of usage of a particular type of service within a healthcare organization.

Reasons for Studying Statistics

Statistics is about using data for decision-making, which is required in every area of our lives. To make decisions, we must have information. In healthcare settings, information is often incomplete. As a result, we must learn to estimate the characteristics of a complete population using statistics based on a subset or sample of the population.

Most organizations keep statistics to make decisions about their business. For example, an organization may use statistics to determine its markets; that is, to identify who is buying its products or using its services to decide how it can increase the availability and variety of products and services. Healthcare organizations use statistics to determine the use and cost of services as well as outcomes of patients. Many examples of healthcare data and statistics will be presented in this text.

Healthcare Operations Needs

In the healthcare industry, there are compelling reasons to collect and analyze data and compute statistics. For example, statistics kept on activities in the healthcare facility indicate why patients come to the facility and the costs of taking care of them. Patient care statistics and comparison of the values for different providers may be used to measure the quality of care provided. Many accrediting agencies require a data analysis system as part of accreditation, and many third-party payers require facilities to collect performance data. Organizational leadership also may use statistics for prioritizing needed services and to identify areas where efficiency and effectiveness might be increased. For example, laboratory data may show that most outpatients come in for blood work early in the day, so the lab may add more staff in the morning hours. Additionally, healthcare facilities are interested in the types of patients they have with respect to their diagnoses in order to maintain the optimum physician specialty and other professional staff mix they need to treat their patients.

Public Health Needs

Government agencies also need to maintain statistics on and about the population in order to provide services. For example, the **CDC**, a division of the Department of Health and Human Services (HHS), is recognized as the lead agency responsible for protecting the health of the US population by providing credible information to help individuals make the right healthcare decisions and promoting quality of life through the prevention and control of disease, injury, and disability (CDC 2019). The organization compiles and uses health statistics, such as birth and death statistics, to understand the conditions of life and health in our country.

CMS is the division of HHS that is responsible for administering the Medicare program and the federal portion of the Medicaid program. CMS also publishes information on death rates among Medicare patients, and patients in diagnosis and procedure categories. Researchers use this information for studies, which may lead to improvement in patient care and services.

The **Agency for Healthcare Research and Quality (AHRQ)**, a part of HHS, tries to make healthcare safer; of higher quality; and more accessible, equitable, and affordable. For example, AHRQ publishes research-based fact sheets for patients and consumers on a variety of issues, such as patient safety and reducing errors when a patient is in the hospital. AHRQ also works within HHS and with other partners to make sure that the data and statistics are understood and used. AHRQ conducts research on the elderly, children, and various healthcare conditions to provide information to consumers and other HHS agencies so they may meet their objectives. For example, their work around how to reduce readmissions is intended to help hospitals by providing tools to identify causes of readmissions and aid in the development of prevention strategies (AHRQ 2017).

The **World Health Organization (WHO)**, an international organization founded by the United Nations (UN), is the directing and coordinating authority on international health within the UN's system. WHO provides leadership on critical health matters, works to support countries to ensure all of their citizens have accessible and safe healthcare, and helps prevent the spread of communicable diseases, especially vaccine-preventable diseases. They support good health through the continuum of life and are working toward reducing quality of life disparities among countries. WHO supports healthcare research in maternal, child, and adolescent health; malaria; tuberculosis; HIV; Ebola; and other global healthcare issues (WHO 2019). For example, in 1988, WHO helped launch the Global Polio Eradication Initiative to help protect all children from polio. As a result of this immunization initiative, the number of polio cases has dropped by 99 percent. Today, 80 percent of the world's population lives in polio-free regions (WHO 2019).

Importance of Data

To obtain the knowledge they need to make decisions, organizations first must determine what data to collect. Data are raw facts and figures that can pertain to a process or activity that an organization is interested in measuring. Information is derived from data for the purpose of making decisions. The data used to calculate these statistics must be valid and reliable. Validity answers the question of whether one measured what one intended to measure, and reliability means that there is some consistency or ability to replicate results. For example, if a supervisor is checking the coding work of a new employee, the codes assigned should be the same for the supervisor as they were for the employee for the results to be considered reliable.

Descriptive Statistics Versus Inferential Statistics

The primary focus of descriptive statistics is to organize and describe the features of data in a study. **Descriptive statistics** describe what the data show about the characteristics of a group or population; in other words, they may be used to describe a particular population. For example, it might be necessary to know the average age of patients or which service is used most in a given facility. A database including the age of each patient may be used to calculate the descriptive statistic average age. **Inferential statistics**, on the other hand, help organizations make inferences or decisions about a larger group of data by drawing conclusions from a small group of the population. The smaller group selected from the population is called a sample. The results obtained from the sample, if gathered carefully, are assumed to be representative of the entire population. Both types of statistics are used in healthcare.

Sources of Healthcare Statistics

Healthcare data are derived from both primary and secondary data sources. It is important to understand the source of the data prior to using it to compute statistics for use in decision-making.

Primary Data Sources

In healthcare, **primary data source** refers to the record that was developed by healthcare professionals in the process of providing care or services to a patient. Health records are one of the most important primary sources of health statistics because they contain a systematic record of a patient's medical history and care.

The patient's health record contains administrative data, such as admission and discharge dates, patient data, and billing data, as well as clinical data. Notes from physicians, such as orders, progress notes, operative reports, history and physical examination, and a discharge summary, may be included. Nurses' documentation includes their notes and assessments on admission and throughout the hospital stay and medication records. Reports from clinical departments in the facility, such as laboratory, blood bank, radiology, pharmacy, rehabilitation services, and dietary services, may also be included in the health record.

Hospital departments also keep statistics on the activities they perform for patients. For example, the laboratory department may keep data on the number of lab tests performed. The radiology department may keep track of the number of chest and hip x-rays. The physical therapy department may use statistical data, such as the number of patient visits, to decide whether to hire additional physical therapists or add physical therapist assistants to their staff. These reports may be used in turn by the managers of the departments for productivity measurement and combined with other departments to produce a report of activity for the entire facility. The administration of a hospital might ask staff to keep data on the number of patients transferred to another hospital for procedures the facility does not offer in order to determine the need for that service at the facility.

Another example of a primary source of data is vital statistics. The National Vital Statistics System (NVSS) is part of the National Center for Health Statistics (NCHS) of the CDC. These data are provided to the NCHS throughout the

50 states; Washington, DC; New York City; and the five territories of the US—Puerto Rico, the US Virgin Islands, Guam, American Samoa, and the Commonwealth of the Northern Mariana Islands. **Vital statistics** refers to a special group of statistics that record important events in our lives, such as birth, marriage, death, divorce, and fetal death (CDC 2019). Healthcare facilities are interested in births and deaths, fetal deaths, and induced terminations of pregnancy to drive quality improvement initiatives. Facilities generally are responsible for completing certificates for births, fetal deaths, abortions, and occasionally, death certificates. All states have laws that require this data. The certificates are reported to the individual state registrars and maintained permanently. State vital statistics registrars compile the data and report them to the NCHS.

The NCHS has developed standard certificates and procedures that states and territories must use to facilitate the reliable collection of data. The standard certificates represent the minimum basic data set necessary for the collection and publication of comparable national, state, and local vital statistics data. The standard forms are revised about every 10 to 15 years, and the latest adoption to the 2003 revisions of the US Standards Certificate of Live Birth were completed in 2015.

The NCHS is currently working on the development of an e-Vital Standards Initiative (NCHS 2015) that will provide support for the development of vital statistics standards to enable an exchange of data regarding births and deaths from a healthcare facility's electronic health record system directly to the state registrar and then to the NCHS.

Data from the states and territories provide important information for use in medical research and are extremely valuable in estimating population growth areas of the country and essential in planning and evaluating maternal and child health programs. The NCHS prepares and publishes national statistics based on vital statistics data because the figures are important in the fields of social welfare and public health. Because of their many uses, the data on these certificates must be complete, reliable, and accurate.

Censuses

Another primary source of health data is the census. A **census** is defined as a survey of a population. The US government conducts a population census; that is, a count of the people residing in the US and their location. The US Constitution requires that a population census be taken decennially (every 10 years), mainly to determine the number of congressional representatives in the states.

Over the years, Congress has authorized gathering more information about each person. The census now is used in many ways. For instance, the amount of government money given to school districts is based partly on the number of children in a district. Congress also has requested that other types of censuses be taken periodically. These include a census of the types of businesses and industries in the US; for example, farms and fisheries and construction, foreign trade, manufacturing, and energy companies. Aggregated census data, or data that have been clustered together, are available to the public. Healthcare researchers use the US census when they want to determine statistics about the population at large. For example, if researchers want to show the rate of maternal deaths in a population, they must know information about the size of the population, which the US census provides.

Healthcare facilities also have a census, which is the count of patients present at a specific time and place. A hospital **inpatient** is a patient who is provided with room, board, and continuous general nursing services in an area of an acute-care facility where patients generally stay at least overnight. In hospitals, this census is referred to as the **inpatient census**. The hospital census is a source of primary data. Ambulatory care facilities also may keep a census. An **ambulatory care facility** is a healthcare facility that provides preventive or corrective healthcare services on a nonresident basis in a provider's office, clinic setting, or outpatient setting. Patients treated in a hospital setting such as the emergency department or clinic are classified as **outpatient**. The census for this setting usually represents the number of visits or encounters during a specified period, usually one day. A **visit** is a single encounter with a healthcare professional that includes all the services supplied during the encounter. An **encounter** is defined as the direct personal contact between a patient and a physician or other person authorized by state licensure and, if applicable, by medical staff bylaws to order or furnish healthcare services for the diagnosis or treatment of the patient.

Secondary Data Sources

Secondary data sources are data derived from primary sources and may be reported by someone other than the primary user. For example, the disease and operation index is a secondary source of data. The disease index is a listing of patients discharged with a specific diagnosis code, and an operation index is similar to the disease index, but the patients are listed by the operation or procedure code. All data in the index comes from a primary data source, the health record. Registries are also considered secondary data sources. A registry is a listing of patients who share a common characteristic. For example, data from patients' health records may be used to create a cancer or trauma registry. This is a listing of patients in the facility who have been diagnosed with cancer and will include their treatment information as well as follow-up information.

Exercise 1.1

Identify the following as either a primary or a secondary data source:

Type of Healthcare Data	Type of Data Source
1. Productivity reports pulled from patient visit report	
2. Tumor registry	
3. State vital statistics	
4. Hospital census	
5. Hospital disease index	
6. Patient health record	
7. Health insurance data pulled from national census	

Users of Health Statistics

All healthcare entities and third-party payers collect and use statistics. Following are examples of individuals and organizations that collect statistics and how they use statistics:

- **Hospital leadership:** Inpatient facilities use health statistics to help address staffing issues and to determine the types of services to provide. For example, if the number of patients in the intensive care unit is increasing, the hospital administration may want to consider adding beds and staff to meet the growing need. Conversely, if a request is made to the hospital administration for new facilities and equipment that cannot be substantiated by the statistics, it is unlikely the request will be granted. Quality management departments in healthcare facilities collect data to determine how the facility is performing regarding patient care and how it can improve their patient care services. Leaders also use statistics to determine if they have the correct mix of medical specialties to treat the citizens in their communities.

- **Healthcare department managers:** Individual department managers in healthcare organizations use statistics to implement their department goals. For example, a manager needs to know if he or she is staying within budget. If not, the manager will need to investigate.

- **Cancer registries:** A cancer registry may be maintained by a separate department or may be a function of the health information department. States may also have a state cancer registry that is responsible for collecting data about cancer. A cancer registry collects data about the diagnosis, treatment, and follow-up of cancer patients. These statistics are important in tracking cancer survival rates. Facilities may choose to undergo accreditation through the American College of Surgeons Commission on Cancer (ACS 2019). This is an evaluation by an independent team to determine whether the facility's cancer registry meets their standards, which guide treatment and ensure patient-centered care. Statistics must show the facility is providing high-quality care and follow-up to its cancer patients. Physicians and researchers conduct research studies to learn about the biology of cancer, investigate new treatments and tests, and learn how to prevent cancers from occurring.

- **Nursing facilities:** Long-term care (LTC) or **nursing facilities** may use statistics to determine the types of payers their patients have. These statistics also are helpful in demonstrating to the public the types of patients being cared for and the quality of care given. For example, an LTC facility will collect data on the number of patients who are incontinent. This will tell the facility if protocols need to be established for patients in order to help them void. The American Health Care Association, a nonprofit association of LTC associations, publishes statistics on the trends in nursing home care.

- **Home health (HH):** HH agencies provide care to elderly, disabled, and convalescent patients in their homes. This is also called home care. These agencies keep statistics to determine the types of services used by their patients and their outcomes. For example, a HH agency would need to know the number of nursing visits, HH aide visits, physical therapy treatments, and patients using various types of equipment, such as oxygen machines or other respiratory aids. Additionally, agencies will report patient outcomes, such as the number of patients who have improved, the number of patients who were compliant with taking their medications, or the number of patients who had to be readmitted to a hospital.

- **Hospice: Hospice** programs provide interdisciplinary programs of palliative care and supportive services that address the physical, spiritual, social, and economic needs of terminally ill patients and their families. These services may be given in either the home or an inpatient setting. A hospice needs to know types of illnesses in order to match the appropriate caregiver with each patient.

- **Mental health facilities:** These may be inpatient or outpatient facilities. These facilities use health statistics to determine whether they are providing the proper services for patients in the community. Because the economic burden of psychiatric illness is great, the CDC collects data about mental illness and its impact on the country.

- **Drug and alcohol facilities:** These programs may be inpatient, ambulatory, or a combination of the two. Statistics are important in this area to show the success rates of these facilities' clients. The National Institute on Drug Abuse and the National Institute on Alcohol Abuse and Alcoholism are centers in the National Institutes of Health that each collect statistics to conduct research.

- **Outpatient facilities:** These include physician clinics, surgery centers, emergency centers, and the like. Outpatient facilities often use statistics to determine whether they are providing the proper level of care to the community.

- **Managed care organizations (MCOs):** An MCO is a type of healthcare organization that delivers medical care and manages all aspects of care or payment for care by controlling access to providers of care and negotiating discounted payment rates to providers of care. MCOs use statistics to determine whether they are providing an appropriate level of care and preventive services to their members. Additionally, MCOs contract with healthcare facilities to provide specific services to their members at a prenegotiated rate. The MCO pays the agreed-upon amount each time a member uses the service.

- **Healthcare researchers:** Researchers depend on healthcare statistics to conduct research and help develop solutions to healthcare problems. Some examples include research in managed care, health law and regulations, mergers and acquisitions of healthcare facilities, physician practice issues, different types of illness and risk factors, telehealth issues, pharmaceutical research, drug and alcohol research, and so on. Healthcare statistics can also help researchers understand our quality of life.

- **Accreditation agencies:** These organizations use healthcare statistics to determine the most common diagnoses and procedures and whether the resources are available to treat patients with those diagnoses.

- **Federal government:** The US government collects data for public health issues. For example, the CDC reports data on births, deaths, birth defects, cancer, and HIV/AIDS, just to name a few of the categories of data. CMS uses data collected by quality improvement organizations for its quality improvement projects. Legislators and other policymakers use healthcare statistics when working on new laws, conducting program oversight, and considering the amount of the budget that should be allotted to federal health agencies.

Because health information management (HIM) professionals have a broad knowledge of healthcare facilities as well as immediate access to a wide range of clinical data, they are in the best position to collect, prepare, analyze, and interpret healthcare data. HIM professionals must learn acceptable terminology, definitions, and computational methodology if they are to provide the basic and most frequently used health statistics. One important point to remember is that health statistics are dependent upon accurate reporting by those individuals responsible for the task.

Chapter 1   Matching Quiz

Match the definitions with the terms.

Definitions:

a. A type of healthcare organization that delivers medical care and manages all aspects of care or payment for care by controlling access to providers of care and negotiating discounted payment rates to providers of care

b. A comprehensive term for facilities that provide nursing care and related services for residents requiring medical, nursing, or rehabilitative care

c. The direct personal contact between a patient and a physician or other person authorized by state licensure law and, if applicable, by medical staff bylaws to order or furnish healthcare services for the diagnosis or treatment of the patient

d. A group of federal agencies that oversees health promotion and disease control and prevention activities in the US

e. An interdisciplinary program of palliative care and supportive services that addresses the physical, spiritual, social, and economic needs of terminally ill patients and their families

f. Data related to births, deaths, marriages, and fetal deaths

g. An umbrella term that refers to the medical and nonmedical services provided to patients and their families in their places of residence

h. Record developed by healthcare professionals in the process of providing patient care

i. The UN's specialized agency created to ensure the attainment or the highest possible levels of health by all peoples

j. Data derived from the primary patient record, such as an index or registry

Terms:

1. _____ Secondary data source
2. _____ Nursing facility
3. _____ Hospice
4. _____ Vital statistics
5. _____ MCO

6. _____ Encounter
7. _____ CDC
8. _____ WHO
9. _____ Home health
10. _____ Health record

Chapter 1   Review

Select the best answer to the following questions:

1. The CDC is the lead agency that _____.
   a. Accredits and licenses acute hospital facilities in the US
   b. Is responsible for providing vital statistics to various agencies, such as the NCHS
   c. Develops and updates ICD-10 for the world
   d. Is responsible for protecting the health of the people of the US

2. The type of statistics that make conclusions about a population by drawing conclusions from a sample is called _____.
   a. Descriptive statistics
   b. Inferential statistics
   c. Generalized statistics
   d. Mathematical statistics

3. Which of the following is a primary source of data?
   a. Inpatient census
   b. Vital statistics collected by the NCHS
   c. Health record
   d. a, b, and c
   e. b and c only

4. The division of HHS that is responsible for administering the Medicare program is the _____.
   a. CDC
   b. CMS
   c. AHRQ
   d. WHO

5. A secondary data source includes _____.
   a. Vital statistics
   b. The health record
   c. The physician's index
   d. A videotape of a counseling session

6. Which user of statistics has the primary job of supporting terminally ill patients and their families?
   a. Home health agencies
   b. Nursing facilities
   c. Hospice
   d. MCOs

7. The NCHS keeps statistics on _____.
   a. The licensing information on all healthcare providers in the 50 states
   b. Cancer and other deadly diseases in the 50 states and the US-owned territories
   c. Vital statistics, such as births, deaths, and fetal deaths, in North America
   d. Vital statistics, such as births, deaths, and fetal deaths, in the 50 states and US territories

8. Which of the following is *not* a primary source of data?
   a. Health record
   b. Vital statistics
   c. Hospital census
   d. Disease and operation index

9. To be useful, the data used to calculate statistics must be _____.
   a. Fair and exact
   b. Valid and reliable
   c. Honest and justified
   d. Simple and clear

10. To be reliable, statistical data must _____.
    a. Be reproducible
    b. Be applicable to what is being measured
    c. Be collected from one source only
    d. Have multiple meanings

11. Which of the following is a secondary use of a patient health record?

    a. Determining the results of a diagnostic test

    b. Identifying patients that have a cancer diagnosis

    c. Recording the health and physician information during an office visit

    d. Submitting diagnoses and procedures for claim submission

12. Facilities may choose to pursue accreditation for their cancer registry with the _____.

    a. American College of Physicians

    b. American Cancer Society

    c. American College of Surgeons

    d. National Institutes of Health

13. The type of patient who receives care in a hospital-based clinic or department is called a(n) _____.

    a. Inpatient

    b. Outpatient

    c. Hospice patient

    d. MCO patient

14. The number of inpatients present in a healthcare facility at any given time is called a(n) _____.

    a. Survey

    b. Census

    c. Sample

    d. Enumeration

15. An international organization founded by the UN that is the directing and coordinating authority on international heath is called the _____.

    a. CDC

    b. AHRQ

    c. NCHS

    d. WHO

CHAPTER

2 | Mathematics Review

Learning Objectives

At the conclusion of this chapter, you should be able to do the following:

- Calculate using decimals, ratios, proportions, rates, and percentages
- Differentiate between a numerator and denominator
- Perform rounding of numbers
- Determine the proper methods to convert among fractions, decimals and percentages
- Compute the average or mean

Key Terms

Average
Decimal
Denominator
Fraction
Mean

Numerator
Percentage
Proportion
Quotient
Rate

Ratio
Rounding
Whole number

Numbers may be expressed in a variety of ways for use in calculating statistics. As discussed in the previous chapter, data and statistics are needed to help healthcare organizations make decisions. The following sections explain and review fractions, quotients, decimals, proportions, how to round numbers, percentages, ratios, rates, and averages. We will use these statistics in subsequent chapters.

Most healthcare data are collected and tabulated using software. There are a number of spreadsheet products available in the market that may be used for this purpose: Microsoft Excel, Google Sheets, and Apple Numbers. The formatting and basic functionality are very similar among these data tools. The examples in this text will be presented using Microsoft Excel. Excel is the most utilized spreadsheet program in the market and is considered an industry standard by many. Some basic concepts of spreadsheets will be introduced in this chapter and expanded upon in subsequent chapters.

Fractions

A **fraction** is one or more parts of a whole. Figure 2.1 shows two circles; the first circle is split into two equal parts, and the second shows one part of the circle larger than the other part. The fraction of the first circle is ½; the fraction of the second circle (in darker color) is ¾. The top number is called the **numerator** and the bottom number is called the

Figure 2.1. Fractions of a circle

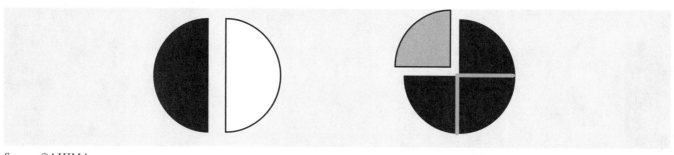

Source: ©AHIMA

denominator. The denominator tells us how many equal parts a whole is broken into. For example, if we have a fraction of ½, the denominator is 2. That indicates there are two equal parts that make up the whole. The numerator tells us how many parts of the whole we have selected. In the fraction ½, 1 of the two equal parts were selected. In figure 2.1, the first circle shows one part shaded black of the two equal parts. We can say that ½ or one out of the two parts is shaded black. The second circle in figure 2.1 depicts three out of four equal parts is selected and shaded in black. This represents ¾ of the circle.

Example 2.1: Of the 40 patients with diabetes seen last month in a physician's clinic, 20 were Caucasian, 10 were African American, and 10 were Asian American. The following fractions show the number of patients of each race compared with the total number of patients who visited the clinic: Caucasian, $\frac{20}{40}$; African American, $\frac{10}{40}$; and Asian American, $\frac{10}{40}$. Fractions should be converted to their simplest form. The simplest form of a fraction is when the numerator and denominator do not have any common factors.

Each fraction can be converted by dividing both top (numerator) and bottom (denominator) by a common factor. In this example, 10 is a factor of both the numerator and the denominator: Caucasians, $\frac{2}{4}$; African American, $\frac{1}{4}$; and Asian American, $\frac{1}{4}$. The first fraction can be further simplified with the common factor of 2; thus, $\frac{2}{4}$ can be expressed as $\frac{1}{2}$.

QUICK
TIP

Factors are numbers that you multiply together to get another number. For example, 2 and 3 are factors of 6 (2 times 3 equals 6). If two numbers can be formed by using some of the same factors, those are called common factors. For example, 2×3=6 and 2×5=10, therefore 2 is a common factor of both 6 and 10.

Exercise 2.1

Find the simplest form of each of the following fractions:

1. $\frac{20}{40}$

2. $\frac{4}{6}$

3. $\frac{12}{54}$

4. $\frac{8}{12}$

5. $\frac{16}{28}$

Quotient

A **quotient** is the number obtained by dividing the numerator of a fraction by the denominator. This number may be expressed in decimals. As a simple example, consider the fraction ½ (one half). Using your calculator, divide 1 by 2. The result is 0.5. This is a decimal representation of the quotient found by dividing the numerator 1 by the denominator 2.

> **Example 2.2:** The 14 members of your health information class decide to participate in your college's information day. The booth is going to be open for 21 hours over a three-day period. To find out how many hours each student would need to attend to the booth, you would divide the numerator (21 hours) by the denominator (14 students). This could be expressed as a fraction, 21/14, or 3/2 when simplified by removing the common factor of 7 from the numerator and denominator. This is difficult to interpret in terms of hours per student. If we restate the fraction 3/2 as the quotient 1.5, we can easily see that the number of hours per student is 1.5.

It is important to keep track of the units of measurement for data. The numerator and denominator in fractions may have different units. In example 2.2, the numerator is measured in "hours" and the denominator is measured in "students." The resulting quotient is measured in "hours per student" or "units of numerator per units of denominator" in general.

QUICK TIP

Decimals

A **decimal** is a quotient derived from a fraction where the denominator is a multiple of 10. These fractions are sometimes called decimal fractions, but that term is rarely used in practice. The portion of the decimal to the left of the decimal point (.) is called a **whole number**. The most common use of decimals in the real world is the accounting of dollars and cents. If a syringe costs $2.49, we interpret that as 2 dollars and 49 cents. If we just consider the numeric portion of the cost, it is really a whole number with a decimal. The whole number is the 2, the number to the left of the decimal point. The decimal is the fractional portion to the right of the decimal point, 0.49. We convert 0.49 to 49 cents quickly, but we can also think of 49 cents as 49/100 of a whole dollar. The decimal fraction is then 49/100 that can be expressed as the decimal 0.49.

Decimal fractions are typically expressed as decimals (no one says "49/100 cents"). The notation indicates a value that is less than one. In 14.37, for example, the digits to the right of the decimal point (3 and 7) are called decimal digits. The digit "3" in this example is in the tenths position and "7" is in the hundredths position. The decimal point is used to separate the fraction (.37) of a whole number from the whole number itself (14). The decimal point is not ordinarily used in whole numbers (for example, 14.0) unless the healthcare facility has a reason for doing so. Figure 2.2 displays the interpretation of digits to the left (whole numbers) and right (fractional portions) of the decimal point for a sample number measured to the ten thousandth place.

Figure 2.2.   Illustration of whole number and decimal positions

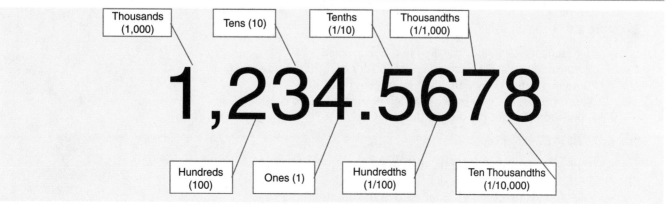

Decimal numbers without a value to the left of the decimal point are typically written with a leading zero to call attention to the decimal point. For example, .5 is typically written as 0.5.

Example 2.3: Identify the following decimal positions in the number 3.492.

3 – ones position
4 – tenths position
9 – hundredths position
2 – thousandths position

Rounding Numbers

Rounding is a process of approximating a number to a level of precision that is meaningful for the application. Numbers may be rounded to the nearest 10, 100, and so on. In healthcare facilities, rounding is commonly used when expressing data because staff must manage statistics measured as both parts of a whole number, as in length of stay, and in whole numbers, as in the number of patients or census.

Rounding can occur in either whole or decimal numbers. The level of rounding is expressed using the names of the whole number and decimal positions found in figure 2.2. When rounding to the nearest digit, examine the digit to the right of the level of rounding. If that digit is 0, 1, 2, 3, or 4, then round down. If that digit is 5, 6, 7, 8, or 9, then round up. One important rule to remember in rounding is that only the digit to the right of the position of the level of rounding should be considered. These concepts are best explained through a series of annotated examples.

The determination of rounding up or down when the digit to be rounded is 5 is not a uniform rule. For this text, we will round up. You may encounter other texts or even situations in practice where the rule may differ. For example, in this text 25 is rounded to the nearest 10 which is 30, but you may find other references that state 25 should be rounded to 20 (the nearest even number).

Example 2.4: Rounding to the nearest whole number or one:

   a. 1.9 rounds to 2 since 9 is in the tenths place.
   b. 1.905 rounds to 2 since 9 is in the tenths place and since we only consider the 9 when rounding.
   c. 0.5 rounds to 1 since 5 is in the tenths place.
   d. 0.1 rounds to 0 since 1 is in the tenths place.
   e. 9.496 rounds to 9 since 4 is in the tenths place.

Example 2.5: Rounding to the nearest ten:

   a. 31 rounds to 30 since the digit in the ones place is 1.
   b. 31.9 also rounds to 30 since we only consider the 1 in determining the rounding.
   c. 35 rounds to 40 since the digit in the ones place is 5.
   d. 439 rounds to 440 since the digit in the ones place is 9.
   e. 2,257.92 rounds to 2,260 since the digit in the ones place is 7.

Example 2.6: Rounding to the nearest hundred:

   a. 4,325 rounds to 4,300 since the digit in the tens place is 2.
   b. 4,325.99 rounds to 4,300 since we only consider the 2 in the tens place.
   c. 5,990 rounds to 6,000 since the digit in the tens place is 9.
   d. 79,320.95 rounds to 79,300 since the digit in the tens place is 2.
   e. 99 rounds to 100 since the digit in the tens place is 9.

Example 2.7: Rounding to the nearest thousand:

   a. 45,025 rounds to 45,000 since the digit in the hundreds place is 0.
   b. 96,591 rounds to 97,000 since the digit in the hundreds place is 5.
   c. 42,984.9 rounds to 43,000 since the digit in the hundreds place is 9.
   d. 43,400 rounds to 43,000 since the digit in the hundreds place is 4.
   e. 1,632.01 rounds to 2,000 since the digit in the hundreds place is 6.

Example 2.8: Rounding to the nearest tenth:

   a. 1.39 rounds to 1.4 since the digit in the hundredths place is 9.
   b. 2.91 rounds to 2.9 since the digit in the hundredths place is 1.
   c. 9.3694 rounds to 9.4 since the digit in the hundredths place is 6.
   d. 0.98 rounds to 1.0 since the digit in the hundredths place is 8.
   e. 0.06 rounds to 0.1 since the digit in the hundredths place is 6.

QUICK TIP

Example 2.8d is interesting. Because the 8 is in the hundredths place, 9 should be rounded up to 10. This is achieved by rounding the 0.98 up to 1.0. When the digit to be rounded up is a 9, then the digit to the left must be incremented (ones or whole number in this case).

Example 2.9: Rounding to the nearest hundredth:

   a. 6.395 rounds to 6.40 since the digit in the thousandths place is 5.
   b. 3.209 rounds to 3.21 since the digit in the thousandths place is 9.
   c. 65.591 rounds to 65.59 since the digit in the thousandths place is 1.
   d. 0.009 rounds to 0.01 since the digit in the thousandths place is 9.
   e. 0.999 rounds to 1.00 since the digit in the thousandths place is 9.

Exercise 2.2

Find the quotient in the following fractions. Round to two decimal places.

1. $\dfrac{2}{5}$

2. $\dfrac{3}{4}$

3. $\dfrac{7}{8}$

4. $\dfrac{107}{98}$

5. $\dfrac{54}{65}$

Exercise 2.3

Round the following numbers to the nearest 10.

1. 42

2. 338

3. 217

4. 6,989

5. 8,532

Round the following numbers to the nearest hundred.

6. 156

7. 321

8. 3,807

9. 4,357

10. 8,175

Round to the nearest whole number.

11. 38.1

12. 55.69

13. 14.7

14. 625.23

15. 100.5

Round to the nearest tenth or one decimal place.

16. 19.76

17. 34.623

18. 172.87

19. 99.98

20. 125.969

Round to two decimal places.

21. 8.36801

22. 14.5264

23. 0.87642

24. 27.99999

25. 15.90176

When asked to provide an answer to one decimal (or more) and the resulting answer is a whole number, add 0's after the decimal point. For example, rounding 10 to one decimal is 10.0 and rounding 10 to two decimals is 10.00.

QUICK
TIP

Percentage

The ratio of a part to the whole is often expressed as a **percentage**. A percentage is a value computed on the basis of the whole divided into 100 parts. It may help to remember that percent means "per 100" when interpreting percentages. Percentages should be labeled with either the percent sign (%) or the word "percent" after the number value is stated. For example, 0.34 would be written as $\frac{34}{100}$ and is equal to 34 percent. Percentages are a useful way to make fair comparisons because the calculation of a percent essentially standardizes each value to be scaled to "per 100".

Example 2.10: If 20 patients died in Hospital A last month, and 50 patients died in Hospital B during the same period, one might conclude that it would be better to use the services at Hospital A because Hospital A had fewer deaths. However, that conclusion would be wrong if Hospital A had 100 discharges during the month and Hospital B had 500 discharges for the same period.

Hospital A: 20/100 = 20% deaths
Hospital B: 50/500 = 10% deaths

In this case, the percent of deaths allows us to compare Hospital A and Hospital B on the same scale of deaths "per 100." Not all percentages are whole numbers. For example:

$$\frac{1}{8} = 0.125 = 12.5\%$$

Percentages can be rounded to various levels just as decimals are. For example, if we wanted to round 12.5 percent to the nearest whole percent, the rounded value would be 13 percent (round digits 5 and up to the next number).

Common Transformations of Fractions, Decimals and Percentages

Numbers may be expressed in a different format based on the context in which they are used. The same value may be expressed as a fraction (1/2), decimal (0.5), or percentage (50 percent). The following section contains guidance on how to convert between these formats.

Converting a Fraction to a Percentage

To convert a fraction to a percentage, divide the numerator by the denominator and multiply by 100.

Example 2.11: Convert $\frac{1}{2}$ to a percentage.
Step 1: Divide 1 by 2.

$$1 \div 2 = 0.5$$

Step 2: Multiply by 100.

$$0.5 \times 100 = 5\%$$

Converting a Decimal to a Percentage

To convert a decimal to a percentage, simply multiply the decimal by 100. The calculation changes the position of the decimal point two digits to the right.

Example 2.12: Convert the decimal 0.29 to a percentage.

$$0.29 \times 100 = 29\%$$

Converting a Percentage to a Fraction

To convert a percentage to a fraction, eliminate the percent sign and multiply the number by $\frac{1}{100}$. A simpler method is to place the number in the numerator and 100 in the denominator.

Example 2.13: Convert 5 percent into a fraction.
Step 1: Eliminate the percent sign and multiply the value by 1/100.

$$5 \times \frac{1}{100} = \frac{5}{100}$$

Step 2: Express the fraction in simplest form. Since 5 is a factor of both the numerator and denominator, the simplest form is:

$$\frac{5 \div 5}{100 \div 5} = \frac{1}{20}$$

Example 2.14: Convert 23 percent into a fraction.
Step 1: Eliminate the percent sign and multiply the value by 1/100.

$$23 \times \frac{1}{100} = \frac{23}{100}$$

Step 2: Express the fraction in simplest form. There are no common factors for 23 and 100. Therefore, 23/100 is the simplest form for this fraction.

Converting a Percentage to a Decimal

To convert a percentage to a decimal, eliminate the percent sign and divide the remaining number by 100. This is the equivalent of moving the decimal point two places to the left. Hint: If the percentage is less than 10, place a 0 in front of the value and place the decimal point in front of the 0.

Example 2.15: Convert 76 percent to a decimal.
Step 1: Eliminate the percent sign: 76.
Step 2: Divide the number by 100.

$$76 \div 100 = 0.76$$

Example 2.16: Convert 4 percent to a decimal.
Step 1: Eliminate the percent sign: 4.
Step 2: Divide the number by 100.

$$4 \div 100 = 0.04$$

Example 2.17: Convert 109 percent to a decimal.
Step 1: Eliminate the percent sign: 109.
Step 2: Divide the number by 100.

$$109 \div 100 = 1.09$$

The decimal point in whole numbers is often not displayed, but it is still present. For example, 76, 76., and 76.0 are all equivalent numbers. When the decimal point is not displayed, it is sometimes confusing to visualize moving it to the left or right for the percent-to-decimal and decimal-to-percent conversions. It may be helpful to actually write the whole number with the decimal point present for these conversions.

Using Excel to Convert Fractions to Decimals and Percentages

Using spreadsheet software such as Excel is very convenient when converting fractions to quotients and decimals or percentages. First, let's look at the anatomy of a spreadsheet to understand how we may use that tool to help with this type of calculation. You can think of a spreadsheet as a table with rows and columns.

In figure 2.3, the rows of the spreadsheet are labeled by the numbers 1 through 5. The columns are labeled with letters A through C. Excel spreadsheets can be very large. The most recent version of Excel can hold up to 1,048,576 rows by 16,384 columns. The cells are referenced by their row and column. The upper left cell is referred to as cell A1. The cell below A1 is A2 and the cell to the right of A1 is B1. Figure 2.4 shows the cells with their labels.

The cells in a spreadsheet may hold either values or calculation instructions. For example, if we wanted to calculate the value in example 2.2 using Excel, we could put the numerator (21 hours) in cell A2, the denominator (14 students) into cell B2, and then the formula to calculate the value of dividing the numerator by the denominator in cell C2. Figure 2.5 shows the values that should be keyed into each cell.

Figure 2.3.   Spreadsheet example

Figure 2.4. Display of cell references in spreadsheet

	A	B	C
1	A1	B1	C1
2	A2	B2	C2
3	A3	B3	C3
4	A4	B4	C4
5	A5	B5	C5
6	A6	B6	C6

Figure 2.5. Excel calculation example

	A	B	C	D
1	Hours	Students	Hours per Student	
2	21	14	=A2/B2	<< Keyed Values
3	21	14	1.5	<< Results

Notice that the cells A1, B1, and C1 are used as title or label cells. They are not part of the calculation but are important to include so that the units and interpretation of the various values can be conveyed to the reader. The value in C2 is a calculation or formula. All calculation cells in a spreadsheet must begin with an equal sign or "=." This is a signal to Excel that a calculation should be performed as opposed to simply displaying the values keyed into the cell.

In addition to performing calculations, Excel has a number of formatting options that can make rounding and converting to percentages very easy.

Example 2.18: Suppose General Hospital's health information management (HIM) staff of 48 includes 20 staff members with RHIT credentials, 5 staff members with RHIA credentials, and the remaining staff with no credentials. What percentage of the HIM staff has an RHIT credential? Round to the nearest tenth of a percent.

Let's walk through the steps in calculating a percent by hand:

1. Determine the numerator and denominator:
   a. Numerator – number of RHITs
   b. Denominator – total staff
2. Divide numerator by denominator.
3. Multiply by 100 to convert to a percentage.
4. Round to the nearest whole percent.

The steps in Excel are quite similar, but the conversion to a percentage and rounding may be completed via formatting. Steps (displayed in figure 2.6):

1. Put the labels of each column in cells A1, B1, and C1.
2. Enter the numerator (20) into cell A2.
3. Enter the denominator (48) into cell B2.
4. Enter the formula "=A2/B2" into cell C2.

Figure 2.6.   Example 2.18 steps 1–4

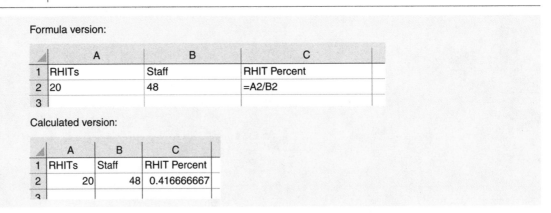

Formula version:

	A	B	C
1	RHITs	Staff	RHIT Percent
2	20	48	=A2/B2
3			

Calculated version:

	A	B	C
1	RHITs	Staff	RHIT Percent
2	20	48	0.416666667
3			

Figure 2.7.   Format menu

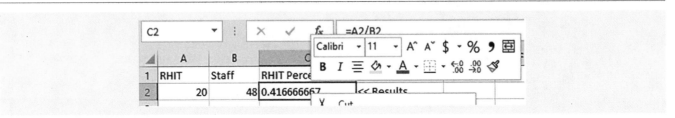

Figure 2.8.   Results for example 2.4

	A	B	C
1	RHIT	Staff	RHIT Percent
2	20	48	41.7%

5. Format the value in C2 as a percent.
   a. Highlight the value in cell C2 by clicking on the cell.
   b. Right click on the cell to display the format menu in figure 2.7.
   c. Select the "%" icon from the format menu.
   d. Excel will round the nearest whole percent by default.
   e. Right click on the percentage value to display the format menu once again.
   f. Click once on the "increase decimal" icon (left pointing arrow with zeroes).

The resulting value is 41.7 percent as displayed in figure 2.8. Repeat the calculation using your calculator to check the answer.

Exercise 2.4

Complete the following conversions.

Convert the following fractions to percentages (round to one decimal place):

1. $\dfrac{5}{8}$

2. $\dfrac{3}{5}$

3. $\dfrac{2}{4}$

4. $\dfrac{7}{12}$

5. $\dfrac{3}{15}$

Convert the following decimals to percentages (round to one decimal place):

6. 0.28

7. 0.07

8. 0.1254

9. 0.4299

10. 0.9981

Convert the following percentages to fractions:

11. 42%

12. 58%

13. 78%

14. 75%

15. 20%

Convert the following percentages to decimals:

16. 12%

17. 27%

18. 0.5%

19. 7.5%

20. 3.4%

21. A family practitioner in your local physician's clinic saw 150 adults in one week for their annual physical examinations. Of those 150 patients, 67 received the flu vaccine. Express the rate of the flu vaccine administration in percent. Round to one decimal place. Perform this calculation using a calculator and repeat the calculation using Excel. (Hint: Follow the steps in example 2.18.)

22. The physician practice you work for needs a new paper shredder. They want a cross-cut shredder that can cut 20 sheets at a time. It must be strong enough to destroy staples and small paper clips with a waste bin of at least eight gallons. You did some investigation and secured five offers from different companies. The shredders are all of equal quality. Set up an Excel spreadsheet using the information here. Which company is giving you the best deal?

Hint: Calculate the discounted price and then add in the shipping and handling where appropriate. Calculate the discounted price by subtracting the discount dollar amount from the list price.

	List Price	Discount	Discount Amount	Discounted Price	Shipping and Handling
Company A	$600.00	20%			Free $00.00
Company B	$625.00	30%			$25.00
Company C	$551.00	15%			$33.00
Company D	$584.00	25%			$30.00
Company E	$579.00	20%			Local $00.00

23. Using the information found in the scenario below, complete the following tables using Excel.

Forty patients were seen in the Hematology/Oncology Clinic last Tuesday. Twenty patients had sickle-cell anemia, 12 patients had hemophilia, 6 patients had Ewing's sarcoma, and 2 patients had Wilms' tumor.

Express in counts, decimals (round to two places), and percentages (round to whole percent) the number of patients with each condition compared with the number of patients who visited the clinic last Tuesday.

	Count	Decimal	Percentage
Sickle cell			
Hemophilia			
Ewing's			
Wilms'			
Total			

Ratios

A **ratio** is a number found by dividing one quantity by another; also, a general term that can include a number of specific measures such as proportion, percentage, and rate. Ratios typically express the relationship of one quantity to another. To calculate ratios, one quantity is compared to another. The number can be greater than 1 or less than 1. Ratios may be expressed in a fractional form, but they have a different interpretation than fractions. Fractions are essentially numbers: ½ is a fraction and its representation might be ½, 0.5, or even 50 percent, as we demonstrated earlier in the chapter. It is an expression of a part of a whole. Ratios are a comparison of two subsets.

> **Example 2.19:** If seven men and five women were in a group, the ratio of men to women would be $\frac{7}{5}$. This ratio also may be written as 7:5 and verbalized as 7 to 5.

Notice in example 2.19 that the ratio of men to women is a different value than the percentage of men. The fraction of men in this case would be the number of men divided by the total in the group or 7/12. We may express this as a decimal, 0.58, or a percentage, 58 percent.

Ratios should be expressed in their simplest form just like fractions, and they may be applied to a particular situation by multiplying the numerator and denominator by the same factor. Suppose we wanted to recruit a focus group of 36 members and wanted to maintain the ratio of men to women of 7:5 found in example 2.19. Table 2.1 shows how the ratio of men to women can be maintained for focus groups of various sizes.

Table 2.1. Focus groups of various sizes

Focus Group Size	Number of Men	Number of Women
12	7	5
24 (multiply by 2)	14	10
36 (multiply by 3)	21	15
48 (multiply by 4)	28	20

> **Example 2.20:** If an HIM department of 16 staff includes 6 RHIAs and 10 RHITs, what is the ratio of RHIAs to RHITs?

The ratio of RHIAs to RHITs is 6 to 10 or 6:10 or 6/10. All of these are equivalent expressions of the same ratio. Notice that 2 is a factor of both 6 and 10. This ratio should be expressed in its simplest form:

$$\frac{6}{10} = \frac{6 \div 2}{10 \div 2} = \frac{3}{5} \text{ or } 3:5 \text{ or "3 to 5"}$$

Exercise 2.5

1. Express the following ratios in their simplest form.
    a. 8:96
    b. 3:15
    c. 8:16
    d. 12:72
    e. 5:7

2. A group of 15 men and 20 women have diabetes. Express the ratio of men with diabetes to women with diabetes. Calculate it to its simplest form.

3. Your college bookstore reported that of the 1,000 books sold during enrollment, 320 were HIM books. Express the ratio of HIM books to the total number of books sold. Calculate it to its simplest form.

4. There are 12 instructors in your HIM program. Five of these are male instructors, and the rest are female. Express the ratio of male instructors to female instructors. Calculate it to its simplest form.

5. Of the 12 instructors in the previous example, three have a master's degree and the rest have a bachelor's degree. Express the ratio of bachelor's degree prepared instructors to master's degree prepared instructors. Calculate it to its simplest form.

6. Community Hospital reported 16 births this past month. Four were male. What is the ratio of male births to female births? Calculate it to its simplest form.

Proportions

A **proportion** is a type of ratio in which x is a portion of the whole $(x + y)$. In a proportion, the numerator is always included in the denominator. A proportion may be expressed as a percentage, a decimal, or a fraction.

> **Example 2.21:** If 2 women out of a group of 10 over the age of 50 have had breast cancer, what is the proportion of women who have had breast cancer in the over-50 age group? Express the proportion as a decimal.
>
> Step 1: Find the size of the whole group: 10.
> Step 2: Find the number of women who had breast cancer: 2.
> Step 3: Calculate the proportion as portion/whole.
>
> $$\frac{\textit{Portion of women over 50 that had breast cancer}}{\textit{Number in group of women over 50}} = \frac{2}{10}$$
>
> Step 4: Convert to a decimal.
>
> $$\frac{2}{10} = 2 \div 10 = 0.2$$

Table 2.2 shows a sample computerized statistical report provided by the information systems (IS) department of an acute-care facility and illustrates how the department uses proportions expressed as percentages to understand which days admissions peak. Examining this table, we can see that less than 10 percent of the patients are admitted on Mondays or Saturdays. This type of report can guide staffing levels during high- and low-volume days.

Table 2.2. Administrator's semiannual reference report

Administrator's Semiannual Reference Report Admissions by Day of Week 7/1/20XX–12/31/20XX		
Day	**Number of Patients**	**Percent of Patients**
Sunday	1,283	18.7
Monday	577	8.4
Tuesday	1,126	16.4
Wednesday	1,301	18.9
Thursday	1,240	18.0
Friday	702	10.2
Saturday	645	9.4
Totals	6,874	100.0

Exercise 2.6

1. A school district wants to know the proportion of students who have deferrals for mandated vaccines. District School #1 has 237 students. Of the 237 students, 225 students are up to date on their vaccines. There are 12 students with deferrals. What is the proportion of students with deferrals who have not been vaccinated? Round to two decimal places.

2. At Community Clinic, 50 patients were seen in one day. Of those, 6 have type 2 diabetes mellitus. What is the proportion of people in the group who have diabetes? Express as a decimal and round to two decimal places.

3. At Community Clinic, Dr. Clark treats only diabetic patients. He has 650 active patients. Of those, 458 have attended his specialized training session for newly diagnosed diabetes. What proportion of Dr. Clark's patients have undergone his training? Express as a decimal and round to two decimal places.

4. At Community Clinic, Dr. Simpson, an interventional cardiologist, saw 270 patients last quarter. Of those, he performed stent procedures on 182 patients. What is the proportion of Dr. Simpson's patients who have had stent procedures? Express as a decimal and round to two decimal places.

5. Dr. Rutan, an internist at Community Clinic, asked that 14 of the 35 patients he saw last week get their x-rays and lab work completed the day before their appointments. What is the proportion of Dr. Rutan's patients who had preliminary work completed prior to their appointments? Express as a decimal and round to two decimal places.

Rates

A **rate** is a fraction that is formulated to express the relationship between the numerator and denominator. A measure of time is often an intrinsic part of the denominator. For example, number of patients treated per day or charts coded per shift are rates that are used in healthcare. Healthcare facilities calculate many types of rates to determine how they are performing compared to benchmark or best practice value.

The term *rate* is often used loosely to refer to rate, proportion, percentage, and ratio. Indeed, many books and organizations use these terms interchangeably. For this reason, it is important to be aware of how any measure reported is defined and calculated. For rates, proportions, and ratios, the numerator and denominator must be clearly defined and documented to communicate the interpretation of the value to the reader.

The basic rule of thumb for calculating rates is to indicate the number of times something *actually* happened in relation to the number of times it *could have* happened (actual/potential or part/base). The number of times the event occurred is the part that we would like to measure; the number of times the event could have occurred is the base that we use for comparison. The formula for determining rates is as follows:

$$Rate = \frac{Part}{Base}, \text{ or } R = \frac{P}{B}$$

Example 2.22: If 10 of the 35 patients visiting a physician's office received a flu vaccine, what is the vaccine rate for that set of patients? Round to two decimal places.

Step 1: Determine the event to be measured: flu vaccines.
Step 2: Determine the number that actually happened (part): 10.
Step 3: Determine the number that could have happened (base): 35
Step 4: Calculate the rate:

$$Vaccine\ Rate = \frac{10}{35} = 10 \div 35 = 0.285\ round\ to\ 0.29$$

All calculations should be checked to make sure they are reasonable in the context of the calculation. Misplaced decimal points are a common source of mathematical errors. For example, a hospital death rate of 25 percent should seem unreasonable because it indicates that one of every four patients treated at this hospital died. Thus, the decimal placement in this calculation should be checked. The correct death rate for this hospital may be 2.5 percent or 0.25 percent, which would be more realistic.

Averages

An **average** or **mean** is the value obtained by dividing the sum of a set of numbers by a count of the number of values in the set. The term *average* with no other qualifier is generally referred to as the arithmetic mean to distinguish it from the mode or median. (This is covered in more detail in chapter 10.)

The symbol $\bar{X}$ (pronounced "ex bar") is used to represent the mean in this formula.

$$\bar{X} = \frac{Sum\ of\ all\ values}{Count\ of\ value}$$

Example 2.23: Let's say that you completed six medical terminology tests. Your scores are 82, 78, 94, 56, 91, and 85. According to the calculation displayed below, your average score on the medical terminology tests is 81.

$$\bar{X} = \frac{82 + 78 + 94 + 56 + 91 + 85}{6} = \frac{486}{6} = 81$$

There are several different types of averages used in healthcare. The arithmetic mean or average is presented here. Other types of averages may be encountered in healthcare and will be presented in later chapters.

Excel may be used to calculate averages also. To solve example 2.23 using Excel, follow these steps:

Step 1: Enter the test values into column A as displayed in cells A2 through A7 in figure 2.9.

Step 2: Key the formula displayed in cell B8 in figure 2.9 into cell A8. Notice that this is a formula and therefore must start with an "=" sign so that Excel knows to evaluate the formula. The Excel function is called "average" and the cells in the parentheses are the cells that we want to average. The range of cells is written as A2:A7. Excel interprets this as cells A2 through A7.

Figure 2.9. Calculating an average using Excel

	A	B
1	Test Scores	
2	82	
3	78	
4	94	
5	56	
6	91	
7	85	
8	81	<<=average(A2:A7)

Exercise 2.7

1. Community Hospital reported the following birth weights, in pounds, for babies born January 30, 20XX: 6.9, 3.7, 7.7, 6.6, 7.3, 5.5, 9.9, 7.0, 5.5, and 7.7. What was the average birth weight for the day? Round to two decimal places.

2. A patient's temperature for five days after surgery taken at 7:00 a.m. each morning was recorded as 101.7, 100.4, 98.9, 100.2, and 98.6. What was the patient's average temperature after surgery? Round to two decimal places.

3. A patient's blood sugar was recorded for seven days at 8:00 a.m. and recorded as the following: 164, 155, 172, 145, 138, 136, and 142. What was the patient's average blood sugar at 8:00 a.m.? Round to a whole number.

4. A patient's systolic blood pressure was recorded from February 1 through February 7 at 6:30 a.m. each morning as the following:

February 1	130
February 2	135
February 3	132
February 4	126
February 5	120
February 6	122
February 7	124

    Create an Excel spreadsheet to calculate the patient's average systolic blood pressure at 6:30 a.m. Round to a whole number.

5. There are five health record analysts in the HIM department where you are working. Their hourly wages are: $13.87, $14.02, $15.56, $15.75, and $16.32. What is the average salary for the health record analysts? Perform this calculation both by hand and using Excel. Round to two decimal places.

Chapter 2   Matching Quiz

Match the definitions with the terms.

Definitions:

a. One or more parts of a whole
b. A type of ratio in which x is a portion of the whole (x + y).
c. An integer with no fractional or decimal parts

d. A measure used to compare an event over time; a comparison of the number of times an event did happen (numerator) with the number of times an event could have happened (denominator)

e. The relation of one part to the whole with respect to magnitude, quantity, or degree

f. The value obtained by dividing the sum of a set of numbers by the number of values in the set.

g. The part of a fraction below the line signifying division that functions as the divisor of the numerator and indicates into how many parts the unit is divided

h. The number resulting from the division of one number by another

i. A quotient derived from a fraction where the denominator is a multiple of 10

j. The process of approximating a number

Terms:

1. _____ Numerator
2. _____ Rate
3. _____ Fraction
4. _____ Average
5. _____ Denominator

6. _____ Whole number
7. _____ Proportion
8. _____ Decimal
9. _____ Rounding
10. _____ Quotient

Chapter 2   Review

Complete the following exercises.

1. Convert the fraction $\frac{1}{5}$ to a quotient and then a percentage.

2. Round the following percentages to two decimal places.
   a. 16.981%
   b. 13.655%
   c. 0.569%
   d. 98.990%
   e. 98.999%

3. Round the following percentages to one decimal place.
   a. 0.698%
   b. 53.123%
   c. 0.075%
   d. 34.337%
   e. 3.876%

4. Complete the following conversions:
   a. Convert $\frac{1}{6}$ to a percentage with two decimal places.
   b. Convert 0.65 to a percentage with two decimal places.
   c. Convert 34% to a fraction. Calculate it to its simplest form.
   d. Convert 34% to a decimal.

5. Convert the following fractions to their simplest form:

   a. $\dfrac{3}{9}$

   b. $\dfrac{4}{8}$

   c. $\dfrac{1}{5}$

   d. $\dfrac{3}{5}$

   e. $\dfrac{124}{248}$

6. Recreate the following table in Excel. Use an Excel formula to calculate each percentage to verify that the calculations are correct. If any are incorrect, note which ones and provide the correct answers.

Community Hospital Administrator's Semiannual Reference Report Discharges by Day of Week January 1, 20XX to June 30, 20XX		
Day	**Number of Patients**	**Percent of Patients**
Sunday	1,187	19.1%
Monday	755	11.3%
Tuesday	1,085	16.3%
Wednesday	1,031	15.5%
Thursday	1,024	17.0%
Friday	808	12.1%
Saturday	773	11.6%
Totals	**6,663**	**100.0%**

7. A physician on your staff performed 44 cardiac catheterizations last month. Thirty-four of those treated were male. What is the ratio of male patients to female patients who had cardiac catheterizations? What is the proportion of males? Round to one decimal point.

8. It was reported in your department meeting that over the past year your hospital decreased the number of employees by 4 percent. Last year there were 389 people employed; how many fewer employees are there this year? Round to a whole number.

9. Your manager needs to purchase a computer for the new receptionist in your department. The usual price is $1,100. The local supply company gives the facility a 13 percent reduction on all items they purchase. What price will your manager pay?

10. Your beginning salary as an analyst in the HIM department is $14.50 per hour. You are due to receive a 3.4 percent cost-of-living raise in your next paycheck. Your performance evaluation is coming up in one month, and you believe you should get an additional 5 percent increase based on your excellent performance. What should your hourly wage be after your next paycheck, and what do you anticipate it will be after your performance evaluation?

11. Last year, you purchased equipment in the HIM department for $14,250. You have been told that the equipment you bought has depreciated in value by 20 percent. What is the value of the equipment now?

12. You just scored 40 points out of a possible 50 on your health information test. What percentage of available points did you earn?

13. Last year, the number of hospitals in your state decreased from 320 to 240. What is the percentage of decrease?

14. Use Excel and the data in the following table to determine the average birth weights and average age of mother. Round to one decimal place.

Community Hospital Births March 1 through March 31, 20XX			
Birth	**Birth Weight in Pounds**	**Mother's No.**	**Mother's Age**
1	5.6	1	18.5
2	6.7	2	19.3
3	5.9	3	15.5
4	6.0	4	34.2
5	3.9	5	25.6
6	9.2	6	29.7
7	10.3	7	24.8
8	11.3	8	26.6
9	6.9	9	17.3
10	7.1	10	26.5
11	5.9	11	24.7
12	5.7	12	23.2
13	5.2	13	21.4
14	6.9	14	22.9
15	10.2	15	31.5
Totals			

For the following questions, refer to the following Quarterly Coding Professional Accuracy Report.

15. Are the calculations of the percentage of records accurately coded for each coder and the total correct?

16. Coding professional D determined her accuracy rate for the quarter to be 95.9 percent. She would like you to recalculate her accuracy rate because she thinks it is incorrect in the report.

Community Hospital
Quarterly Coding Professional Accuracy Report
January through March, 20XX

	January			February			March			Total		
	# Records	# Correct	% Correct	# Records	# Correct	% Correct	# Records	# Correct	% Correct	# Records	# Correct	% Correct
Coding professional A	560	504	90.0%	544	495	91.0%	270	243	90.0%	1,374	1,242	90.4%
Coding professional B	540	503	93.1%	523	491	93.9%	531	494	93.0%	1,594	1,488	93.4%
Coding professional C	500	440	88.0%	445	401	90.1%	493	435	88.2%	1,438	1,276	88.7%
Coding professional D	620	583	94.0%	588	570	96.9%	584	551	94.3%	1,792	1,704	95.1%
Coding professional E	480	408	85.0%	432	392	90.7%	465	397	85.4%	1,377	1,197	86.9%
Totals	2,700	2,438	90.3%	2,532	2,349	92.8%	2,343	2,120	90.5%	7,575	6,907	91.2%

CHAPTER

3

Patient Census

Learning Objectives

At the conclusion of this chapter, you should be able to do the following:

- Perform the calculations of the following healthcare utilization statistics: inpatient admission, inpatient census, complete master census, daily inpatient census, inpatient service day, total inpatient service days, and admission and discharge on the same day (A&D)
- Differentiate between an interhospital (interfacility) transfer and an intrahospital transfer
- Calculate daily census and inpatient service days using the admission and discharge data provided
- Calculate census and inpatient service days with data given for newborns and transfers

Key Terms

Admission date	Discharge	Interhospital transfer
Average daily inpatient census	Discharge date	Intrahospital transfer
Census day	Inpatient admission	Newborn
Complete master census	Inpatient census	Patient care unit (PCU)
Daily inpatient census	Inpatient service day	Patient day

Hospitals keep track of patient census statistics to determine when they have the largest number of patients and when that number drops. They can then tell when the busiest times of the year are to determine increasing staffing, whether there are any patient care units being overburdened by a large number of patients, and which units have a decrease in patients. Resources allocated to those units may change throughout the year to accommodate the units with more patients. Policies regarding low census staffing may be enforced when needed, and staff may be asked to take time off. Hospital administration also reviews the census by individual physician and patient care units because they are interested in understanding trends in the patient admission process and the factors that may be driving those trends.

Inpatient Census

Hospital management uses census data for various purposes, including planning, budgeting, and staffing. The accounting of patients in the hospital is an important statistic tracked by hospital leaders. An **inpatient admission** is when an acute care facility's formal acceptance of a patient who is to be provided with room, board, and continuous nursing service in an area of the facility where patients generally stay at least overnight. The **inpatient census** indicates the number of patients admitted to and assigned to an inpatient bed in the facility at a particular point in time.

A staff member, usually a member of the nursing staff, on each **patient care unit (PCU)** is designated to count the patients on that unit each day. A PCU is an organizational entity of a healthcare facility organized both physically and functionally to provide care. For example, the intensive care unit (ICU) would be considered a PCU. In some facilities, PCUs may be designated by location, such as 2-West or 3-North, or by specialties such as oncology, neurology, or surgery.

The inpatient census-taking time is usually at midnight but may occur at any time as long as the time is consistent for the entire facility; that is, each PCU conducts the census at the same time. Around midnight is a good time to take the census because patients are usually in their beds. It would be difficult to account for all patients at 8:00 a.m., for example, because they might be in an exam room, with radiology, in surgery, with their healthcare provider, or just taking a walk in the hospital.

The necessary data are first entered into the computer as admissions, discharges, or intrahospital transfers and then verified at the designated time by the responsible person on each PCU. In this context, an **admission date** is the day a patient first enters the hospital as an inpatient. A **discharge date** is the day the patient leaves the hospital. Discharges include patients who are sent home, those who die in the hospital, and interhospital transfers. **Interhospital transfers** are events when a patient leaves one hospital and is immediately admitted to another hospital or healthcare facility. **Intrahospital transfers** are transfers within the hospital from one PCU to another during an inpatient admission.

Figure 3.1 shows a form for a manual daily census summary for a nursing home. Although most census data are now collected via electronic forms or custom spreadsheets, the contents are essentially the same as displayed in the paper form in figure 3.1.

Figure 3.1.   Daily census summary at Community Manor Nursing Home

To be completed daily at 12:01 a.m. by charge nurse			Community Manor Nursing Home Daily Census Summary	
Hall: ____A ____B ____C ____D			**Date** _____	
Initial admits—New residents			Date	Time
				a.m.–p.m.
				a.m.–p.m.
				a.m.–p.m.
				a.m.–p.m.
Discharged to home or transfer			Date	Time
				a.m.–p.m.
				a.m.–p.m.
				a.m.–p.m.
Transfer to hospital	Location		Date	Time
				a.m.–p.m.
				a.m.–p.m.
				a.m.–p.m.
				a.m.–p.m.
Out on leave—Pass	Date Left	Time	Returned	Time
		a.m.–p.m.		a.m.–p.m.
		a.m.–p.m.		a.m.–p.m.
		a.m.–p.m.		a.m.–p.m.
Deceased			Date	Time of Death
				a.m.–p.m.
				a.m.–p.m.
				a.m.–p.m.
Return from hospital stay			Date	Time
				a.m.–p.m.
				a.m.–p.m.
				a.m.–p.m.
				a.m.–p.m.
Charge nurse: _____				

Source: ©AHIMA

Complete Master Census

In addition to reporting the head count to the central collection area, each PCU reports, the number of patients admitted, discharged, and transferred into or out of the PCU that day. This is commonly referred to as the admission discharge and transfer (ADT) system in a facility. The transfers tabulated in the ADT system are intrahospital transfers. The central collection area then uses the census from all the units to compile a total census for the facility, sometimes referred to as the **complete master census**. The complete master census shows the names of patients present at a particular point in time and their location. In most facilities this is a computerized process that is linked with the facility's master patient index, billing system, and other electronic health record systems.

The spreadsheet template presented in figure 3.2 may be used to calculate the inpatient census.

Figure 3.2.   Inpatient census template

	A	B
1	**Data Element**	**Value**
2	Starting inpatient census (@ 12:01 am)	
3	Admissions (Not discharged same day)	
4	Discharges (Not admitted same day)	
5	Ending inpatient census (Midnight)	=B2+B3-B4

Example 3.1: The number of patients in General Hospital at midnight on May 1 is 230. Two patients are admitted and 40 patients are discharged on May 2. What is the inpatient census for General Hospital on May 2?

Manual calculation: 230 + 2 – 40 = 192

Using Excel:

	A	B
1	**Data Element**	**Value**
2	Starting inpatient census (@ 12:01 am)	230
3	Admissions (Not discharged same day)	2
4	Discharges (Not admitted same day)	40
5	Ending inpatient census (Midnight)	192
6		

Exercise 3.1

Answer the following questions.

1. A PCU has a count of 20 patients at 1:00 a.m. on September 1, and 30 patients at the same time on September 2. Could the counts have been different if the PCU had taken a census at 12:01 a.m. on both days?

2. Would you accept the different PCUs in the hospital taking censuses at different times as long as each unit is consistent within itself?

3. A patient transferred at 5:00 p.m. to unit A from unit B is counted in unit A's 12:01 a.m. census as one additional patient present. Would that patient still be included in unit B's 12:01 a.m. census?

4. What term is used to describe a patient who is transferred from one PCU to another within the same facility?

5. On July 1, your community hospital has 124 inpatients who are staying overnight in their facility. In addition, 231 patients have come into the hospital for various tests and treatments. Which of these patients would be included in the inpatient census, the 124 patients, the 231 patients, or the 355 patients?

Figure 3.3. Spreadsheet template for daily inpatient census calculations

	A	B
1	**Data Element**	**Value**
2	Starting inpatient census (@12:01 am)	
3	Admissions (Not discharged same day)	
4	Admitted & Discharged Same Day	
5	Discharges (Not admitted same day)	
6	Daily inpatient Census	=B2+B3+B4−B5

Figure 3.4. Example daily inpatient census calculation

	A	B
1	**Data Element**	**Value**
2	Starting inpatient census (@12:01 am)	20
3	Admissions (Not discharged same day)	0
4	Admitted & Discharged Same Day	1
5	Discharges (Not admitted same day)	0
6	Daily inpatient Census	21

Daily Inpatient Census

The **daily inpatient census** is a statistic that measures the number of patients admitted to the hospital or unit at any time during a given day. Therefore, it includes the number of inpatients present at census-taking time each day, plus any inpatients who were both admitted and discharged after the census-taking time the previous day. Thus, a patient admitted to the hospital at 8:00 a.m. on June 1 and discharged at 10:00 p.m. that same day would not be present for the midnight head count. Therefore, he or she would not appear on the census report. However, the patient must be accounted for separately in some manner. For an example, in an ICU, a patient could be admitted at 8:00 a.m. and consume a high volume of services and staff time before passing away. This resource intensity would not be visible on the midnight census but is critically important in determining staffing. Figure 3.3 displays an example spreadsheet template that is useful when calculating daily inpatient census.

Example 3.2: Twenty patients are on a PCU. One patient was admitted at 10:00 a.m. and discharged at 7:00 p.m. If there are no other discharges, the daily inpatient census for this day is 21. The patient that was admitted and discharged on that day is added to the 20 patients already on the unit.

Manual Calculation: 20 + 1 = 21
Figure 3.4 shows how to use the Microsoft Excel template in figure 3.3.

Exercise 3.2

1. The census at 12:01 a.m. on June 1 is 110. Three patients were admitted on June 1 at 6:00 a.m. and discharged later that same day. One patient admitted at 6:00 a.m. died at 5:30 p.m. the same afternoon. What is the PCU's daily inpatient census for June 1?

2. Which statistic is more useful in understanding the patients served at a facility, census or daily inpatient census? Why?

3. Community Hospital's census at 12:01 a.m. on September 19 was 327. On that day, 12 patients were admitted and 10 patients were discharged. Calculate the inpatient census for September 19.

4. Community Hospital's Critical Care Unit (CCU) census at 12:01 a.m. on December 2 was 14. Four patients were admitted to the CCU on December 2, one patient was transferred to the medicine unit, and one patient died. Calculate the inpatient census for the CCU for December 2.

5. The census in the telemetry unit at Community Hospital on May 1 was 26 patients. Two patients were admitted after stent insertions and three patients were transferred into the unit from the ICU. On the same day, four patients were discharged and one patient was transferred to the ICU. One patient was admitted at 7:00 p.m. and was discharged and transferred at 9:00 p.m. to another facility. What will the daily inpatient census of the telemetry unit be for May 1?

Inpatient Service Days

An **inpatient service day** is a unit of measure denoting the services received by one inpatient in one 24-hour period or any portion of that 24-hour period. The 24-hour period is the time between the census-taking hours on two successive days. The usual 24-hour reporting period begins at 12:01 a.m. and ends at midnight. One inpatient service day is counted for each inpatient admission when a patient is admitted and discharged on the same day because they received services during that stay. Failure to account for this time will result in lost credit for the services provided to that patient.

There are a number of important issues concerning inpatient service days. These include the following:

- One unit of one service day is not usually divided or reported as a fraction of a day.
- The day of admission is counted as an inpatient service day, but the day of discharge is not. Therefore, no patient admitted to an inpatient unit can have a zero-service day stay.

An inpatient service day may also be referred to as a **patient day**, inpatient day, bed occupancy day, or **census day**. The operative word here is service; that is, the number of patients who received service on a particular day. Using the full term "inpatient service day" reflects the hospital function of providing services to patients each day and more clearly defines the quantity counted. If 20 patients are provided services in one 24-hour period, the number of inpatient service days for that calendar day is 20. Although inpatient service days and the daily inpatient census are used for two different purposes, the calculation is the same for both statistics. The daily inpatient census is a statistic representing the number of patients (people) that were present in the hospital at any time during the day, while the inpatient service day is a statistic measured in days. Therefore, the template displayed in figure 3.2 may also be used to determine the inpatient service days with one minor change in the title listed in cell A6. The revised inpatient service day template is presented in figure 3.5.

Figure 3.5. Spreadsheet template to calculate inpatient service days

	A	B
1	**Data Element**	**Value**
2	Starting inpatient census (@12:01 am)	
3	Admissions (Not discharged same day)	
4	Admitted & Discharged Same Day	
5	Discharges (Not admitted same day)	
6	Inpatient Service Days	=B2+B3+B4-B5

Exercise 3.3

Differentiate among census, inpatient census, daily inpatient census, and inpatient service days. If a facility has 129 inpatient service days, would 129 also be the daily inpatient census or inpatient census?

Total Inpatient Service Days

The term **total inpatient service days** refers to the sum of all inpatient service days for each of the days during a specified period of time. For example, if the inpatient service days for June 1, 2, and 3 are 100, 105, and 101, the total for the three days is 306. Typically, total inpatient service days are calculated monthly, quarterly, semiannually, or annually.

Example 3.3: Given the following inpatient service days for Community Hospital, a 75-bed facility, what is the total number of inpatient service days provided during these 10 days in June?

Date	1-Jun	2-Jun	3-Jun	4-Jun	5-Jun	6-Jun	7-Jun	8-Jun	9-Jun	10-Jun
Inpatient Service Days	70	71	72	68	69	71	73	74	69	70

Total inpatient service days = 70+71+72+68+69+71+73+74+69+70 = 707 days

Be sure to note the units of measure for each statistic calculated. Total inpatient service days are measured in days. Census statistics (daily, inpatient, master) are measured in people or patients.

QUICK TIP

Exercise 3.4

Complete the following exercises.

1. The time for taking the inpatient census must always be _____.
   a. Variable
   b. Consistent
   c. 12:00 p.m.
   d. 11:59 a.m.

2. Patient day or inpatient day is more correctly termed _____.
   a. Inpatient service day
   b. Daily inpatient census
   c. Total inpatient service day(s)
   d. Census

3. The inpatient census at 12:01 a.m. is 24. Two patients were admitted at 1:00 p.m. One patient died at 3:15 p.m., and the other patient was discharged at 10:00 p.m. The inpatient service days for that day are _____.

   a. 22

   b. 24

   c. 25

   d. 26

4. The difference between the census and the daily inpatient census is that any patients admitted and discharged the same day are added to _____.

   a. The census to calculate the daily inpatient census

   b. The 12:01 a.m. (or other designated time) head count to calculate the daily census

   c. Both a and b

   d. Neither a nor b

5. Which of the following should be used when calculating the number of inpatients who received service on a particular day?

   a. Inpatient census

   b. Daily inpatient census

   c. Total inpatient service days

   d. Census

Calculation of Inpatient Service Days

The calculation of inpatient service days is the measurement of services received by all inpatients in one 24-hour period (the time between the census-taking hours on two successive days). The usual reporting period begins at 12:01 a.m. and ends at 12:00 a.m. (midnight). Moreover, one inpatient day must be counted for each inpatient admitted and discharged on the same day between two successive census-taking hours.

The definitions of census, inpatient service day, and total inpatient service days provide clues for actual computation. The sample shown in table 3.1 includes all of a hospital's inpatient care units. A summary of all such units helps the administration review the hospital's overall level of activity.

Table 3.1. Sample inpatient service days display

Sample Inpatient Service Days	
Number of patients in hospital at 12:01 a.m. on November 1	257
Plus the number of patients admitted on November 1	+ 45
Subtotal	302
Minus the number of patients discharged (including deaths) on November 1	− 24
Number of patients in hospital at 11:59 p.m. on November 1 (subtotal)	278
Plus the number of patients both admitted and discharged on November 1	+ 4
Total inpatient service days for November 1	282

 Sometimes you may be asked by administration to exclude PCUs such as ICUs and obstetrical units from the inpatient service days. Units such as these are often studied separately because the intensity of service on these units varies greatly from the intensity of services provided on medical and surgical units.

QUICK
TIP

Table 3.2 shows a sample of how hospital administration can use inpatient service days data to determine performance. Figure 3.6 demonstrates that the spreadsheet template from figure 3.5 may be used to perform the same calculation.

Table 3.2. Year-to-date inpatient service days

Community Medical Center **September 20XX** **Year-to-Date Inpatient Service Days**					
Service	**Actual**	**Budget**	**Actual - Budget**	**Prior Year**	**Actual - Prior Year**
Medicine	13,762	15,000	–1,238	15,608	–1,846
Surgery	8,953	13,500	–4,547	11,634	–2,681
ICU	3,874	3,500	374	3,623	251
Step-down	679	1,500	–821	1,278	–599
Rehabilitation	1,646	2,500	–854	2,136	–490
Obstetrics	1,730	2,200	–470	2,188	–458
Psychiatry	1,002	1,800	–798	872	130
Newborn	1,689	1,800	–111	2,099	–410
Neonatal ICU	2,875	3,900	–1,025	2,643	232
Pediatrics	645	1,000	–355	833	–188
Total	**36,855**	**46,700**	**–9,845**	**42,914**	**–6,059**

Figure 3.6. Sample inpatient service days calculation using spreadsheet template in figure 3.5

	A	B
	Data Element	**Value**
1		
2	Starting inpatient census (@ 12:01 am)	257
3	Admissions (Not discharged same day)	45
4	Admitted & Discharged Same Day	4
5	Discharges (Not admitted same day)	24
6	Inpatient Service Days	282

Hospital statistics are often tabulated separately for adults and children and newborns. Newborns (NB) are defined to be an inpatient who was born in a hospital at the beginning of the current inpatient hospitalization.

QUICK TIP

This medical center's analysis of its inpatient service days can be examined to determine how well the facility is doing year to date and to compare its performance with the previous year. This can lead to discussions by hospital leadership concerning marketing of their services or examination of whether there are enough practitioners in those services.

Before beginning the actual calculation of census data and inpatient service days, it is important to understand the calculation of transfers. The calculation of transfers occurs on the PCU census. Transfers in and out of the unit are shown as subdivisions of patients admitted to and discharged from the unit.

The hospital may be referred to as the "house," as in "How many patients are in the house?" This refers to the number of patients in the hospital.

QUICK TIP

The census for the next day must begin with the 11:59 p.m. census data and not inpatient service days. Calculate under the assumption that the patients admitted and discharged on the same day and the transfers are not newborns.

QUICK TIP

Example 3.4: Figure 3.7 displays census calculation data in a format frequently used by hospitals. Key to abbreviations used in this example

Abbreviation	Definition
A/C	Adults and children
NB	Newborns (born during the hospital stay)
Adm	Admissions (includes transfers into the hospital)
Bir	Births
Trf	Intra-hospital Transfers—may be into a unit (in) or out of a unit (out).
Dis	Discharges (including transfers out of hospital and deaths)
A/D	Admitted and discharged on same day

Transfers may also be abbreviated as TX and discharges may also be abbreviated as DC.

In this example, a patient head count at 12:01 a.m. on June 1 shows 48 adult and child inpatients and two newborns. This type of display allows a unit manager to view the flow of patients into and out of the unit. The last three columns are discussed later in this chapter. Note that the end census of 49 A/C patients and 1 NB may be used as the starting census for the next day.

Figure 3.7. Example census tracking table

	Start		Activity into unit					Activity out of unit			End			Serv	
	12:01 a.m. Census		Adm		Trf	Total		Dis	Dis	Trf	11:59 p.m. Census			Serv Days	
Day	A/C	NB	A/C	Bir	in	A/C	NB	A/C	NB	out	A/C	NB	A/D	A/C	NB
1-Jun	48	2	2	1	1	51	3	1	2	1	49	1	1	50	1

The following points are important to keep in mind:

- The terms *transfers in* and *transfers out* refer to intrahospital transfers, that is, transfers between inpatient units within the hospital. Transfers in and out of the hospital (called interhospital or interfacility transfers) are included in admissions and discharges.

- Transfers in and out of any specific medical care unit may or may not be equal, but they must be equal for the overall hospital summary. Every patient transferred into a unit on any given day must have been transferred out of another unit. Failure of these data to balance may mean that a unit neglected to report transfers correctly.

- Newborns are considered separately for all computations based on census data. They should be reported separately unless otherwise directed by administration, medical staff, or other persons using the statistical data produced. Births are considered newborn admissions.

- The census at the close of one day (11:59 p.m.) is the inpatient census at the beginning of the next day and is commonly referred to as the number of patients remaining.

Summary of Census Data

The process of verifying the data obtained by the process of calculating census statistics on a daily basis is called the monthly or yearly summary of census data, meaning a concise summary of the data. The total number of patients admitted and born during the month or year is added to the patients-remaining census with which the month or year began. From this sum, the number of discharges (including deaths) during the month or year is subtracted. The resulting data are the number of patients remaining at the end of the month or year. This number should equal the actual head count at 11:59 p.m. the last night of that month or year. Table 3.3 shows a sample monthly census summary. Notice

Table 3.3.   Sample monthly census summary

Community Hospital	Adults and Children	Newborns
Number of patients in hospital at 12:01 a.m. on October 1	48	2
Add the number of patients admitted in October	+ 100	+ 7
Subtotal	148	9
Subtract the number of patients discharged (including deaths) in October	− 110	− 5
Number of patients in hospital at 11:59 p.m., October 31	38	4

that patients admitted and discharged on the same day are not included in the monthly census calculations in table 3.3. The monthly census is intended to measure the patients actually present at the census-taking time and not the patients actually served during the month. This demonstrates the key difference between census calculations and inpatient service days.

When you summarize monthly or annual census data, you are verifying that the columns have been added correctly. This procedure also verifies that no error was made in the original data on one or more lines. This verification is accomplished by taking the 12:01 a.m. inpatient census at the beginning of the period, adding total admissions and transfers in, and subtracting total discharges and transfers out. The resultant data represent the ending census on the last day of the period (month or year).

Exercise 3.5

Complete the following exercises.

1. Using the data given in example 3.4, create a spreadsheet to calculate the census for June 2. Then, fill in the blanks in the table below.

	12:01 a.m. Census		Adm		Trf	Total		Dis	Dis	Trf	11:59 p.m. Census			Serv Days	
Day	A/C	NB	A/C	Bir	in	A/C	NB	A/C	NB	out	A/C	NB	A/D	A/C	NB
6/1	48	2	2	1	1	51	3	1	2	1	49	1			
6/2			3	1	2			4	1	2					

2. What data will you use to begin June 3, and why?

3. Fill in the blanks in the table below. What are the inpatient service days for June 2 and 3?

	12:01 a.m. Census		Adm		Trf	Total		Dis	Dis	Trf	11:59 p.m. Census			Serv Days	
Day	A/C	NB	A/C	Bir	in	A/C	NB	A/C	NB	out	A/C	NB	A/D	A/C	NB
6/1	48	2	2	1	1	51	3	1	2	1	49	1	1	50	1
6/2	49	1	3	1	2	54	2	4	1	2	48	1	1		
6/3			1	1	1			3	0	1			0		

4. Would a newborn ever be considered an A/D?

5. At this point, you have inpatient service days for three successive days. The total of these data, excluding newborns, for June 1, 2, and 3 is 145 (50 + 49 + 46). What will you need to know and do to get the hospital total inpatient service days for the entire month of June?

Exercise 3.6

Using the information supplied for June 1, fill in the blanks in the table below.

Day	12:01 a.m. Census A/C	12:01 a.m. Census NB	Adm A/C	Adm Bir	Trf in	Total A/C	Total NB	Dis A/C	Dis NB	Trf out	11:59 p.m. Census A/C	11:59 p.m. Census NB	A/D	Serv Days A/C	Serv Days NB
6/1	230	12	20	4	3			19	3	2			1		
6/2			21	4	1			19	4	1			0		
6/3			23	6	0			24	5	0			3		
6/4			25	5	1			23	4	1			1		
6/5			24	4	2			18	3	2			2		

Exercise 3.7

Two hundred and fifty adults and children were in the hospital at 12:01 a.m. on August 1. There were 23 newborns at 12:01 a.m. on August 1. During August, the following data were compiled:

Admissions:	
Adults and children	1,353
Newborns	73
Discharges (including deaths):	
Adults and children	1,348
Newborns	65

1. What would the inpatient census for adults and children be on August 31 at 11:59 p.m.?

2. What would the inpatient census be for newborns on August 31?

3. Can the inpatient service days be calculated with the information supplied in the previous question? Explain why or why not.

4. The surgery unit in Community Hospital has reported the following data. Do these data look correct? Explain your answer.

Day	12:01 a.m. Census	Adm	Trf in	Total	Dis	Trf out	11:59 p.m. Census	A/D	Serv Days
8/1	20	4	2	26	2	8	16	1	16

5. On March 1, the telemetry unit at Community Hospital has reported the 15 patients on the unit at 12:01 a.m. During March, the following data were collected:

Admissions	240
Discharges (including deaths)	232

What would the inpatient census be on March 31 at 11:59 p.m. in the telemetry unit?

Exercise 3.8

This exercise consists of two worksheets for calculating a month's inpatient census and inpatient service days. Using the data provided for May 1, complete the first worksheet. If your findings do not match the data for May 31, you have made an error either in your column additions or on one or more of the horizontal lines above the total. You must correct this error to ensure the validity of the monthly totals. If the column additions are correct, continue on to the second worksheet for the recap. Use a spreadsheet to complete these worksheets.

Worksheet 1

Day	12:01 a.m. Census A/C	NB	Adm A/C	NB	Trf in	Total A/C	NB	Disch A/C	NB	Trf out	11:59 p.m. Census A/C	NB	A/D	Serv Days A/C	NB
1	165	3	29	0	8	202	3	10	0	7	185	3	0		
2	185	3	24	4	7			12	3	6			1		
3			18	3	3			16	2	2			0		
4			17	2	5			15	2	4			0		
5			13	0	1			12	1	3			0		
6			20	0	6			19	2	4			0		
7			21	0	14			17	0	12			0		
8			27	1	10			23	3	8			3		
9			23	4	6			22	3	14			2		
10			22	2	8			15	1	10			1		
11			17	3	7			14	4	5			3		
12			19	3	6			17	2	4			0		
13			14	1	4			12	2	2			0		
14			15	4	5			19	3	7			0		
15			20	14	8			13	0	6			1		
16			23	3	6			15	4	2			0		
17			17	1	3			13	3	1			1		
18			15	0	2			21	1	6			2		
19			17	0	7			25	3	2			1		
20			13	2	3			27	4	4			0		
21			12	1	5			21	2	5			3		
22			10	0	1			17	4	1			2		
23			9	2	4			18	1	4			0		
24			23	4	3			12	3	2			2		
25			15	2	4			22	2	3			1		
26			13	3	2			9	1	4			0		
27			21	1	3			29	1	0			2		
28			29	2	5			22	4	4			3		
29			23	4	1			25	3	2			1		
30			15	1	4			21	2	3			0		
31			16	4	2			18	3	2			3		
Totals															

Worksheet 2

Recap of Monthly Data for Adults and Children: May 20XX Enter numbers from worksheet 1		
12:01 a.m. Census A/C		165
Admissions Adult and Children	+	_____
Transfers in	+	_____
Total A/C	=	_____
Discharges Adult and Children	–	_____
Transfers out	–	_____
11:59 p.m. Census A/C on May 31	=	
Recap of Monthly Data for Newborns:		
12:01 a.m. Census NB		
Newborn Admissions	+	_____
Total NB	=	_____
Discharges NB	–	_____
11:59 p.m. Census NB on May 31	=	
Serv Days A/C (total inpatient service days excluding newborns) _____		
Serv Days NB (total newborn service days) _____		
Total inpatient service days _____		

Average Daily Inpatient Census

The **average daily inpatient census** is the average or mean number of inpatients present in the hospital each day for a given period of time. The total inpatient service days for any period (usually a month or a year) represent the inpatient service days for all the calendar days in that period. The formula for calculating the average daily inpatient census is:

$$Ave\ Daily\ Inp\ Census = \frac{Total\ inpatient\ service\ days\ (excluding\ newborns)}{Total\ number\ of\ days\ in\ the\ period}$$

 When calculating the average daily inpatient census for a month, you need to know how many days there are in each month.

QUICK
TIP

Example 3.5: If a hospital had 6,653 inpatient service days for adults and children and 155 inpatient service days for newborns for the month of May, what was the average daily inpatient census in May? Round to the nearest whole number.

$$Ave\ Daily\ Inp\ Census = \frac{Total\ inpatient\ service\ days\ (excluding\ newborns)}{Total\ number\ of\ days\ in\ May}$$

$$Ave\ Daily\ Inp\ Census = \frac{6,653}{31} = 214.61\ rounded\ to\ 215\ patients$$

As mentioned earlier, adults and children are calculated separately from newborns unless otherwise directed by the hospital's administration. Newborn census data can distort statistics related to resource use. For example, it costs less to maintain a newborn nursery than it does to staff other PCUs. If the average daily inpatient census is consistently low over a specified period, it may be appropriate to close PCUs to reduce expenses.

 Whether to round to a whole number is the individual hospital's decision. There is a difference between working with data representing people (because you cannot have a portion of a person) and working with percentages that represent numbers. Many facilities use a whole number when calculating the census and fractions with other healthcare statistics. (Refer to chapter 2 to review rounding.)

QUICK
TIP

Example 3.6: A 150-bed hospital reports 3,489 inpatient service days for December. Calculate the average daily inpatient census for December. Round to the nearest whole number.

$$Ave\ Daily\ Inp\ Census = \frac{Total\ inpatient\ service\ days\ (excluding\ newborns)}{Total\ number\ of\ days\ in\ December}$$

$$Ave\ Daily\ Inp\ Census = \frac{3,489}{31} = 112.54\ rounded\ to\ 113\ patients$$

Again, this number is important to administration because they will want to know how many patients are being served each month to determine staffing and supply needs for practitioners and to monitor the overall financial performance of the facility.

Average Daily Newborn Census

The formula for calculating the average daily newborn census follows the same pattern as the formula for calculating the average daily inpatient census of adults and children.

$$Ave\ Daily\ NB\ Census = \frac{Total\ newborns\ inpatient\ service\ days}{Total\ number\ of\ days\ in\ the\ period}$$

Example 3.7: A hospital with 20 bassinets had 552 newborn inpatient service days during April. What was the average newborn daily census in April? Round to the nearest whole number.

$$Ave\ Daily\ NB\ Census = \frac{Total\ newborns\ inpatient\ service\ days}{Total\ number\ of\ days\ in\ April}$$

$$Ave\ Daily\ NB\ Census = \frac{552}{30} = 18.4\ rounded\ to\ 18\ newborns$$

Assume all exercises in this text do not occur on a leap year. A leap year is a year in which an extra day is added to the calendar at the end of February, giving February 29 days. Therefore, regular years have 365 days; leap years have 366. Leap years only occur on an even-numbered year, so if the example is an odd year, one not need consider a leap year as a possibility.

Average Daily Inpatient Census for a Patient Care Unit

The hospital's administration often finds it helpful to know the average use of a specific medical care unit (for example, to know whether additional beds are needed for the ICU). Statistics are the basis for decision-making. The formula for calculating the average daily inpatient census for a care unit is the same used in the overall average daily inpatient census. The difference here is that the inpatient service days specific to the PCU measured should be included in the numerator.

Example 3.8: A hospital with a 24-bed CCU reports 740 inpatient service days for July. Calculate the average daily inpatient census. Round to the nearest whole number.

$$Ave\ Daily\ Inp\ Census\ for\ CCU = \frac{Total\ inpatient\ service\ days\ for\ the\ CCU}{Total\ number\ of\ days\ in\ July}$$

$$Ave\ Daily\ Inp\ Census\ for\ CCU = \frac{740}{31} = 23.87\ rounded\ to\ 24\ patients$$

Do not confuse the terms regarding the census and inpatient service days. Inpatient census refers to patients present at the census taking time. Some healthcare facility staff may just say "census"—they are referring to the inpatient census. The average inpatient census is the mean number of hospital inpatients present in the hospital each day for a given period. The inpatient service days include any patients who were admitted and discharged on the same day.

Exercise 3.9

Complete the following exercises.

1. Community Hospital has 200 beds and 25 newborn bassinets. The total inpatient service days for May were 5,297 for adults and children and 486 for newborns.
   a. What is the average daily inpatient census for adults and children? Round to a whole number.
   b. Determine the average daily newborn census. Round to a whole number.

2. A 150-bed, 15-bassinet hospital has 4,350 inpatient service days for adults and children and 360 newborn service days during June.
   a. What is the average daily inpatient census, excluding newborns? Round to a whole number.
   b. Determine the average daily newborn census. Round to a whole number.

3. Calculate the average daily newborn census for a 125-bed, 10-bassinet hospital with 3,001 inpatient service days for adults and children and 298 inpatient service days for newborns during February (not a leap year). Round your answer to a whole number.

4. If you need to calculate the average daily inpatient census of the surgical unit, where can you obtain the surgical unit's inpatient service days?

5. Community Hospital's burn unit has 12 beds. The inpatient service days for the burn unit in December were 358. What is the average daily inpatient census for the burn unit during December? Round your answer to a whole number.

Chapter 3 Formulae for Calculation of Bed Occupancy Statistics

Statistic	Numerator	Denominator
Inpatient bed occupancy rate	Total number of inpatient service days for a given period	Total number of inpatient bed count days for the same period
Newborn bassinet occupancy rate	Total number of newborn inpatient service days for a given period	Total number of bassinet bed count days for the same period
Bed turnover rate (direct Formula)	Number of discharges (including deaths) for a period	Average bed count during the period
Bed turnover rate (indirect Formula)	Occupancy rate x number of days in period	Average length of stay for period

Chapter 3   Matching Quiz

Match the definitions with the terms.

Definitions:

a. The day that a patient first enters the hospital as an inpatient.
b. The mean or average number of hospital inpatients present in the hospital each day for a given period of time
c. The number of inpatients present at census-taking time each day plus any inpatients who were both admitted and discharged after the census-taking time the previous day
d. The number of inpatients occupying a bed in a healthcare facility at any given time

e. A change in medical care unit or medical staff unit during an inpatient stay

f. An organizational entity within a healthcare facility organized both physically and functionally to provide care

g. A unit of measure equivalent to the services received by one inpatient during one 24-hour period

h. The sum of all inpatient service days for each of the days during a specified period of time

Terms:

1. _____ Inpatient census   5. _____ Intrahospital transfer

2. _____ PCU   6. _____ Average daily inpatient census

3. _____ Total inpatient service days   7. _____ Admission day

4. _____ Daily inpatient census   8. _____ Patient day

Chapter 3   Review

1. What is an intrahospital transfer?

2. Differentiate between the terms *inpatient census* and *daily inpatient census*.

3. Is it possible that the transfers into a PCU may not equal the transfers out of the same PCU on the same day?

4. When must transfers in and transfers out be equal?

5. At 11:59 p.m. on February 1, the Community Hospital census was 427. On February 2, 37 patients were admitted, 33 were discharged, and 2 were admitted and discharged that day. In their CCU, the census on February 1 was 16. On February 2, six patients were admitted, four were discharged, and one was admitted who died later that day in the CCU. Answer the following questions and round the answers to whole numbers.

   a. Calculate the hospital inpatient census for February 2.

   b. Calculate the hospital daily inpatient census for February 2.

   c. Calculate the CCU inpatient census for February 2.

   d. Calculate the CCU inpatient service days for February 2.

6. In 20XX, a hospital had 175 beds for adults and children from January 1 through June 30. On July 1, the hospital increased its beds to 250 and the number remained at 250 through December 31. During the first six months, 30,875 patient days of service were provided to the hospital's adults and children. During the past six months, 36,982 days of service were provided. Answer the following questions and round the answers to whole numbers. This is a non-leap year.

   a. What was the average daily inpatient census for the first six months?

      A. 169

      B. 170

      C. 171

      D. 172

   b. What was the average daily inpatient census for the entire year?

      A. 184

      B. 185

      C. 186

      D. 187

c. The same hospital provided 12,345 newborn days of service in its 35-bassinet nursery during the year. What was the average daily newborn census?

    A. 31

    B. 32

    C. 33

    D. 34

d. The same hospital's new surgery unit has 50 beds. During July, the unit provided 1,705 days of service. What was the average daily inpatient census for the surgery unit in July?

    A. 52

    B. 53

    C. 54

    D. 55

e. Do you think the hospital's administration provided enough beds for the new surgery unit?

7. Using the statistics from the following monthly report from the nursing administration of Community Hospital, an acute-care facility, use Excel to calculate the current month's (November) average daily inpatient census for each nursing unit and the totals. Note: This facility's policy is to round to a whole number.

	Community Hospital Inpatient Statistical Report Average Daily Inpatient Census by Nursing Unit November 20XX			
	Unit	Number of Beds	Inpatient Service Days	Average Daily Inpatient Census
A	Medicine/Surgery	40	1,108	
B	Pediatrics	40	997	
C	Obstetrics	25	733	
D	Rehabilitation	15	400	
E	CCU	20	592	
F	Surgical ICU (SICU)	15	445	
G	Medicine ICU (MICU)	20	585	
Total Adult and Children		175		
I	Newborn Nursery	20	588	
J	Special Care Nursery	10	201	
K	Neonatal ICU (NICU)	10	285	
Total Nursery				

8. Community Hospital reported the following for the month of July 20XX. Round your answers to whole numbers.

Community Hospital July 20XX		
	Adults and Children	Newborn
Beginning census on July 1	92	6
Admissions	301	54
Discharges and Deaths	286	50
Inpatient Service Days	3,198	300

   a. Calculate the average daily inpatient census for adults and children.

   b. Calculate the average daily inpatient census for newborns.

   c. What will the census for adults and children be at 11:59 p.m. on July 31?

   d. What will the nursery census be at 11:59 p.m. on July 31?

9. Metropolitan Hospital has a large, busy rehabilitation unit. The 30-bed unit reported the following inpatient service days for the week of April 6. Use the information that follows to determine the average daily inpatient census for the week of April 6 through April 12. Round to three digits after the decimal.

Metropolitan Hospital Rehabilitation Unit Inpatient Service Days April 6–April 12, 20XX	
Day	**Inpatient Service Days**
April 6	29
April 7	28
April 8	29
April 9	26
April 10	27
April 11	28
April 12	29

10. Children's Hospital reported the following statistics for March 20XX. Use an Excel spreadsheet to calculate the average daily inpatient census for each unit and the total. Round each calculation to a whole number.

Children's Hospital Inpatient Service Days March 20XX			
Unit	**Number of Beds**	**Inpatient Service Days**	**Average Daily Inpatient Census**
Pediatrics Surgical	30	833	
Hematology Oncology	20	566	
Neurology/Neurosurgical	30	756	
Renal/Gastroenterology/Endocrinology	20	555	
Respiratory	30	897	
Cardiac Medicine/Surgical	20	589	
Infant Care Unit	10	281	
Pediatric Intensive Care	20	540	
Total	180		

11. Community Hospital has 15 bassinets with 286 newborn inpatient service days during October. What is the average daily census for October? Round to a whole number.

12. The planning committee for Metropolitan Hospital is studying the activity of their burn unit, which has 15 beds. During the third quarter of the year (July, August, and September), there were 1,356 inpatient service days. What is the average daily census for this period? How could this information be important to the planning committee at Metropolitan Hospital? Round to a whole number.

13. University Hospital is a 765-bed facility with 250,415 inpatient service days for the past year. What was their average daily census for the period? Round to a whole number.

14. In February 20XX (a leap year), Children's Hospital reported they had 500 inpatient service days in their neurosurgery unit. What was the average daily inpatient census? Round to a whole number.

15. Of the 500 inpatient service days in the above example, 386 were Dr. Smith's patients. What percentage of inpatient service days did Dr. Smith have in the neurosurgery unit? Round to one decimal place.

CHAPTER 4

Inpatient Bed Occupancy

Learning Objectives

At the conclusion of this chapter, you should be able to do the following:

- Determine the beds that are included in a bed count
- Analyze the bed occupancy percentage
- Summarize the direct and indirect bed turnover rate
- Formulate the direct and indirect bed turnover rate
- Construct the percentage of occupancy for a period when there has been a change in the number of beds during that period

Key Terms

Bed capacity
Bed count
Bed count day
Bed occupancy percent
Bed occupancy ratio
Bed turnover rate

Certificate of need (CON)
Hospital inpatient bed
Hospital newborn bassinet
Inpatient bed occupancy rate
Newborn bassinet count
Newborn bassinet count day

Observation patient
Occupancy ratio
Percent of occupancy
Total bed count days

Healthcare facilities are licensed by the state to operate with a specific number of beds. When a new facility wants to open its doors for patient care, or when an existing hospital wants to add services or major medical equipment, hospital administration may need to apply to the state for a **certificate of need (CON)** to prove that patient care beds or equipment is needed in the area. A CON is state-directed program that requires healthcare facilities to submit detailed plans and justifications for the purchase of new equipment, new buildings, or new service offerings that cost in excess of a certain amount. CON programs are designed to promote healthcare cost containment and prevent duplication of services and equipment, such as Gamma Knife surgical equipment. Even though the federal mandate to require a CON has been repealed, 35 states, the District of Columbia, and Puerto Rico have maintained their CON programs. States that have kept their CON programs are also responsible for reviewing the needs of outpatient and long-term care facilities and other free-standing facilities (National Conference of State Legislatures 2019). Even the fifteen states that do not require a CON have some mechanisms to regulate costs and duplication of services. When granted a CON, the facility is licensed for the specific number of beds requested and is responsible for reporting its actual bed count. Hospitals may not staff all the beds included in their licensed number. Staffing is based on the number of occupied beds that the hospital typically experiences.

Percentage of Occupancy

One of the indicators of a facility's financial well-being is the **percentage of occupancy**. From a facility's perspective, a high percentage of occupancy indicates a positive financial outlook. Conversely, a low percentage of occupancy can mean that the facility may need to work to attract more patients or reduce the number of staffed beds. Percentage of occupancy can also reveal the health of a community. For example, in winter months, a hospital that has a high percentage of occupancy may reflect that there are many cases of influenza or respiratory illnesses in the community.

Factors affecting occupancy include the number of available beds, volume of elective surgeries, the size of the emergency department (ED), and the number of hospitals in the immediate area. Understanding the impact of occupancy rate has become increasingly important in healthcare, as cost containment efforts receive more recognition.

Inpatient Bed Count

A **bed count**, also called an inpatient bed count or staffed beds, is the number of hospital inpatient beds staffed and available for use, both occupied and vacant, on any given day. A bed count may be reported for the entire hospital or for any of its units.

The term **hospital inpatient bed** refers to accommodations with supporting services, such as food, laundry, and housekeeping, for hospital inpatients. It excludes those for the newborn nursery but could include incubators and bassinets in neonatal intensive care units (NICU) for premature or sick newborn infants.

Bed capacity is used to denote the number of beds that a facility has been designed and constructed to house, rather than the actual number of beds set up and staffed for use. Unlike the business industry, hospital space tends to be expressed in terms of beds and not square footage. However, there is no required methodology when reporting bed-related statistics. To avoid confusion, it is preferable to use bed count as the reported bed-related statistic. This is an important consideration because regulatory agency surveyors often verify bed count and location against licensed beds and appropriate staffing levels. The bed count may be used in various reports, from those prepared for accrediting agencies to those for regulatory agencies. In a hospital, the number of available beds in the facility or a unit may remain constant for long periods of time. At times, however, the number can change. For example, a significant number of beds may be unavailable for use during a major remodeling or renovation project, but the number will increase after the project is completed. Beds located in treatment areas such as examining rooms, emergency services, physical therapy, labor rooms, and recovery rooms are excluded from the bed count.

 During a disaster, natural or otherwise, regular beds may be occupied, so additional beds would be set up in alcoves, hallways, offices, or other areas that are not considered patient rooms. These beds do not become a part of the regular bed count, which can result in a percentage of occupancy over 100 percent.

QUICK
TIP

Labor and Delivery Room and Newborn Bassinets

An obstetrics patient may be admitted directly to a bed in the labor and delivery area room bed instead of to a postpartum bed where she may spend most of her hospital stay. Beds in the labor and delivery area are accounted for separately and not included in the bed count because they are used only temporarily before the patient delivers. Postpartum beds are included in the bed count because they are staffed beds that are available for an inpatient stay.

Newborn beds, called bassinets, are tabulated separately from the bed count. The **newborn bassinet count** is the number of **hospital newborn bassinets**, both occupied and vacant, on any given day. A hospital newborn bassinet includes incubators and isolettes in the newborn nursery with supporting services (such as food, laundry, and housekeeping) for hospital newborn inpatients.

Emergency Department Beds

Emergency department beds are normally considered outpatient beds. In some instances, however, the hospital provides observation beds in the ED. If observation beds meet the qualifications of being set up, equipped, and staffed for inpatient use, they may be counted in the bed count depending on facility preference or state-licensing compliance. A patient that is in observation status is considered an outpatient even if they occupy a bed that is staffed for inpatient use. These patients would not be counted as part of the inpatient census although the beds are counted as inpatient beds.

Observation Patients

A patient under observation, an **observation patient**, is one who presents with a medical condition that imposes a significant degree of instability and disability and who needs to be monitored, evaluated, and assessed to determine whether he or she should be admitted for inpatient care or discharged for care in another setting. A patient can occupy a special bed set aside for this purpose or a bed in any unit of the hospital (that is, the ED, a medical unit, or obstetrics). Hospital policy determines the terms to describe and classify outpatients who occupy hospital beds and information systems to track these patients.

Exercise 4.1

1. In the event of a disaster, extra beds may be set up to meet the immediate needs of the situation. Would these beds be part of the bed count? Explain your answer.

2. Compare and contrast the terms bed count and bed capacity.

Bed Count Days

A **bed count day** is a unit of measure denoting the presence of one inpatient bed that is set up and staffed for use in one 24-hour period. Both occupied and unoccupied beds are included in the bed count day. The term **total bed count days** refers to the sum of inpatient bed count days for each of the days during a specified time period. Bed count days also may be referred to as the maximum number of patient days or potential days at a facility.

> **Example 4.1:** A hospital has an inpatient bed count of 100. What would the bed count be for June?
>
> During June, the bed count days would be 100 (number of beds) × 30 (the number of days in June) or 3,000.

We can also use this statistic for newborn bassinets. A **newborn bassinet count day** is a unit of measure denoting the presence of one newborn bassinet (either occupied or vacant) set up and staffed for use in one 24-hour period. The term total bassinet count days refers to the sum of newborn bassinet count days for each of the days in the period under consideration.

> **Example 4.2:** A hospital has a bassinet count of 15. What would the bed count days be for April?
>
> The bed count days in April would be 15 (number of bassinets) × 30 (the number of days in April) or 450.

All the rates in this text can be determined by remembering this general rule: A rate is the number of times something has happened compared with the number of times something could have happened. In the context of bed-related statistics, the number of times "something happened" is expressed in terms of inpatient service days. The number of times "it could have happened" is expressed in terms of bed count days (bed count multiplied by the number of calendar days). Refer to chapter 2 for a more complete discussion on rates.

Inpatient Bed Occupancy Ratio or Percentage

Occupancy percentages also are referred to as rates or ratios. The **bed occupancy ratio** is the proportion of beds occupied, defined as the ratio of inpatient service days to bed count days during a specified period of time. The inpatient service days are used to represent the actual occupancy (number of times something happened), and the bed count represents the possibility for occupancy (number of times it could have happened). The formula for determining bed occupancy ratio is:

$$Bed\ Occupancy\ Ratio = \frac{Total\ inpatient\ service\ days\ in\ a\ period}{Total\ bed\ count\ days\ in\ the\ period}$$

Synonymous terms for bed occupancy ratio are occupancy rate, **inpatient bed occupancy rate**, and **occupancy ratio**. The ratio is usually expressed as a percentage by multiplying the ratio by 100 and may be called **percent of occupancy** or **bed occupancy percent**. This statistic may be calculated for any specified day or as a daily average for any period of time.

Example 4.3: On September 1, 207 inpatient service days were provided in a 225-bed hospital. Making the appropriate substitutions in the previously stated formula, the bed occupancy ratio for September 1 is calculated as follows:

$$Bed\ Occupancy\ Ratio = \frac{207}{225} = 0.92$$

The bed occupancy ratio for September 1 is 0.92. The bed occupancy percent is 92 percent (0.92×100). This simply means that on September 1, 92 percent of the beds were occupied.

Example 4.4: A hurricane hit a small coastal town on November 17. The local hospital is licensed for 70 beds. All 70 beds were occupied; an additional 10 beds (disaster beds) were set up in the facility and occupied. The calculation for the percentage of occupancy for November 17 would be:

$$Bed\ Occupancy\ Ratio = \frac{80}{70} = 1.143\ or\ 114.3\%$$

Notice in example 4.4 the 10 disaster beds are not included in the bed count days in the denominator of the occupancy rate. Only the licensed beds are included in the calculation of the bed occupancy ratio. This situation results in an occupancy percentage higher than 100 percent.

 Always verify that the value calculated makes sense in the context. In practice, any time an occupancy percentage is greater than 100 percent you should investigate to verify that there is some sort of special circumstance causing that value and not a calculation error.

Bed occupancy ratios may be calculated for individual patient care units (PCUs). Excel is an excellent tool to use in this situation. Example 4.5 demonstrates the process of using Excel to calculate bed occupancy ratios.

Example 4.5: Community Hospital has four PCUs with the bed counts listed in table 4.1. Use the October patient service days and bed counts listed in table 4.1 to calculate the bed occupancy ratio for each unit and the facility total for the month. Report both the ratio (round to two decimal places) and the percent values (round to one decimal).

Table 4.1.   Community Hospital bed statistics

PCU	October Bed Count	October Inpatient Service Days
Medicine	24	587
Surgery	16	432
Psychiatry	4	124
Obstetrics	6	169

Excel spreadsheet formula version:

	A	B	C	D	E
1	Bed Statistics for October				
2	Bed Statistics for October	Bed Count	Inpatient Service Days	Bed Occupancy Rate	Percentage Occupancy
3	Medicine	24	587	=C3/(B3*31)	=C3/(B3*31)
4	Surgery	16	432	=C4/(B4*31)	=C4/(B4*31)
5	Psychiatry	4	124	=C5/(B5*31)	=C5/(B5*31)
6	Obstetrics	6	169	=C6/(B6*31)	=C6/(B6*31)
7	Total	=SUM(B3:B6)	=SUM(C3:C6)	=C7/(B7*31)	=C7/(B7*31)
8					

Notice that the calculation in D3 includes the bed count times the number of days in October (31) in the denominator. Recall that is the formula for total bed count days for October.

Excel spreadsheet calculated version:

	A	B	C	D	E
1	Bed Statistics for October				
2	Bed Statistics for October	Bed Count	Inpatient Service Days	Bed Occupancy Rate	Percentage Occupancy
3	Medicine	24	587	0.79	78.9%
4	Surgery	16	432	0.87	87.1%
5	Psychiatry	4	124	1.00	100.0%
6	Obstetrics	6	169	0.91	90.9%
7	Total	50	1312	0.85	84.6%
8					

Notice that the formulae used in columns D and E are identical. The conversion from the ratio displayed in column D and the percentage displayed in column E is achieved using the formatting feature in Excel.

Steps to perform the formatting from a ratio to a percentage:

1. Right click on the cell to be formatted (cell E3, for example).

2. Select "Format Cells."

3. Select "Percentage" and set "Decimal places" to 1 as displayed below:

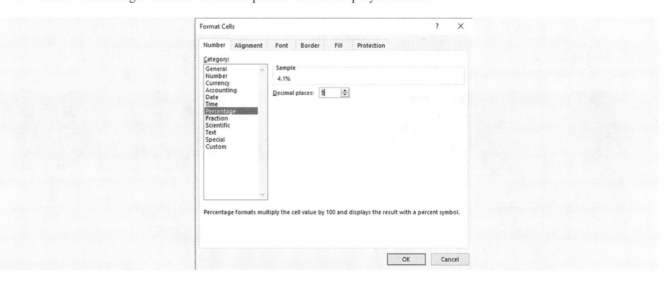

Exercise 4.2

Use the information in the following table to calculate the percentage of occupancy for each day of the month and for the entire month using an Excel spreadsheet. Round to one decimal place.

		Community Hospital April 20XX 80 beds			
Date	**Inpatient Service Days**	**Percentage of Occupancy**	**Date**	**Inpatient Service Days**	**Percentage of Occupancy**
1	75		16	56	
2	77		17	71	
3	72		18	78	
4	79		19	57	
5	73		20	52	
6	74		21	53	
7	76		22	50	
8	60		23	55	
9	69		24	58	
10	54		25	68	
11	59		26	64	
12	63		27	80	
13	65		28	70	
14	66		29	62	
15	67		30	61	

Exercise 4.3

Use the information in the following table to calculate the percentage of occupancy for each unit of Children's Hospital as well as the total percentage of occupancy. Perform the calculations by hand. Verify the calculations using an Excel spreadsheet. Round to one decimal place.

	Children's Hospital June 20XX		
Unit	**Number of Beds**	**Inpatient Service Days**	**Percentage of Occupancy**
Pediatrics Surgical	30	833	
Hematology Oncology	20	566	
Neurology/Neurosurgical	30	756	

(continued on next page)

Children's Hospital June 20XX			
Unit	Number of Beds	Inpatient Service Days	Percentage of Occupancy
Renal/Gastroenterology/Endocrinology	20	555	
Respiratory	30	897	
Cardiac Medicine/Surgical	20	589	
Infant Care Unit	10	281	
Pediatric Intensive Care	20	540	
Total			

Change in Bed Count

Occasionally, a hospital changes its bed count during a period of time. This expansion or reduction would only impact the bed count used in occupancy statistics if it is a permanent change and not designed to meet a temporary or emergency situation.

Example 4.6: General Hospital changed its official bed count from 50 to 75 on May 15 and provided a total of 1,700 inpatient service days for the month of May. What were General Hospital's bed count days for May? What was the occupancy rate? Round to one decimal place.

Since the bed count changed on May 15, the bed count must be calculated as two components: the 50 beds available for the first 14 days in May and the 75 beds available for the last 17 days in May (recall that May has 31 days).

$$Bed\ Count\ Days = 14 \times 50 + 17 \times 75 = 700 + 1275 = 1975$$

The bed count days for May are 1,975. Now, compute the bed occupancy ratio. The calculation is:

$$Bed\ Occupancy\ Ratio = \frac{Total\ inpatient\ service\ days\ in\ a\ period}{Total\ bed\ count\ days\ in\ the\ period}$$

$$Bed\ Occupancy\ Ratio = \frac{1700}{1975} = 0.861$$

The bed occupancy ratio for May is 0.861 or 86.1 percent (multiply 0.861×100).

The midperiod change in bed count demonstrated in example 4.6 creates a much more complicated calculation. Calculating the bed occupancy ratio based on the 50 beds available at the beginning of May would result in an occupancy percentage of:

$$Bed\ Occupancy\ Ratio\ (based\ on\ 50\ beds) = \frac{1700}{31 \times 50} = \frac{1700}{1550} = 1.097\ or\ 109.7\%$$

If 75 beds had been used for the entire month, the calculation would be:

$$Bed\ Occupancy\ Ratio\ (based\ on\ 75\ beds) = \frac{1700}{31 \times 50} = \frac{1700}{2325} = 0.731\ or\ 73.1\%$$

Obviously, there is a significant difference in the results. This example illustrates how easy it can be to present an inaccurate statistical picture. Because many administrative decisions are made based on statistical presentations, the health information management practitioner has an important responsibility in providing accurate data and statistics. Although occupancy statistics are typically calculated via computer systems, they must be validated to ensure they reflect the current bed count.

Exercise 4.4

Community Hospital began the year 20XX, a non-leap year, with 102 beds. On March 1, it expanded the number of beds to 116. From April 1 through June 30, the hospital reported 120 beds. The hospital increased to 124 beds from July 1 through October 31. Finally, the hospital completed its expansion process on November 1 to end the year with 130 beds. Use these data and calculations via an Excel spreadsheet to answer the questions below. Round to one decimal place.

1. Calculate the percentage of occupancy for each month.

2. Calculate the percentage of occupancy for each quarter (January through March, April through June, July through September, and October through December).

3. Calculate the percentage of occupancy for the year.

Community Hospital Annual Statistics, 20XX			
Month	**Bed Count (A/C)**	**Inpatient Service Days**	**Percentage of Occupancy**
January	102	2,765	
February	102	2,897	
March	116	2,987	
April	120	3,123	
May	120	3,078	
June	120	3,245	
July	124	3,459	
August	124	3,598	
September	124	3,634	
October	124	3,687	
November	130	3,760	
December	130	3,792	

Exercise 4.5

Use the statistics in the following report generated for University Hospital to create an Excel spreadsheet and calculate the percentage of occupancy for the month of January. Round to one decimal place.

University Hospital January 20XX			
PCU	**Inpatient Service Days**	**Bed Count**	**Percentage of Occupancy**
Medicine	3,752	130	
Rehabilitation/Neurology	600	35	
Orthopedics/Trauma	485	20	
Medicine/Surgical Oncology	1,803	60	
Pediatrics	2,142	80	

(*continued on next page*)

University Hospital January 20XX			
PCU	**Inpatient Service Days**	**Bed Count**	**Percentage of Occupancy**
Critical Care			
Medicine ICU	1,603	55	
Surgical ICU (Adult)	1,584	55	
Transplant	895	30	
Surgical ICU (Pediatrics)	923	40	
Total			

Newborn Bassinet Occupancy Ratio or Percentage

Typically, newborn occupancy ratios are computed using the same methodology as adult and children beds. If every bassinet were full every day in the period, the hospital would have the maximum potential bassinet occupancy or newborn bassinet count days. The formula for determining newborn bassinet occupancy is:

$$Newborn\ Bassinet\ Occupancy = \frac{Total\ newborn\ inpatient\ service\ days\ in\ period}{Total\ newborn\ bassinet\ count\ days}$$

Example 4.7: During July, a hospital with a bassinet count of 30 provided 874 newborn inpatient service days of care. Calculate the newborn occupancy percentage. Round to one decimal place.

$$Newborn\ Bassinet\ Occupancy = \frac{874}{30\ beds \times 31\ days\ in\ July} = \frac{874}{930} = 0.940\ or\ 94.0\%$$

Exercise 4.6

Use the statistics in the following report generated for Community Hospital to create an Excel spreadsheet. Complete the following three calculations (assume a non-leap year). Round to one decimal place.

1. Calculate the percentage of occupancy for each month.

2. Calculate the percentage of occupancy for each quarter (January through March, April through June, July through September, and October through December).

3. Calculate the percentage of occupancy for the year.

Community Hospital Annual Statistics 20XX		
Newborn bassinet count: January–March: 10 April–June: 15 July–September: 20 October–December: 30		
Month	**Newborn Inpatient Service Days**	**Percentage of Occupancy**
January	270	
February	256	

(*continued on next page*)

Community Hospital Annual Statistics 20XX		
Month	**Newborn Inpatient Service Days**	**Percentage of Occupancy**
March	300	
April	309	
May	315	
June	350	
July	410	
August	451	
September	475	
October	655	
November	730	
December	779	

Bed Turnover Rate

The **bed turnover rate** refers to the number of times a bed, on average, changes occupants during a given period. The bed turnover rate is useful because two PCUs may have the same percentage of occupancy, but the turnover rates may be different. For example, if a unit such as an obstetrics unit has a high turnover rate, this could be an indication that the unit can accommodate more patients because the patients have a shorter length of stay (LOS). Conversely, a rehabilitation unit might have a low turnover rate because the patients in that unit have a longer LOS. The bed turnover rate is a measure of the frequency of bed use and can be used to measure the efficiency of a unit. The bed turnover rate demonstrates the net effect of changes in occupancy rate and LOS.

The length of stay for patients is calculated to be the number of days they are an inpatient. See chapter 5 for a full discussion of length of stay.

QUICK
TIP

Following are two formulae for determining bed turnover rate:

$$\text{Bed Turnover Rate (direct formula)} = \frac{\text{Number of discharges (including deaths) for a period}}{\text{Average bed count during the period}}$$

$$\text{Bed Turnover Rate (indirect formula)} = \frac{\text{Occupancy rate} \times \text{Number of days in a period}}{\text{Average length of stay during the period}}$$

Using a good bit of algebra, we can show that both formulae are mathematically equivalent. The choice used in practice depends on the underlying statistics that are readily available at the time the calculation is performed. Administrators of short-stay hospitals place an emphasis on bed turnover rate as a measure of hospital service use and efficiency, especially when it is related to occupancy and LOS. When occupancy goes up and LOS goes down, or vice versa, the bed turnover rate can improve recognition of the net effect of these changes.

Turnover rates can be used in comparing one facility with another or in comparing utilization rates for different time periods or for different units of the same facility. For example, the occupancy rate for one hospital can be essentially the same in two time periods, but the turnover rate may be lower because of a longer LOS in one time period. In other words, bed turnover rate can be a measure of intensity of service.

Exercise 4.7

Calculate the turnover rate for Community Hospital using both the direct and indirect calculation. Any differences in the results are due to rounding the statistics used in the calculation. Perform the calculation by hand and using Excel to demonstrate the impact of rounding.

Community Hospital
Annual Statistics, 20XX
Non-Leap Year
200 Beds

Patients discharged (includes deaths): 7,054
Average length of stay: 9 days
Bed occupancy rate: 85 percent

1. Apply the direct formula for the turnover rate. Round to one decimal place.

2. Apply the indirect formula for the turnover rate. Round to one decimal place.

Chapter 4 Formulae for Calculation of Bed Occupancy Statistics

Statistic	Numerator	Denominator
Inpatient bed occupancy rate	Total number of inpatient service days for a given period	Total number of inpatient bed count days for the same period
Newborn bassinet occupancy rate	Total number of newborn inpatient service days for a given period	Total number of bassinet bed count days for the same period
Bed turnover rate (direct Formula)	Number of discharges (including deaths) for a period	Average bed count during the period
Bed turnover rate (indirect Formula)	Occupancy rate x number of days in period	Average length of stay for period

Chapter 4   Matching Quiz

Match the definitions with the terms.

Definitions:

a. The number of available hospital inpatient beds

b. A unit of measure that denotes the presence of one newborn bassinet, either occupied or vacant, set up and staffed for use in one 24-hour period

c. The sum of inpatient bed count days for each of the days in a period

d. A state-directed program that requires healthcare facilities to submit detailed plans and justifications for the purchase of new equipment, new buildings, or new service offerings that cost in excess of a certain amount

e. A patient who presents with a medical condition with a significant degree of instability and disability and who needs to be monitored, evaluated, and assessed to determine whether he or she should be admitted for inpatient care or discharged for care in another setting

f. The number of available newborn bassinets

g. Percent of occupancy, percentage of occupancy, or occupancy ratio

h. A unit of measure denoting the presence of one inpatient bed set up and staffed for one 24-hour period

i. The number of beds that a facility has been designed and constructed to house

j. The average number of times a bed changes occupants during a given period of time

Terms:

1. _____Certificate of need
2. _____Newborn bassinet count day
3. _____Observation patient
4. _____Bed capacity
5. _____Bed count/Inpatient bed count

6. _____ Bed turnover rate
7. _____ Total bed count days
8. _____ Bed occupancy ratio
9. _____ Newborn bassinet count
10. _____ Bed count day

Chapter 4   Review

Community Hospital compiled the following annual statistics for 20XX (non-leap year). Use the table provided to answer questions 1, 2, and 3 that follow. Round to one decimal place.

Community Hospital Annual Statistics, 20XX		
	Inpatient Service Days	**Bed Count**
January–June	34,872	175
July–December	31,894	200
December 31 only	201	200
Newborn	12,732	40

1. The inpatient occupancy rate (without newborns) for 20XX was _____.
   a. 37.4%
   b. 90.8%
   c. 99.2%
   d. 97.5%

2. The newborn bassinet occupancy rate for 20XX was _____.
   a. 84.7%
   b. 85.2%
   c. 86.2%
   d. 87.2%

3. The bed occupancy rate for December 31 was _____.
   a. 87.3%
   b. 99.5%
   c. 100.0%
   d. 100.5%

The following table is a report of the first quarter of 20XX (January through March) from a 400-bed medical center regarding its insurance categories. In this example, deaths are included in discharges. Round all to one decimal place. This is a non-leap year. Create an Excel spreadsheet to complete the table and use the results to answer questions 4, 5, and 6.

Community Medical Center Inpatient Service Days and Number of Discharges by Insurance Category January–March 20XX					
Insurance Category	Inpatient Service Days	Number of Discharges	Occupancy Rate	Bed Turnover Rate (Direct Formula)	Average Daily Inpatient Census
Third-party contracts	5,849	598			
Medicare	9,427	1,450			
Medicaid	13,604	2,011			
No insurance	2,598	480			
Total					

4. Calculate the occupancy rate for the following:
   a. Total
   b. Medicare
   c. Third-party contracts

5. Use the direct formula to calculate the bed turnover rate for the following:
   a. Total
   b. Medicare
   c. Third-party contracts

6. What is the total average daily inpatient census for this period of time?

7. The following table is a report of the annual inpatient service days of Community Hospital for 20XX. The hospital has an inpatient bed count of 250 and a bassinet count of 30. Create an Excel spreadsheet to calculate the percentage of occupancy for each month for adults and children and for newborns. Calculate statistics for January to verify the spreadsheet is set up properly. This is a non-leap year. Round to one decimal place.

Community Hospital Annual Statistics, 20XX				
	Inpatient Service Days		Percentage of Occupancy	
Month	Adults/Children	Newborn	Adults/Children	Newborn
January	7,250	874		
February	6,532	788		
March	7,354	820		

(continued on next page)

Community Hospital Annual Statistics, 20XX				
	Inpatient Service Days		Percentage of Occupancy	
Month	Adults/Children	Newborn	Adults/Children	Newborn
April	7,365	895		
May	7,235	866		
June	7,132	756		
July	7,501	875		
August	7,523	796		
September	7,196	856		
October	7,362	878		
November	7,065	821		
December	7,175	801		
Total				

8. Community Hospital, a 120-bed facility, reported that in March there were 545 discharges (including deaths). Using the direct formula, what was the bed turnover rate for March?

9. Which of the following beds should be counted in the bed count?
   a. A hospital inpatient bed
   b. A labor room bed
   c. An observation bed
   d. An extra bed set up during a disaster

10. On October 1, a hurricane hit a small coastal community that has a community hospital licensed for 50 beds. Hospital staff set up 10 additional beds around the facility and used 3 labor room beds and 2 treatment room beds in order to help take care of patients. Which of the following would be the denominator used to determine the percentage of occupancy for October 1?
    a. 50
    b. 60
    c. 63
    d. 65

11. The 15-bed surgical intensive care unit at Memorial Hospital had 400 inpatient service days during March. What is the percentage of occupancy? Round to one decimal place.

12. On February 12, a fire occurred at a local dry-cleaning plant, and the inpatient service days for the local hospital (120 beds) was reported to be 130. What is the bed occupancy rate for February 12? Round to one decimal place.

13. What is the bed occupancy rate for the 15-bassinet Children's Hospital NICU during March if the inpatient service days were 400? Round to one decimal place.

14. During January through June (non-leap year), a 50-bed hospital had 9,001 inpatient service days. What is the percentage of occupancy? Round to one decimal place.

15. During the period July through December, the same hospital as above added 25 beds making its total bed count 75. During July through December there were 12,765 inpatient service days. Calculate the percentage of occupancy. Round to one decimal place, for the following:
    a. July through December
    b. January through December

CHAPTER 5

Length of Stay

Learning Objectives

At the conclusion of this chapter, you should be able to do the following:

- Analyze the length of stay for adults, children, and newborns
- Assess the total length of stay for a group of discharged patients
- Interpret the relationship between length of stay and utilization management

Key Terms

Admission date	Discharge days	Medicare severity diagnosis-related
Average length of stay (ALOS)	Duration of inpatient stay	groups (MS-DRGs)
Case management	Inpatient days of stay	Military time
Days of stay	Leave of absence	Total length of stay
Discharge date	Length of stay (LOS)	Utilization management (UM)

Length of stay (LOS) is a key indicator of the expected amount of resources used in a healthcare facility for inpatient care. The longer the LOS, one would assume the more resources used by the inpatient. Consequently, a shorter LOS would equate to fewer resources. LOS is used to benchmark performance based on diagnoses, Medicare severity diagnosis-related groups (MS-DRGs), physicians, and other hospitals.

Length of Stay

The **LOS** is the total number of patient days for an inpatient episode, calculated by subtracting the date of admission from the date of discharge. The healthcare facility uses LOS data in **utilization management (UM)**. UM is a program that evaluates the facility's efficiency in providing necessary services in the most resource-effective manner, while also evaluating the level of care required. This program may also be referred to as **case management**. The goal of the UM program is to eliminate over- and underutilization of services. Part of the UM evaluation process involves reviewing LOS for continued medical necessity for patients currently admitted to the hospital. For example, is it more appropriate to continue to treat the patient in an acute-care facility or to transfer the patient to a subacute or rehabilitation facility?

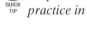 *Length of stay calculations include two very similar acronyms. LOS refers to the length of stay for a particular patient or a listing of length of stays. ALOS represents the average length of stay. It is a statistic that is used to summarize the LOS for the typical or average patient.*

LOS data also are used in financial reporting; for example, to compare patients within the same MS-DRG. **MS-DRGs** are payment groups, designed for the Medicare population, that recognize severity of illness, resource use, and patient complexity. Patients are assigned to an MS-DRG based on diagnosis, surgical procedures, age, and other administrative information. Patient complexity refers to the patient's characteristics, including physical, mental, social, and financial issues, that will determine resources required to care for the patient. MS-DRGs can measure the physical and mental issues that impact the care patients require, but do not address the social and financial issues impacting a patient's care and recovery. Managing medically complex patients takes more healthcare practitioner time and uses more resources, including lab, x-ray, and medications, than a patient with fewer problems. For example, patient A has congestive heart failure as a principal diagnosis and secondary diagnoses of dementia and smoking. Patient B has congestive heart failure as a principal diagnosis and secondary diagnoses of Parkinson's disease, dementia, atrial fibrillation, high blood pressure, atrial blockage, smoking, and medication noncompliance. Even though the principal diagnoses are the same, patient B would most likely consume more resources than patient A.

Patients who have similar clinical characteristics and costs to treat are assigned to an MS-DRG, which is often linked to a fixed payment amount. The average length of stay (ALOS) for discharges assigned to an MS-DRG can be compared to the overall healthcare facility's ALOS to determine whether there are too many extreme values, also known as outliers. The **ALOS** is the average number of days that inpatients discharged during the period under consideration stayed in the hospital. This is discussed in more detail later in this chapter. LOS data for patients with the same diagnosis or procedure treated by various physicians are compared to evaluate any extremes. For example, it is important for hospital administration to be aware of physician differences in LOS because these may be indicative of different types of treatment for the same condition provided by different physicians.

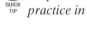 *Each hospital stay is assigned to an MS-DRG by using a software tool called a grouper. Inpatient payment to hospitals is often determined by the MS-DRG. Therefore, reporting statistics based on MS-DRG is a common practice in hospitals.*

Discharge Days

Chapter 3, *Patient Census,* introduced the concept of inpatient service days, which are compiled while the patient is hospitalized. This chapter discusses **discharge days**, which are days calculated after the patient has been discharged from the hospital. Discharge days, **days of stay**, **inpatient days of stay**, and **duration of inpatient stay** are other terms used for LOS.

A discharge occurs at the end of the patient's inpatient stay. Patients may leave the hospital to go home, to go to another facility for further care, against medical advice (AMA), or by dying while in the hospital. Death is considered a discharge. That is why the discharge statistic presented in chapter 3 included deaths. Some patients are transferred to other facilities to continue their care. Hospital staff may refer to these patients as transfers or external transfers, but they are counted as discharges.

In general, every day that a patient is in the hospital is counted as a day except the day of discharge. The LOS for an inpatient is determined by subtracting the **admission date** from the **discharge date**. The admission date is the year, month, and day of inpatient admission, beginning with a hospital's formal acceptance of a patient who is to receive healthcare services while receiving room, board, and continuous nursing services The discharge date is the year, month, and day that an inpatient was formally released from the hospital and room, board, and continuous nursing services were terminated The day of admission is counted in computing the number of discharge days or LOS, but the day of discharge is not. This ensures that no patient admitted to the hospital has a zero LOS. If the patient is admitted and discharged on the same day, then the LOS would be one day.

Hospital length of stay is calculated using the same method as the stay at a hotel. The stay starts on the check-in day and does not count the checkout day. Hotels will charge for one "night" even if the check-in and checkout are on the same day.

Example 5.1: A patient is admitted to the hospital on March 27 and discharged on March 30. What is that patient's LOS?

To calculate the patient's LOS, subtract March 27 from March 30. Subtracting dates is most easily done by viewing a calendar and counting the days between March 27 and March 30—remembering to include March 27 (admission day).

Method 1: Figure 5.1 is a calendar view of March 2019 that demonstrates the determination of the LOS for this patient: three days.

Method 2: If a calendar is not available, calculate the LOS by listing the dates from admission to discharge and counting all the dates except the date of discharge:

3/27 (admission), 3/28, 3/29

Method 3: If the admission and the discharge are in the same month, then the calculation of LOS may also be accomplished by subtracting the day portion of the admission and discharge dates (30 − 27 = 3 days).

Figure 5.1.   Calculation of LOS for example 5.1

2019 CALENDAR YEAR	MARCH CALENDAR MONTH		MONDAY FIRST DAY OF WEEK			
Monday	Tuesday	Wednesday	Thursday	Friday	Saturday	Sunday
25	26	27	28	01	02	03
04	05	06	07	08	09	10
11	12	13	14	15	16	17
18	19	20	21	22	23	24
25	26	Day 1 Admission 27	Day 2 28	Day 3 29	30 Discharge	31

Example 5.2: Calculate the LOS for a patient admitted on March 30 and discharged on April 4. Use the methods listed below.

In this case, the admission and discharge dates are in different months (March and April). The calendar and listing methods used in example 5.1 may be applied here, but we can only use the third method if we divide the LOS calculation into parts based on the month of the stay.

Method 1: Calendar view
Figure 5.2 shows a calendar view that facilitates the LOS calculation: five days.

Method 2: Listing the dates

Dates included in the stay are 3/30 (admission), 3/31, 4/1, 4/2, 4/3: five days.

Method 3: Segment into months

Since the admission date and discharge date are in different months, the subtraction of the days must be segmented by month and then added together. When using this method, one day must be added to represent the day that transitions one month to the next.

March LOS: 31 – 30 = 1 day
March/April transition: 1 day
April LOS: 4 – 1 = 3 days
Total LOS = 1 + 1 + 3 = 5 days

Methods 1 and 2 become unwieldy to apply to longer lengths of stay.

Figure 5.2. Calculation of LOS for example 5.2

Example 5.3: Calculate the LOS for a patient that is admitted on September 25 and discharged on December 15. Utilize method 3 as demonstrated in table 5.1.

Table 5.1. LOS calculation for example 5.3

Month	Dates	LOS
September	25 to 30	30 – 25 = 5
Transition from September to October	9/30 to 10/1	1
October	1 to 31	31 – 1 = 30
Transition from October to November	10/31 to 11/1	1
November	1 to 30	30 – 1 = 29
Transition from November to December	11/30 to 12/1	1
December	1 to 15	15 – 1 = 14
Total		5+1+30+1+29+1+14=81 days

In situations where the number of months becomes unwieldy, method 4 may be used to calculate LOS.

Method 4: Use Excel date functions to calculate LOS
Using example 5.3, enter the admission and discharge dates into cells A2 and B2. The calculated LOS of 81 days is displayed in figures 5.3 and 5.4.

Figure 5.3. Using Excel to calculate LOS—formula view

	A	B	C
1	Admission Date	Discharge Date	LOS
2	25-Sep	15-Dec	=B2-A2

Figure 5.4. Using Excel to calculate LOS—calculated view

	A	B	C
1	Admission Date	Discharge Date	LOS
2	25-Sep	15-Dec	81

If a computer with Excel installed is available for the calculation of LOS, then method 4 is the quickest method to perform the calculation. It is important to understand the other methods so you can calculate LOS in situations where a computer is not available.

 Subtracting the admission date from the discharge date in Excel is an efficient method for calculating LOS, but if the admission date and the discharge date are the same, the calculation will result in a zero-day stay. By convention, the LOS is never zero, and a same-day admission and discharge should be a one-day stay. This may be addressed by using the "if" function in Excel.

QUICK TIP

Exercise 5.1

Calculate the LOS for the following discharged patients in an acute-care facility using the method listed.

Date Admitted	Date Discharged	Method	LOS
7/9	7/10	2	
9/12	9/22	1	
3/10	3/24	2	
6/17	7/18	4	
10/20	11/25	3	

Exercise 5.2

Use Excel (method 4) to calculate the LOS for the following discharged patients in this long-term care facility.

Date Admitted	Date Discharged	LOS
1/1/2009	11/01/2014	
4/07/2012	12/31/2013	
6/28/2011	1/23/2012	
2/1/2012	3/15/2013	
10/30/2013	7/07/2014	

Calculating Length of Stay in an Outpatient Setting

Since patients in the outpatient or clinic setting do not spend the night at the facility, the LOS is calculated based on arrival time and departure time. LOS in the outpatient setting may be segmented into portions of the patient's encounter that may be tracked for analysis of patient flow bottlenecks and efficiency. Some common time segments that may be tracked are: arrival or check-in to exam room, exam room to first provider, or provider completion to checkout or departure.

 The LOS components of an outpatient visit may only be tracked if there is a method to record the time that each event occurs. Electronic health records will support this type of tracking, but the clinical and administrative staff must
QUICK
TIP *be trained to record the times.*

Example 5.4: If a patient arrived at an outpatient clinic at 8:05 a.m. and was taken to the exam room at 8:22 a.m., calculate the LOS utilizing the clinic arrival to exam room methodology for this patient.

Since the hour portion of the time is the same for both time points, subtract the minutes portion to calculate the LOS:

LOS = exam room time – arrival time = 8:22 a.m. – 8:05 a.m. = 22 – 5 = 17 minutes

Example 5.5: If a patient arrived at an outpatient clinic exam room at 8:22 a.m., and the physician entered the exam room at 8:50 a.m., calculate the LOS utilizing the arrival to exam room to physician contact methodology for this patient.

As in example 5.4, the hour portion of the time is the same for both time points. Subtract the minutes portion to calculate the LOS:

LOS = exam room time – arrival time = 8:50 a.m. – 8:22 a.m. = 50 – 22 = 28 minutes

Example 5.6: If the physician in example 5.5 leaves the patient's exam room at 9:05 a.m., calculate the LOS from the physician's arrival to exam room to physician's departure from the exam room.

In this example, the starting time is 8:50 a.m. (the physician arrival time from example 5.5), and the end time is 9:05 a.m. The subtraction of the minutes component of the time will no longer work in this example. A method analogous to method 3 can be applied. If we replace the "months" in method 3 with "hours," the LOS may be calculated by adding together the following components:

LOS from 8:50 a.m. to 8:59 a.m. = 59 – 50 = 9 minutes
LOS from 8:59 a.m. to 9:00 a.m. = 1 minute (hour time component transition)
LOS from 9:00 a.m. to 9:05 a.m. = 5 – 0 = 5 minutes
Total LOS = 9 + 1 + 5 = 15 minutes

Example 5.7: If the patient in examples 5.4 to 5.6 leaves the clinic at 9:10 a.m., what is the total clinic LOS for the patient?

Total LOS

= LOS for arrival to exam room
+ LOS for exam room to physician contact start
+ LOS for physician contact start to physician departure
+ LOS physician departure to patient leaving clinic

The LOS of the physician departure (9:05 a.m.) to patient leaving the clinic (9:10 a.m.) is:

9:10 a.m. – 9:05 a.m. = 10 – 5 = 5 minutes
Total LOS
= 17 minutes (from example 5.4)
+ 28 minutes (from example 5.5)
+ 15 minutes (from example 5.6)
+ 5 minutes (from example 5.7)
= 65 minutes or one hour and 5 minutes or 1:05

Always include the unit of measurement in LOS calculations. In example 5.7, the LOS was over 60 minutes, therefore we should report it in hours and minutes. To convert minutes to hours, divide the number of minutes by 60 and report the remainder portion as minutes. 65/60 = 1 with a remainder of 5: report 1:05 as the LOS. The notation for LOS in hours and minutes is HH:MM where HH represents the hours and MM represents the minutes.

The next two calculations concern the amount of time between two times when one is before 11:59 and one is after 11:59, since this is the time when there is a shift from a.m. to p.m. or p.m. to a.m. The method applied in example 5.3 will still work under these circumstances but taking shortcuts by subtracting the hour and minute components of the time will not result in the correct answer. Many healthcare facilities use times expressed in **military time** format. Military time is measured via a 24-hour clock; therefore, there is no need for a designation of a.m. or p.m. Hours have the numbers 00 (midnight) to 23 (11 p.m.). The minute and second components of military time are the same as the more familiar civilian time format. Times after 12 noon are expressed by adding 12 to the time expressed in traditional or civilian p.m. format. For instance, 1:00 p.m. in civilian time is expressed as 1300 hours (thirteen hundred hours) in military time, and 8:29 p.m. in civilian format is expressed as 2029 hours (twenty twenty-nine hours). Notice that there is no colon listed when writing military time and the unit "hours" is attached to the time.

Should midnight be expressed as 0000 hours or 2400 hours in military time? In practice, 0000 is used most often and is the standard for computer equipment and digital watch and clock displays.

Example 5.8: A patient arrived at the physician's office at 11:47 a.m. and was taken to the exam room at 1:27 p.m. Calculate the patient's LOS in the waiting room.

LOS = exam room time – arrival time = 1:27 p.m. – 11:47 a.m.
Break the LOS calculation into hour components:
LOS from 11:47 a.m. to 11:59 a.m. = 59 – 47 = 12 minutes
LOS hour transition from 11 to 12 = 1 minute
LOS from 12:00 p.m. to 12:59 p.m. = 59 – 0 = 59 minutes
LOS hour transition from 12 to 1 p.m. = 1 minute
LOS from 1:00 p.m. to 1:27 p.m. = 27 – 0 = 27 minutes
LOS = 12 + 1 + 59 + 1 + 27 = 100 minutes
Or 1 hour and 40 minutes or 1:40

Note that this calculation could also be completed by first converting the start and end time to military time: 1147 hours to 1327 hours. The calculation would be carried out the same way:

LOS = exam room time – arrival time = 1327 hours – 1147 hours
Break the LOS calculation into hour components:
LOS from 1147 to 1159 = 59 – 47 = 12 minutes
LOS hour transition from 11 to 12 = 1 minute
LOS from 1200 to 1259 = 59 – 0 = 59 minutes
LOS hour transition from 12 to 13 = 1 minute
LOS from 1300 to 1327 = 27 – 0 = 27 minutes
LOS = 12 + 1 + 59 + 1 + 27 = 100 minutes
Or 1 hour and 40 minutes or 1:40

Example 5.9: A patient arrives at the outpatient clinic at 11:21 a.m. and departs the clinic at 2:33 p.m. What is the patient's LOS at the clinic?

Step 1: Convert the start and end times to military time: arrival at 1121 hours and departure at 1433 hours.

Step 2: Break the LOS into hourly components.

Component	Start time	End time	LOS
1100 hour	1121	1159	59 – 21 = 38 min
Transition from 1100 to 1200 hour	1159	1200	1 min
1200 hour	1200	1259	59 – 0 = 59 min
Transition from 1200 to 1300 hour	1259	1300	1 min
1300 hour	1300	1359	59 – 0 = 59 min
Transition from 1300 to 1400 hour	1359	1400	1 min
1400 hour	1400	1433	33 – 0 = 33 min

Step 3: Add up the hourly components:
38+1+59+1+59+1+33 = 192 = 3 hours 12 minutes or 3:12

If a computer with Excel installed is available, then the calculation of outpatient LOS is much easier to accomplish. Enter times in Excel using either the civilian or military format. If times are entered in military format, a colon must be inserted between the hour and minute component. For example, 1325 hours should be entered as 13:25. This lets the Excel program know you are entering a time and not simply the number 1325.

Example 5.10: Use Excel to calculate the LOS for the patient in example 5.9.

Figure 5.5 shows the formula version of the Excel workbook with time expressed in both military and civilian time format.

Figure 5.5. Example LOS calculation based on time—formula view

	A	B	C	
1	Patient Arrival Time	Patient Departure Time	LOS	
2	11:21	14:33	=B2-A2	
3	11:21 AM	2:33 PM	=B3-A3	
4				

Figure 5.6. Example LOS calculation based on time—calculated view

	A	B	C
1	Patient Arrival Time	Patient Departure Time	LOS
2	11:21	14:33	3:12
3	11:21 AM	2:33 PM	3:12 AM

Figure 5.7. Using time format in Excel

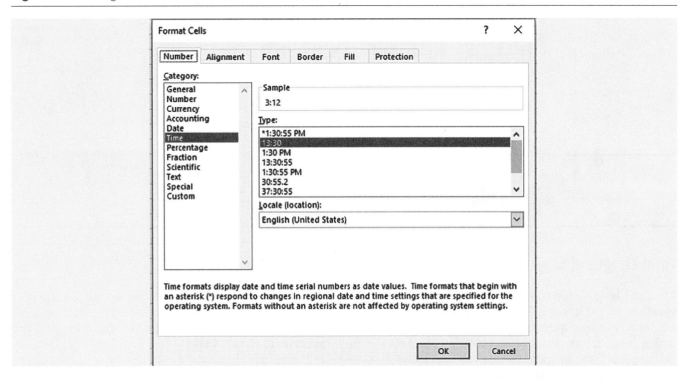

Figure 5.6 shows the calculated LOS for both time formats. Notice that Excel put the units "AM" in the civilian time version of the calculation. This may be removed by formatting the cell as time with no AM or PM designation. To do this, right click on cell C3 and select "Format Cells" from the menu that appears. Make the format selections highlighted in figure 5.7 and click on "OK." Now cells C2 and C3 should be identical.

Exercise 5.3

1. Calculate the time it takes to see patients in this physician's office.

Patient	Check-In Time	Time Seen by Physician	Time between Checking In at Reception and Being Seen by Physician
Patient 1	8:00 a.m.	8:17 a.m.	
Patient 2	1:22 p.m.	2:05 p.m.	
Patient 3	10:30 a.m.	11:43 a.m.	
Patient 4	1:30 p.m.	3:00 p.m.	
Patient 5	2:15 p.m.	2:56 p.m.	

2. Metropolitan Hospital, a very large urban hospital, promises patients that there will be no more than a 60-minute wait between the time they arrive (sign in) at the emergency department until they are triaged. The hospital selected 10 patients at random to check the times. Use Excel to calculate the wait time between arrival and triage.

   a. Calculate the wait time for each patient.

   b. What is the average wait time?

   c. Is the hospital in compliance with its own guidelines?

Patient	Time of Arrival	Time Patient Was Triaged	Wait Time
Patient A	8:00 a.m.	8:23 a.m.	
Patient B	8:23 a.m.	8:56 a.m.	
Patient C	8:56 a.m.	9:20 a.m.	
Patient D	9:45 a.m.	10:46 a.m.	
Patient E	10:20 a.m.	1:45 p.m.	
Patient F	11:20 a.m.	1:50 p.m.	
Patient G	12:15 p.m.	2:40 p.m.	
Patient H	1:05 p.m.	2:56 p.m.	
Patient I	3:27 p.m.	5:05 p.m.	
Patient J	4:05 p.m.	4:56 p.m.	

Total Length of Stay

The **total length of stay,** or **total LOS** is the sum of the days stayed by any group of inpatients discharged during a specified period of time. Total LOS may be referred to as total discharge days. Although the total LOS and inpatient service days may approximate each other over a long period of time, they are not interchangeable. The reason for this is that inpatient service days are counted concurrently, and discharge days are counted post discharge. The patients that are still in an inpatient bed are not counted in the total LOS but are counted in the inpatient service days. This is a subtle but important difference between the two statistics.

Inpatient service days are useful in the analysis of current utilization of hospital facilities related to the entire hospital, a clinical unit, or a service department. They are used to calculate various daily averages and occupancy ratios. The total LOS can be used to perform retrospective analyses comparing LOS for groups of discharged patients with similar characteristics such as age, disease, treatment, clinical service, or day-of-week admission.

Example 5.11: Calculate the LOS for each of the patients in the table below. If no year is specified, assume it is not a leap year and both dates are in the same year. What is the total LOS?

Admitted	Discharged	LOS
1/10	1/31	Admit and discharge in same month, use method 1: 31 − 10 = 21 days
7/8	7/30	Admit and discharge in same month, use method 1: 30 − 8 = 22 days
11/20	11/20	If admit and discharge are same day, then LOS = 1

(*continued on next page*)

Admitted	Discharged	LOS
6/19/2018	10/4/2018	Method 3: June LOS = 30 − 19 = 11 days June to July transition = 1 day July LOS = 31 − 1 = 30 days July to August transition = 1 day August LOS = 31 − 1 = 30 days August to September transition = 1 day September LOS = 30 − 1=29 days September to October transition = 1 day October LOS = 4 − 1 = 3 days 11+1+30+1+30+1+29+1+3 = 107 days

Total LOS = 21 + 22 + 1 + 107 = 151 days

When calculating the LOS for a patient whose stay spans an entire calendar month, the number of days in the month may be used instead of subtracting the first day of the month from the last day and adding in the transition day. For example, in example 5.11, the LOS could be calculated as:
June LOS = 30 − 19 = 11 days
July LOS = 31 days
August LOS = 31days
September LOS = 30 days
September to October transition = 1 day
October LOS = 4 − 1 = 3 days
11+31+31+30+1+3 = 107 days

The method used to determine the LOS in example 5.11 will work for any situation. The method that uses the number of days in the entire month must only be applied in that special situation.

Exercise 5.4

Use the data in the table below and Excel to answer the questions that follow for this group of 15 patients discharged from Community Hospital on October 20, 20XX.

Community Hospital Discharge List October 20, 20XX				
Pt. Name	Age	Clinical Service	Admission Date	LOS
Schulman	71	Surgery	9/18	
Hubbard	40	Medicine	9/12	
Miraboto	35	Obstetrics	10/18	
Tatum	23	Obstetrics	10/18	
Rankins	71	Medicine	9/28	
Lampton	90	Medicine	9/4	
Hruska	45	Surgery	10/5	
Adman	17	Obstetrics	10/19	

(continued on next page)

Community Hospital Discharge List October 20, 20XX				
Pt. Name	**Age**	**Clinical Service**	**Admission Date**	**LOS**
Savage	37	Medicine	9/1	
Beachton	46	Medicine	10/1	
Sanders	14	Obstetrics	10/17	
Pavalchik	62	Surgery	9/26	
Walters	57	Surgery	9/30	
Harding	51	Medicine	10/1	
Clay	82	Medicine	10/10	
Total				

Calculate the following:

a. LOS for each individual patient

b. Total LOS for all patients

c. Total LOS for medicine service patients

d. Total LOS for surgery service patients

e. Total LOS for obstetrics service patients

f. Total LOS for patients 25 years of age and younger

g. Total LOS for patients age 26 to 40 years old

h. Total LOS for patients age 41 to 55 years old

i. Total LOS for patients age 56 to 70 years old

j. Total LOS for patients over age 70

k. What is the percentage of days from medicine? Round to one decimal place.

Average Length of Stay

Recall from earlier in this chapter, the ALOS is the average number of days that inpatients discharged during the period under consideration stayed in the hospital. The default ALOS includes adult and children but excludes newborn stays. The formula to calculate ALOS is:

$$ALOS = \frac{Total\ length\ of\ stay}{Total\ discharges,\ including\ deaths}$$

The formula above does not include newborns. Most hospitals calculate the ALOS for newborns separately because newborns ordinarily stay the same length of time as their mothers. In addition, when compared with many other classifications of patients, normal newborn stays are relatively short. In contrast, newborn stays in the newborn intensive care unit tend to be quite long, sometimes months at a time. Therefore, inclusion of both mothers and newborns would distort the total ALOS.

Example 5.12: Use the statistics in the table below to determine the following calculations for Community Hospital. Round all figures to one decimal place.

Community Hospital Annual Statistics, 20XX		
	Number of Discharges	**Discharge Days**
Total adults and children	15,672	67,392
Total newborns	1,502	3,453
The following services are included in the adults and children statistics above:		
Medicine	9,455	40,780
Surgery	4,650	22,957
Obstetrics	1,567	3,655

1. Calculate the ALOS for adult and children patients.

$$ALOS = \frac{67,392}{15,672} = 4.3$$

2. Calculate the ALOS for newborn patients.

$$ALOS = \frac{3,453}{1,502} = 2.3$$

3. Calculate the ALOS for medicine patients.

$$ALOS = \frac{40,780}{9,455} = 4.3$$

4. Calculate the ALOS for surgery patients.

$$ALOS = \frac{22,957}{4,650} = 4.9$$

5. Calculate the ALOS for obstetrics patients.

$$ALOS = \frac{3,655}{1,567} = 2.3$$

Exercise 5.5

Complete the following exercises.

1. In April, Community Hospital reported 923 discharge days for adults and children and 107 discharge days for newborns. During the month, 192 adults and children and 37 newborns were discharged. Calculate the ALOS for adults and children for the month of April. Round to one decimal place.

2. Use the table in exercise 5.4 to calculate the ALOS using Excel for the following groups of patients:
   a. All patients
   b. Medicine service patients
   c. Surgery service patients
   d. Obstetrics service patients
   e. Patients 25 years of age and younger

   f. Patients age 26 to 40 years old

   g. Patients age 41 to 55 years old

   h. Patients age 56 to 70 years old

   i. Patients over age 70

3. Use the semiannual report below from University Medical Center to calculate the ALOS for each service. Round to one decimal place.

University Medical Center January–June, 20XX			
Clinical Units	**Discharges**	**Discharge Days**	**ALOS**
Medicine	12,280	61,400	
Surgery	10,320	51,762	
Neurology	12,464	68,320	
Oncology	6,228	61,280	
Orthopedics	4,906	20,624	
Rehabilitation	1,926	48,250	
Urology	678	2,698	
Psychiatry	936	22,400	
Ophthalmology	385	804	
Obstetrics/Gynecology	3,528	8,820	
Pediatrics	3,148	18,388	
Total			

Average Newborn Length of Stay

As stated earlier, newborn average LOS is usually calculated separately. The formula to calculate the average newborn LOS (ANLOS) is:

$$ANLOS = \frac{Total\ newborn\ discharge\ days}{Total\ newborn\ discharges,\ including\ deaths}$$

The hospital stay for a newborn is generally just long enough to identify any early healthcare concerns and to determine that the family is able to care for the infant.

Example 5.13

Use the table below and Excel to calculate the ANLOS for newborns in each month, and then calculate the annual ANLOS. Round to one decimal place.

University Hospital Annual Newborn Discharge Statistics 20XX			
Month	**Newborn Discharges**	**Discharge Days**	**ANLOS**
January	103	278	
February	128	427	
March	107	247	

(continued on next page)

University Hospital Annual Newborn Discharge Statistics 20XX			
Month	**Newborn Discharges**	**Discharge Days**	**ANLOS**
April	148	302	
May	152	327	
June	143	396	
July	162	422	
August	163	433	
September	183	568	
October	179	485	
November	164	459	
December	159	407	
Total			

Excel—formula view

	A	B	C	D
1	**Month**	**Newborn Discharges**	**Discharge Days**	**ANLOS**
2	January	103	278	=C2/B2
3	February	128	427	=C3/B3
4	March	107	247	=C4/B4
5	April	148	302	=C5/B5
6	May	152	327	=C6/B6
7	June	143	396	=C7/B7
8	July	162	422	=C8/B8
9	August	163	433	=C9/B9
10	September	183	568	=C10/B10
11	October	179	485	=C11/B11
12	November	164	459	=C12/B12
13	December	159	407	=C13/B13
14	Total	=SUM(B2:B13)	=SUM(C2:C13)	=C14/B14

Excel—calculated view

	A	B	C	D
1	**Month**	**Newborn Discharges**	**Discharge Days**	**ANLOS**
2	January	103	278	2.7
3	February	128	427	3.3
4	March	107	247	2.3
5	April	148	302	2.0
6	May	152	327	2.2
7	June	143	396	2.8
8	July	162	422	2.6
9	August	163	433	2.7
10	September	183	568	3.1
11	October	179	485	2.7
12	November	164	459	2.8
13	December	159	407	2.6
14	Total	1791	4751	2.7

Use the Excel format features to round column D to one decimal place.

Exercise 5.6

Community Hospital compiled the discharge statistics shown in the following July Discharge Statistics table. Notice that the last three days are missing. Prepare an Excel spreadsheet and enter the information from the July discharge statistics table. Then, use the discharge lists for July 29, 30, and 31 to enter the missing data into the appropriate columns for medicine, surgery, obstetrics (OB), and newborn (NB) discharged patients and their corresponding discharge days. Add formulas to an Excel spreadsheet for calculations as needed.

Community Hospital Discharge List July 29, 20XX				
Patient Name	**Age**	**Service**	**Admission Date**	**LOS**
Andres, Michael	47	Medicine	7/21	8
Barty, Stephen	34	Surgery	7/21	8
Christenson, Andrea	17	OB	7/27	2
Christenson, Baby Boy	NB	NB	7/27	2
Denison, William	15	Surgery	7/19	10
Henry, Christopher	67	Surgery	7/17	12
Jackson, Michelle	39	OB	7/25	4
Katon, Marie	41	OB	7/25	4
Williamson, Baby Boy	NB	NB	7/24	5

Community Hospital Discharge List July 30, 20XX				
Patient Name	**Age**	**Service**	**Admission Date**	**LOS**
Adams, Paul	34	Medicine	7/23	7
Butler, Thomas	65	Medicine	7/24	6
Carson, Johnnie	67	Surgery	7/24	6
Daniels, George	45	Medicine	7/22	8
Finley, Joyce	24	OB	7/28	2
Finley, Baby Girl	NB	NB	7/28	2
George, Michael	32	Surgery	7/21	9
Jacquinta, Marlene	29	OB	7/27	3
Jacquinta, Baby Boy	NB	NB	7/27	3
Katosh, Joseph	82	Medicine	7/25	5
Kettison, Jack	78	Medicine	7/18	12
Kettison, Mary	76	Surgery	7/24	6
Laytham, Clint	50	Surgery	7/25	5
Matson, Dorianne	76	Medicine	7/23	7
Nettleson, Andy	43	Surgery	7/24	6
Pierce, Otto	92	Medicine	7/19	11
Ransom, Jackson	54	Medicine	7/28	2
Springer, Mary	32	Surgery	7/27	3
Tatum, Neal	76	Surgery	7/28	2
Wallace, Mattie	19	OB	7/28	2
Zininsky, Maureen	32	OB	7/28	2

Community Hospital Discharge List July 31, 20XX				
Patient Name	**Age**	**Service**	**Admission Date**	**LOS**
Allan, Randy	52	Medicine	7/23	8
Banta, Janet	76	Medicine	7/25	6
Cox, David	56	Surgery	7/27	4
Dunning, Stephen	15	Surgery	7/26	5
Epp, Melvin	65	Medicine	7/26	5
Farmer, Jaimie	19	OB	7/29	2
Finley, Baby Girl	NB	NB	7/28	3
Finney, G. W.	54	Surgery	7/23	8
Fry, Benedict	83	Surgery	7/24	7
Girard, Katherine	73	Medicine	7/25	6
Halford, Harold	65	Surgery	7/26	5
Kilpatrick, Susan	19	OB	7/25	6
Kilpatrick, Baby Boy	NB	NB	7/26	5
Martindale, Amanda	18	OB	7/28	3
Martindale, Baby Boy	NB	NB	7/28	3
Martindale, Baby Boy	NB	NB	7/28	3
Nachtigall, Brian	22	Medicine	7/23	8
Niazi, Baby Boy	NB	NB	7/25	6
Poepperling, Wanda	56	Medicine	7/25	6
Trotman, Baby Girl	NB	NB	7/23	8

July Discharge Statistics												
	Medicine		**Surgery**		**Obstetrics**		**A/C Subtotal**		**Newborn**		**Grand Total**	
Date	**No. Pts.**	**Dis Days**	**No. Pts.**	**Dis Days**	**No. Pts.**	**Dis Days**	**No. Pts.**	**Dis Days**	**No. Pts.**	**Dis Days**	**No. Pts.**	**Dis Days**
1-July	8	40	2	25	5	16			6	23		
2-July	6	36	8	80	3	10			3	10		
3-July	4	21	4	23	1	4			1	4		
4-July	11	47	3	42	4	10			4	10		
5-July	15	77	5	23	3	7			2	5		
6-July	6	52	7	56	2	5			3	7		
7-July	5	71	9	123	6	13			5	10		
8-July	8	63	1	4	3	9			2	13		
9-July	9	72	4	26	2	6			3	9		
10-July	7	34	9	112	3	8			3	8		
11-July	2	9	3	27	1	2			1	2		
12-July	5	28	4	16	2	5			1	3		
13-July	4	29	6	119	2	7			2	7		
14-July	9	26	8	95	2	6			2	6		

(continued on next page)

July Discharge Statistics												
	Medicine		Surgery		Obstetrics		A/C Subtotal		Newborn		Grand Total	
Date	No. Pts.	Dis Days	No. Pts.	Dis Days	No. Pts.	Dis Days	No. Pts.	Dis Days	No. Pts.	Dis Days	No. Pts.	Dis Days
15-July	7	45	4	81	4	8			5	11		
16-July	6	37	2	15	3	8			3	8		
17-July	4	52	9	37	3	10			2	10		
18-July	3	55	6	30	3	9			3	10		
19-July	4	8	4	16	4	10			4	10		
20-July	8	63	3	37	2	6			3	9		
21-July	3	29	5	23	1	3			0	0		
22-July	5	35	8	78	4	9			4	9		
23-July	5	34	4	32	2	4			3	8		
24-July	8	53	1	5	3	6			2	6		
25-July	7	26	2	62	2	2			2	4		
26-July	2	23	3	42	4	12			3	7		
27-July	3	23	4	53	1	5			4	11		
28-July	5	25	2	10	3	10			2	8		
29-July												
30-July												
31-July												
Total												

Leave of Absence Days

Another data element that is significant in some hospitals is the number of leave of absence days. Leaves of absence are rare in the short-term acute-care hospital setting. A **leave of absence** is a physician-authorized absence of an inpatient from a hospital or other facility for a specified period of time occurring after admission and prior to discharge. This means the physician writes an order that the patient can leave the facility and return at a later date. The healthcare facility will hold the bed until the patient returns or it is determined that the patient is absent without leave.

Chapter 5 Formulae for Calculation of Length of Stay Statistics

Indicator	Numerator	Denominator
ALOS	Total LOS (discharge days) for a given period	Total number of discharges, including deaths, for the same period
ALOS for NBs or ANLOS	Total LOS (discharge days) for all NB discharges and deaths for a given period	Total number of NB discharges, including deaths, for the same period

Chapter 5   Matching Quiz

Match the definitions with the terms.

Definitions

a. Time measured in hours numbered to 24 (such as 0100 or 2300) from one midnight to the next

b. The total number of patient days for an inpatient episode, calculated by subtracting the date of admission from the date of discharge

c. The authorized absence of an inpatient from a hospital or other facility for a specified period of time occurring after admission and prior to discharge

d. The date that an inpatient was formally released from the hospital, and room, board, and continuous nursing services were terminated

e. The date of inpatient admission, beginning with a hospital's formal acceptance of a patient, via a physician order, who is to receive healthcare services while receiving room, board, and continuous nursing services

f. The average length of stay for hospital inpatients discharged during a given period of time

g. A program that evaluates the healthcare facility's efficiency in providing necessary care to patients in the most effective manner

h. The sum of the discharge days of any group of inpatients discharged during a specific period of time

i. The time a patient is in an outpatient clinic to receive services

j. Payment groups designed for the Medicare population that recognize severity of illness, resource use, and patient complexity

Terms:

1. _____MS-DRGs
2. _____Utilization management
3. _____Length of stay
4. _____Total length of stay
5. _____Military time

6. _____Leave of absence
7. _____Admission date
8. _____Discharge date
9. _____Average length of stay
10. _____Outpatient LOS

Chapter 5   Review

1. The number of discharge days for a patient admitted January 23 to February 15 is _____.
   a. 21 days
   b. 22 days
   c. 23 days
   d. 24 days

2. Determine the length of stay for the following patients:

Patient	Admitted	Discharged (same year as admission)	LOS
A	6/25	6/25	
B	6/25	7/4	
C	6/25	8/1	
D	6/25	9/2	

Use the information in the table below to answer questions 3, 4, and 5.

3. Use an Excel spreadsheet to determine the length of stay for the following individual patients who were all discharged on July 12 of the same year as the admission year:

Patient	Admitted	LOS
A	7/4	
B	7/5	
C	6/20	
D	3/12	
E	4/17	
F	3/1	
G	6/23	
H	6/25	
I	4/7	
J	5/6	

4. The total length of stay for the patients is _____.
   a. 523
   b. 577
   c. 602
   d. 645

5. The average length of stay for these patients is _____, rounded to one decimal.
   a. 52.3 days
   b. 57.7 days
   c. 60.2 days
   d. 64.5 days

6. When a patient is authorized to be absent from the healthcare facility and plans to return at a later date, this is referred to as (a) _____.
   a. Absent without leave
   b. Leave of absence
   c. Discharge day
   d. Total leave

7. What is the wait time for a patient who arrives at a physician's office at 8:20 a.m. and is seen by the physician at 9:30 a.m.?
   a. 68 minutes
   b. 70 minutes
   c. 1 hour, 5 minutes
   d. 50 minutes

8. Calculate the ALOS for the following Medicare patients. Round to one decimal place.

Community Hospital Medicare Discharge Statistics July 20XX			
Unit	Medicare Discharges	Medicare Discharge Days	ALOS
Medicine	478	3,411	
Surgery	253	2,566	
Rehabilitation	261	4,507	
Skilled Nursing	394	11,132	

Use the information in the table below to answer questions 9 through 12.

Patient arrives at the hospital's surgery center	5:30 a.m.
Patient called back to the prep area	6:12 a.m.
Patient prep completed	7:58 a.m.
Patient taken to surgical suite	8:20 a.m.
Surgery started	8:35 a.m.
Surgery ended	9:50 a.m.
Patient taken to recovery room	10:03 a.m.
Patient taken to hospital room	11:45 a.m.

9. What was the patient's wait time from the time of arrival to the surgery center and being taken to the surgery prep area?
   a. 42 minutes
   b. 43 minutes
   c. 45 minutes
   d. 60 minutes

10. How long was the surgical prep time?
    a. 100 minutes
    b. 103 minutes
    c. 106 minutes
    d. 120 minutes

11. How long was the surgery?
    a. 60 minutes
    b. 65 minutes
    c. 70 minutes
    d. 75 minutes

12. What was the total time from the time of the patient arriving at the hospital to the time the patient was taken to a hospital room?
    a. 5 hours, 15 minutes
    b. 6 hours, 15 minutes
    c. 300 minutes
    d. 400 minutes

Use the table below to answer questions 13, 14, and 15. Round to one decimal place.

Service	Discharges	Discharge Days
Medicine	6,658	37,284
Surgery	7,820	48,481
Obstetrics	2,389	4,790
Newborn	2,214	4,456

13. What is the average length of stay for the medicine service?
    a. 15.6 percent
    b. 5.6 days
    c. 6.9 days
    d. 17.8 days

14. What is the average length of stay for the newborn service?
    a. 2.0 percent
    b. 2.0 days
    c. 2.1 days
    d. 4.9 days

15. What is the average length of stay for all services including newborns?
    a. 2.0 days
    b. 4.7 days
    c. 4.9 days
    d. 5.0 days

CHAPTER 6

Mortality Rates

Learning Objectives

At the conclusion of this chapter, you should be able to do the following:

- Calculate the following mortality rates: hospital, gross, net, postoperative, anesthesia, maternal, newborn, fetal, cancer, crude, and case fatality
- Contrast between general, regional, and local anesthesia
- Differentiate between a direct obstetrical death and indirect obstetrical death

Key Terms

Anesthesia mortality rate
Cancer mortality rate
Cancer registrar
Cancer registry
Case fatality rate
Complication
Dead on arrival (DOA)
Death rate
Early fetal death
Fetal death
Fetal mortality rate
General anesthesia
Gross mortality rate
Hospital live birth

Hospital mortality rate
Infant death
Institutional mortality rate
Intermediate fetal death
Late fetal death
Live birth
Local anesthesia
Maternal death
Maternal mortality rate
Mortality
Mortality rate
Neonatal death
Neonatal period
Net mortality rate

Newborn death
Newborn mortality rate
OB Case Fatality Rate
Obstetrical (OB) discharges
Perinatal death
Postneonatal death
Postoperative mortality rate
Postpartum
Regional anesthesia
Surgical mortality rate
Surgical operation
Surgical procedure

A **mortality rate**, also referred to as a **death rate**, is a rate that measures the risk of death for a defined population. This rate has always been important information for health agencies and hospitals in evaluating the quality of clinical care. Comparison of mortality rates based on certain characteristics, such as socioeconomic status, geography or location, age, and cause of death, is useful to identify disparities in outcomes. Mortality rate information is used by a variety of industries in addition to healthcare. For example, the automobile industry uses mortality rate information to determine the likelihood of drivers and passengers dying in certain car models compared with others. Organizations such as the American Heart Association, the American Cancer Association, and other groups are interested in looking at mortality rates to help bring attention to their causes and to raise money for research. Researchers use mortality rates to show causes of death in certain populations. All of this information can help improve the quality of medical care given to patients. Health information management (HIM) practitioners—and anyone else who relies on statistical information—must remember that numbers count, not only in reports and records, but also in the human equation.

Mortality rate data are also important in helping public health agencies plan for health services. For example, the Centers for Medicare and Medicaid Services (CMS) publishes information on mortality rates among Medicare patients, and patients in particular diagnosis categories, to name a few. CMS is the division of the Department of Health and Human Services that is responsible for developing healthcare policy in the US and for administering the Medicare program and the federal portion of the Medicaid program. CMS also publishes Hospital Compare at Medicare.gov, which provides healthcare consumers information about hospitals in their area, including mortality rates, which can be indicators of the quality of care given to patients. HIM practitioners must understand basic mortality rates and be ready to calculate or verify other data pertaining to mortality.

 The terms "death rate" and "mortality rate" refer to the same statistics. Mortality rate will be used in this chapter, but both terms are used interchangeably in practice. It is important to remember that they are the same statistics, and the same formulae should be used when calculating them.

Guidelines for Calculating Mortality Rates

Consider the following guidelines when calculating mortality rates:

- Mortality rates are typically presented as a percentage rounded to the nearest tenth of a percent or one decimal point.
- Death is a type of discharge. Any data representing total discharges include deaths for that period. Thus, deaths are always assumed to be included in the total discharges in the denominator unless otherwise specified.
- If deaths of newborn inpatients are included in the numerator, all discharges of newborn inpatients must be included in the denominator. Ordinarily, newborns are included in the gross mortality rate (defined below) unless a facility chooses to calculate their mortality rate separately.
- Patients who are **dead on arrival (DOA)** are not included in the gross mortality rate because DOAs are not admitted to the hospital. Patients that arrive at the hospital with no signs of life are considered DOA.
- Patients who die in the hospital while outpatients or in the emergency department are not included in the gross mortality rate, since they were not admitted as an inpatient.

Gross Mortality Rate

The **gross mortality rate** is defined as the number of inpatient deaths for a period of time divided by the total number of live discharges and deaths for the same time period. A synonymous term for gross mortality rate is **hospital mortality rate**.

When computing hospital mortality rates, the concept of number of occurrences versus number of times something could have occurred applies. That is, every patient discharged from the hospital could have possibly died. Therefore, the formula for calculating the hospital mortality rate (gross mortality rate) is the number of inpatient deaths divided by the number of patients discharged including deaths, as shown:

$$Gross\ Mortality\ Rate = \frac{Number\ of\ inpatient\ deaths\ (including\ NB)\ in\ a\ period}{Number\ of\ discharges,\ including\ deaths\ and\ NB,\ in\ a\ period}$$

Example 6.1: If a hospital had 7 deaths and 520 discharges (including deaths) for a month, what is the hospital mortality rate? Round to the nearest tenth.

$$Hospital\ Mortality\ Rate = \frac{7\ deaths}{520\ discharges} = \frac{7}{520} = 0.0134\ or\ 1.3\%$$

The gross mortality rate may also be calculated for subsets of patients, such as a particular disease or service area. This statistic is referred to as a **case fatality rate** or total number of deaths due to a specific illness during a given time period divided by the total number of cases during the same period. It is calculated using the same formula as the gross mortality rate, but the numerator and denominator only include the particular disease or service area of interest. The general formula appears below:

$$Case\ Fatality\ Rate = \frac{Number\ of\ deaths\ for\ patients\ with\ a\ disease\ during\ a\ period}{Number\ of\ patients\ discharged\ with\ a\ disease,\ including\ deaths,\ during\ a\ period}$$

Example 6.2: If a hospital had 40 acute myocardial infarction (AMI) discharges (including deaths) last year and 8 deaths, what is the case fatality rate for AMI? Round to the nearest tenth.

$$AMI\ Case\ Fatality\ Rate = \frac{8}{40} = 0.2\ or\ 20.0\%$$

Example 6.3: If 50 kidney transplant patients were discharged in the past year and two of the discharged patients died, what is the case fatality rate for kidney transplant? Round to the nearest tenth.

$$Kidney\ Transplant\ Case\ Fatality\ Rate = \frac{2}{50} = 0.040\ or\ 4.0\%$$

Example 6.4: The case fatality rate can also be used to examine the mortality rates by physician. If Dr. Howard discharged 600 patients in the past year, and of those patients, 27 died, the formula would be:

$$Dr.\ Howard's\ Case\ Fatality\ Rate = \frac{27}{600} = 0.0450\ or\ 4.5\%$$

Exercise 6.1

1. Use the data in the table that follows to calculate the gross mortality rate at Community Hospital for December. Deaths are not included in the discharges. Round to the nearest hundredth of a percent.

Community Hospital December 20XX Data	
Total adult and children live discharges	645
Total adult and children deaths	4
Total newborn live discharges	87
Total newborn deaths	1

2. The HIM professional reported to the quality improvement committee at Community Hospital that there were 58 patients with influenza discharged from the hospital in January. Of those, 3 died. What is the case fatality rate for influenza for January? Round to the nearest hundredth of a percent.

3. Last year, University Hospital had 15 liver and pancreas transplants. Three of the 15 patients died. What is the case fatality rate for this surgery at University Hospital? Round to the nearest hundredth of a percent.

Exercise 6.2

The table that follows is a sample report for a hospital showing the discharges and deaths for the last quarter of the year. Notice that this report lists the patient discharges and deaths by physicians on the medical staff. Prepare an Excel spreadsheet to calculate the mortality rate for each physician and the total for this quarter. Deaths are not included in the discharges. Round to the nearest hundredth of a percent.

Community Hospital October–December 20XX Discharges and Deaths, by Primary Care Physician			
Physician Number	**No. of Live Discharges**	**No. of Deaths**	**Gross Mortality Rate**
Dr. 097	12	3	
Dr. 123	204	4	
Dr. 256	12	1	
Dr. 372	92	4	
Dr. 431	124	6	
Dr. 537	79	2	
Dr. 638	107	4	
Dr. 725	85	3	
Dr. 800	100	1	
Dr. 901	158	8	
Total			

You may notice when computing your rates that sometimes your answer may be a whole number, such as 6 percent, or there may be a zero (or blank) in the hundredths place, as in 6.1 percent. When asked to compute to two decimal places, always add the zeros required to meet the level of precision (number of decimal places) required. Your answers would read 6.00 percent and 6.10 percent.

Net Mortality Rate

Various reporting or accrediting agencies sometimes request the **net mortality rate**, also referred to as the **institutional mortality rate**. The net mortality rate is the number of inpatients that died more than 48 hours after admission divided by the number of discharges including deaths. This definition removes patient that die within 48 hours of admission from the numerator of the rate. Usually, adult, child, and newborn statistics are kept separately. However, when calculating the net mortality rate, newborn deaths are included in the inpatient deaths along with the adult and children deaths. **Newborn deaths** are infants that die during the same admission as their birth.

The net mortality rate came into use because it was felt that healthcare providers should not be held accountable for a death that occurred less than 48 hours after admission, as they would not have had enough time to directly affect the patient's condition. This figure is not commonly used in practice because of advances in medical care, but is presented for a thorough study of all death-related statistics that may be encountered in healthcare.

The formula for calculating the net mortality rate is:

$$Net\ Mortality\ Rate = \frac{[Number\ of\ inpatient\ deaths] - [Number\ of\ inpatient\ deaths\ within\ 48\ hours\ of\ admission]}{[Total\ number\ of\ discharges\ including\ deaths] - [Number\ of\ inpatient\ deaths\ within\ 48\ hours\ of\ admission]}$$

Notice that the number of deaths within 48 hours of admission are subtracted from both the numerator and denominator when the net mortality rate is calculated.

Example 6.5: Last month, Community Hospital had 255 discharges, including nine deaths. Three of the deaths were patients who were in the hospital less than 48 hours. What is the net mortality rate? Round to the nearest tenth.

$$Net\ Mortality\ Rate = \frac{9-3}{255-3} = 0.0238\ or\ 2.4\%$$

Exercise 6.3

Use the data in the table that follows to calculate the net mortality rate at Community Hospital for April. Discharges do not include deaths. Round to two decimal places.

Community Hospital April 20XX Deaths	
Total adult and children live discharges	409
Total adult and children deaths	7
Deaths < 48 hours	2
Deaths ≥ 48 hours	5
Total newborn live discharges	68
Total newborn deaths	2
Deaths < 48 hours	1
Deaths ≥ 48 hours	1

Exercise 6.4

Use the data in the table that follows. Prepare an Excel spreadsheet to calculate the net mortality rate for each service and the total net mortality rate at Community Hospital for December. In this exercise, deaths are included in the discharges. Round to two decimal places.

Community Hospital December 20XX Deaths				
Service	No. of Discharges (Includes Deaths)	Total Deaths	Deaths < 48 Hours	Net Mortality Rate
Medicine	372	7	3	
Surgery	301	4	3	
Psychiatric	107	4	2	
Rehabilitation	74	6	3	
Total				

Postoperative Mortality Rate

The **postoperative mortality rate**, also called the **surgical mortality rate**, refers to the number of deaths occurring after an operation has been performed. The criteria for computing the postoperative mortality rate includes the ratio of deaths within 10 days after surgery to the total number of patients operated on during that period.

A **surgical operation** is defined as one or more surgical procedures performed at one time for one patient via a common approach or for a common purpose (AHIMA 2017). A **surgical procedure** is any single, separate, systematic process upon or within the body that can be complete in itself; is normally performed by a physician, dentist, or other licensed practitioner; can be performed either with or without instruments; and is performed to restore disunited or deficient parts, remove diseased or injured tissues, extract foreign matter, assist in obstetrical delivery, or aid in diagnosis (AHIMA 2017). It is important to remember that a surgical operation may include more than one procedure. For example, if a patient is undergoing a coronary artery bypass graft (CABG), a procedure is performed to harvest the artery and a second procedure to graft the artery into the heart. These two procedures are performed during the same operative session and therefore would be considered one operation.

The formula for calculating the postoperative mortality rate is

$$Postoperative\ Mortality\ Rate = \frac{Total\ number\ of\ deaths\ within\ 10\ days\ of\ a\ surgical\ operation\ in\ a\ period}{Total\ number\ of\ patients\ experiencing\ a\ surgical\ operation\ in\ a\ period}$$

The postoperative mortality rate may be calculated for a facility or at the specialty or procedure level.

Example 6.6: One hundred and twenty-three patients were operated on in the cardiovascular clinic at University Hospital. Three of those patients died within 10 days of their operations. What is the postoperative mortality rate for the cardiovascular clinic? Round to one decimal place.

$$Postoperative\ Death\ Rate = \frac{3}{123} = 0.0243\ or\ 2.4\%$$

The postoperative mortality rate is limited to patients that die within 10 days of the procedure because other conditions beyond the surgical procedure itself may be the cause of death. Note that the denominator in the postoperative death rate includes patients and not surgical procedures or operations.

Exercise 6.5

Use the information in the table that follows. Prepare an Excel spreadsheet to calculate the postoperative mortality rate for each surgeon at Community Hospital during the semiannual period of July through December. Round to the nearest tenth of a percent.

Community Hospital July–December 20XX Number of Surgery Patients and Deaths, by Surgeon			
Physician Number	**No. of Surgery Patients**	**No. of Deaths within 10 Days after Surgery**	**Postoperative Mortality Rate**
Dr. 102	298	6	
Dr. 237	247	4	
Dr. 391	110	2	
Dr. 518	144	2	
Dr. 637	206	8	
Dr. 802	82	3	
Dr. 900	120	3	
Total			

Exercise 6.6

Use the information in the table that follows to calculate the postoperative mortality rate at Community Hospital during July. Round to the nearest hundredth of a percent.

Community Hospital July 20XX Deaths Surgery Service	
Discharges (does not include deaths)	483
Deaths	9
Within 10 days after surgery	5
More than 10 days after surgery	4
Number of operations	495
Number of patients operated on	480

Exercise 6.7

Use the information in the table that follows. Prepare an Excel spreadsheet to calculate the postoperative mortality rate at Community Hospital for each Medicare severity diagnosis-related group (MS-DRG) listed for January through June and the total for this semiannual period. Round to two decimal places, nearest hundredth of a percent.

Community Hospital January–June 20XX Selected MS-DRGs—Postoperative Deaths Number of Surgery Patients and Deaths Surgery Service				
MS-DRG	MS-DRG Title	No. of Surgery Patients	No. of Deaths within 10 Days after Surgery	Postoperative Mortality Rate
139	Salivary gland procedures	12	1	
217	Cardiac valve & oth maj cardiothoracic proc w card cath w CC	427	5	
239	Amputation for circ sys disorders exc upper limb & toe w MCC	8	2	
327	Stomach, esophageal & duodenal proc w CC	84	3	
338	Appendectomy w complicated principal diag w MCC	6	1	
405	Pancreas, liver & shunt procedures w MCC	62	4	
469	Major joint replacement or reattachment of lower extremity w MCC	212	3	
625	Thyroid, parathyroid & thyroglossal procedures w MCC	207	1	
652	Kidney transplant	27	4	
736	Uterine & adnexa proc for ovarian or adnexal malignancy w MCC	143	4	
Total				

Anesthesia Mortality Rate

The definition of **anesthesia mortality rate** is the ratio of deaths caused by anesthetic agents to the number of anesthetics administered during a specified period of time. Because anesthesia deaths occur so infrequently, some hospitals might choose, instead, to evaluate the relationship between a death and a specific type of anesthetic for a special study.

There are three major types of anesthesia: general, regional, and local. When **general anesthesia** is administered, the patient is unconscious and has no sensations. General anesthesia is given intravenously or inhaled. When **regional anesthesia** is given, the patient may be awake or may be sedated. Regional anesthetics remove the ability to feel any pain or sensations in a specific region of the body. A peripheral nerve block is a type of regional anesthetic that blocks pain and sensations around a specific nerve or group of nerves. These are often used on the hands, arms, feet, legs, or face. Spinal and epidural anesthesia are types of regional anesthesia used near the spinal cord and the spinal nerves and block pain and sensation in an entire region of the body, such as the abdomen, hips, or legs. **Local anesthesia** numbs a small area of the body. This involves an injection of an anesthetic—in this case, a numbing agent—placed directly into the area to block pain.

The formula for calculating the anesthesia mortality rate is:

$$Anesthesia\ Mortality\ Rate = \frac{Total\ deaths\ caused\ by\ anesthetic\ agents}{Total\ number\ of\ anesthetics\ administered}$$

Example 6.7: If anesthetics were given 2,000 times to surgical patients, and one patient death was attributed to anesthesia during the past year, what is the anesthesia mortality rate? Round to the nearest one hundredth, or two decimal places, and report as per 1,000 anesthetics administered.

$$Anesthesia\ Mortality\ Rate = \frac{1}{2,000} = 0.00050\ or\ 0.050\%\ or\ 0.5\ per\ 1,000$$

The anesthesia mortality rate is an example of a statistic that may be very small. It will typically be expressed as a fraction of a percentage or as "per 1,000." Take care in converting to a percentage and be sure to display a "0" in front of the decimal place. Recall that reporting a rate as "per 1,000" requires multiplying the rate by 1,000, and reporting a rate as a percentage requires multiplying by 100.

QUICK TIP

Exercise 6.8

Use the information in the table that follows to calculate the anesthesia mortality rate for University Hospital for January through June. Round to the nearest tenth of a percent.

University Hospital January–June 20XX Surgery Service	
Discharges (does not include deaths)	2,642
Deaths:	59
Within 10 days	12
After 10 days	42
Number of operations	2,645
Number of patients operated on	2,636
Number of anesthetics administered	2,636
Number of deaths due to anesthetic agents	3

Exercise 6.9

Use the information in the table that follows. Prepare an Excel spreadsheet to calculate individually the number of deaths due to the administration of general, regional, and local anesthesia. Round to the nearest hundredth of a percent.

University Hospital January–June 20XX Surgery Service	
Discharges (does not include deaths)	2,642
Deaths	54
Within 10 days	12
After 10 days	42
Number of operations	2,645
Number of patients operated on	2,636
Number of anesthetics administered	2,636
General anesthesia	1,072
Regional anesthesia	1,017
Local anesthesia	547
Number of deaths due to anesthetic agents	7
General anesthesia	4
Regional anesthesia	2
Local anesthesia	1

Maternal Mortality Rate

A **maternal death** is defined as the death of any woman while pregnant or within 42 days of termination of pregnancy from any cause related to or aggravated by pregnancy or its management (regardless of duration or site of pregnancy), but not from accidental or incidental causes (WHO, n.d.). An example of an accidental death would be a motor vehicle accident or a fall down a flight of stairs. Examples of an incidental death would be a suicide or homicide.

The **maternal mortality rate** is a statistic that is tracked closely by public health officials. As with the other statistical rates presented in this text, the numerator includes the event of interest, maternal deaths, and the denominator includes the number of times the event could have occurred. The maternal mortality rate is defined in two contexts. First, at the hospital level the maternal mortality rate is equivalent to the OB case mortality rate. That is, the hospital maternal mortality rate is total number of maternal deaths directly related to pregnancy for a given time period divided by the total number of obstetrical discharges for the same time period.

The maternal mortality rate may also be defined for a community and included as one of the vital statistics reported. In that case, the denominator for the maternal mortality rate is the number of live births. WHO defines a **live birth** as "the complete expulsion or extraction from its mother of a product of conception, irrespective of the duration of the pregnancy, which, after such separation, breathes or shows any other evidence of life - e.g. beating of the heart, pulsation of the umbilical cord or definite movement of voluntary muscles - whether or not the umbilical cord has been cut or the placenta is attached. Each product of such a birth is considered live born" (WHO n.d.). A **hospital live birth** is a live birth that occurs in a hospital.

When reported on a population basis, the of occurrence of events may be rare, and therefore reporting as a percentage may result in a very small number that is difficult to interpret. For example, researchers may use 100,000 to determine how often something occurred per 100,000 people, 10,000 to determine how often it occurred per 10,000 people, and so on. WHO recommends reporting maternal mortality rates per 100,000 live births.

The following vital statistics formula is used for the maternal mortality rate for a community according to WHO recommendation:

$$Maternal\ Mortality\ Rate\ (per\ 100{,}000) = \frac{Number\ of\ maternal\ deaths\ in\ a\ period}{Number\ of\ births\ in\ a\ period} \times 100{,}000$$

When computing the maternal mortality rate, hospitals typically report only direct obstetrical deaths as maternal deaths and include only those deaths that occur during hospitalization. Nonmaternal deaths (deaths resulting from accidental or incidental causes not related to pregnancy or its management) are not included in the maternal mortality rate calculation. A woman who dies after an abortion is considered a maternal death, as is an obstetrical patient who dies in the **prepartum** period (that is, the time period occurring before childbirth—some facilities refer to these as antepartum deaths) of a cause due to pregnancy.

A statistic that is related to the maternal mortality rate is the obstetric (OB) case fatality rate. The denominator of the OB case fatality rate is the number of **obstetrical discharges** Obstetrical discharges are discharges of women while pregnant or within 42 days of termination of the pregnancy. A healthcare facility's service classification system may include a breakdown of obstetrical discharges into delivered, aborted, not delivered, and **postpartum** (the time after childbirth), and all of these should be included in the total obstetrical discharges in the denominator of the formula (and in the numerator if the mother dies).

Many healthcare facilities also differentiate between direct obstetrical deaths and indirect obstetrical deaths. A direct obstetrical death is a death directly related to the pregnancy; for example, a patient who died after a C-section because of a nick to the uterine artery that resulted in hemorrhage. An indirect obstetrical death is not directly due to obstetrical causes, even though the physiologic effects of the pregnancy are partially responsible for the death. An example of an indirect obstetrical death is diabetes. A pregnant woman can have **complications** of diabetes that are aggravated by the pregnancy, but the cause of death is diabetes and not pregnancy. A complication is a medical condition that arises during a hospitalization. The physician is responsible for documenting the cause of death.

The formula for calculating the OB case fatality rate is:

$$OB\ Case\ Fatality\ Rate = \frac{Number\ of\ maternal\ deaths\ in\ a\ period}{Number\ of\ live\ births\ in\ a\ period}$$

Example 6.8: At University Hospital, a mother died from a hemorrhage immediately after delivery. The hospital's annual obstetrics and gynecology discharges are classified as: delivered, 4,782; aborted, 297; not delivered (prepartum), 186; and postpartum within 42 days, 46. The number of live births during that period was 4,782. What is the maternal mortality rate? What is the OB case direct fatality rate? Report the statistic to the three decimals.

$$Maternal\ Mortality\ Rate = \frac{1}{4{,}782} = 0.000209$$

Reported as a Percentage = 0.000209 × 100 = 0.0209%
Reported as per 100,000 = 0.000209 × 100,000 = 21 per 100,000

$$OB\ Case\ Fatality\ Rate = \frac{1}{(4{,}782 + 297 + 186 + 46)} = \frac{1}{5{,}311} = 0.000188$$

$$= 0.019\%\ or\ 19\ per\ 100{,}000$$

 Recall that reporting a rate as a percentage requires multiplying the rate by 100. To report a rate "per 100,000," multiply the rate by 100,000. In general, rates should be reported so that there is a whole number to the left of the decimal point unless otherwise instructed.

Example 6.9: During the year, a community hospital reported 1,307 hospital live births and two maternal deaths after abortions. What is the maternal mortality rate? Report the rate to the nearest tenth per 100,000.

$$Maternal\ Mortality\ Rate = \frac{2}{1{,}307} = 0.00153$$

Reported as per 100,000: 0.00153 × 100,000 = 153.02 or 153.0 rounded to the nearest tenth.

Exercise 6.10

Use the information in the table that follows to calculate Community Hospital's OB case fatality rate for May. These are all direct maternal deaths. Round to two decimal places.

Community Hospital May 20XX Obstetrical Unit	
Maternal discharges (does not include deaths)	
Delivered	227
Aborted	4
Undelivered, prepartum	32
Undelivered, postpartum	17
Deaths	
Delivered	1
Aborted	2
Undelivered, prepartum	1
Undelivered, postpartum	2
Live births	230

Exercise 6.11

Last month, the Women's Hospital reported 123 obstetrical discharges and 5 deaths. (The deaths are included in the discharges.) The causes of the 5 deaths were as follows:

- Injuries due to spousal abuse
- Injuries due to an automobile accident
- Suicide
- Hemorrhage after C-section due to severed uterine artery
- Preeclampsia

Calculate the direct OB case fatality rate for this hospital. Round to two decimal places, or nearest hundredth of a percent.

Exercise 6.12

Use the annual statistics in the table that follows to calculate both the maternal mortality rate and the OB case fatality rate for University Hospital. These are all direct maternal deaths. Deaths are included in the discharges. Round to two decimal places.

University Hospital Annual Statistics, 20XX Obstetrical Service	
Live births	1,040
Maternal discharges and deaths	
Delivered	1,032
Aborted	57
Undelivered, prepartum	92
Undelivered, postpartum	85
Deaths:	
Delivered	3
Aborted	2
Undelivered, prepartum	1
Undelivered, postpartum	1

Exercise 6.13

According to the CDC Wonder database, there were 3,855,500 live births in the US in 2016, and there were 1,231 documented maternal deaths in the US (CDC 2019). What is the maternal mortality rate per 100,000 population? Calculate to the nearest whole number.

Infant Mortality Rate

An **infant death** is the death of a liveborn infant at any time from the moment of birth to the end of the first year of life. Statistical tabulations for vital events related to pregnancy and infants can provide valuable information on reproductive health. They also can provide data on national and international trends.

Infant deaths are divided into newborn, neonatal, post-neonatal and perinatal. The definitions of each of these categories are listed in table 6.1. The infant related time periods are displayed in figure 6.1

Table 6.1.   Definitions describing infant deaths

Type of Death	Definition
Newborn death	Death of a liveborn infant born in the hospital who later dies during the same admission
Neonatal death	Death of a liveborn infant within the **neonatal period**, defined as the first 28 days of life
Postneonatal death	Death of a liveborn infant from 28 days of birth to the end of the first year of life
Perinatal death	Death that occurs from 22 weeks of completed gestation to 7 completed days from the moment of birth (WHO n.d.)

Figure 6.1.   Infant-related time periods

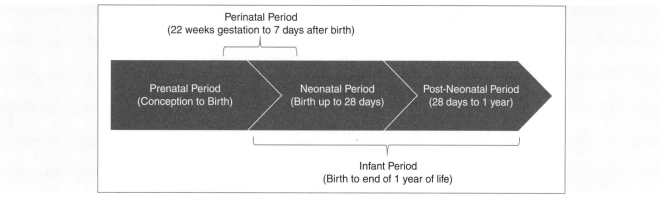

Source: © AHIMA

The formula for calculating the **newborn (NB) mortality rate** is:

$$NB\ Mortality\ Rate = \frac{Number\ of\ NB\ deaths\ for\ a\ period}{Number\ of\ NB\ discharges\ (including\ deaths)\ for\ a\ period}$$

Example 6.10: If University Hospital had 2,567 newborn discharges and 2 newborn deaths in one year, what is the newborn mortality rate? Round to the nearest hundredth of a percent.

$$NB\ Mortality\ Rate = \frac{2}{2,567} = 0.00077 = 0.08\%$$

Neonatal and infant mortality are two statistics that are tracked regularly by public health officials and researchers. The formulae for each rate are:

$$Neonatal\ Mortality\ Rate = \frac{Number\ of\ neonatal\ deaths\ during\ a\ period}{Number\ of\ live\ births\ during\ a\ period}$$

$$Infant\ Mortality\ Rate = \frac{Number\ of\ infant\ deaths\ during\ a\ period}{Number\ of\ live\ births\ during\ a\ period}$$

Infant deaths include both neonatal and perinatal deaths. Review table 6.1 for the formal definition of each term.

QUICK
TIP

Example 6.11: If a hospital had 4,270 births, 3 newborn deaths, and 4,267 newborn discharges, calculate the neonatal mortality rate. Express the answer as a rate per 1,000. Round to two decimals.

$$Neonatal\ Mortality\ Rate = \frac{3}{4,270} = 0.00070$$

Expressed as a rate per 1,000: 0.00070 × 1,000 = 0.70 per 1,000.

Exercise 6.14

1. Use the information in the table that follows to calculate Community Hospital's annual newborn mortality rate. In this exercise, the deaths are included in the discharges. Round to two decimal places.

Community Hospital Annual Statistics, 20XX Newborn Service	
Births	487
Newborn deaths	3
Newborn discharges and deaths	486

2. Use the information in the table that follows to calculate the newborn mortality rate for April at Community Hospital. In this exercise, the deaths are included in the discharges. Round to the nearest hundredth of a percent.

Community Hospital Newborn Unit April 20XX	
Births	52
Discharges and deaths	52
Deaths	2

3. In 2016, there were 23,161 infant deaths in the US, while there were 3,945,875 live births during the same year (CDC 2017) What is the infant mortality rate per 10,000 population? Round to the nearest whole number.

Fetal Mortality Rate

The CDC defines **fetal death** as "the spontaneous intrauterine death of a fetus at any time during pregnancy. Fetal deaths later in pregnancy (at 20 weeks of gestation or more, or 28 weeks or more, for example) are also sometimes referred to as 'stillbirths'" (CDC 2018). The death is indicated by the fact that after such expulsion or extraction, the fetus does not breathe or show any other evidence of life (for example, beating of the heart, pulsation of the umbilical cord, or definite movement of voluntary muscles) as measured via the Apgar score. Typically, hospitals are required to report fetal deaths to a state agency. However, the reporting method varies according to individual state laws, statutes, and regulations.

Because fetal deaths are not considered patient deaths, they are not included in any other calculation of mortality-related statistics and are calculated separately. Determination of whether to include fetal death data in a specific hospital's statistics requires an investigation of the facility's needs by hospital administration, medical staff, and reporting agencies. Fetal deaths are classified by the length of the gestational period and the weight of the fetus, as listed in table 6.2.

The formula for calculating the **fetal mortality rate** is:

$$Fetal\ Mortality\ Rate = \frac{Number\ of\ intermediate\ and\ late\ fetal\ deaths\ for\ a\ period}{Number\ of\ live\ births + intermediate\ and\ late\ fetal\ deaths\ for\ a\ period}$$

Table 6.2.   Classifications of fetal death

Classification	Length of Gestation	Weight
Early fetal death	Less than 20 weeks gestation	500 grams or less
Intermediate fetal death	20 weeks completed gestation, but less than 28 weeks	501 to 1,000 grams
Late fetal death	28 weeks completed gestation	Over 1,000 grams

Example 6.12: During November, a hospital had 207 live births, 1 early fetal death, 2 intermediate fetal deaths, and 3 late fetal deaths. What is the fetal mortality rate? Report the answer to the nearest tenth of a percent.

$$Fetal\ Mortality\ Rate = \frac{5}{207 + 5} = \frac{5}{212} = 0.0235$$

Reported as a percentage: $0.0235 \times 100 = 2.35\%$. Rounded to the nearest tenth: 2.4%.

 Keep in mind that the denominator in the fetal mortality rate formula is not discharges, but instead live births and intermediate and late fetal deaths. Recall that the denominator of a rate should include the number of times an event could happen. Fetal deaths are not a discharge and therefore must be added into the denominator along with live births.

Exercise 6.15

Community Hospital reported the following statistics for the month of February. Calculate the fetal mortality rate. Round to the nearest hundredth of a percent.

Community Hospital February 20XX Newborn Service	
Live births	37
Newborn discharges and deaths	36
Fetal deaths:	
Early	1
Intermediate	4
Late	3

Exercise 6.16

Use the information in the table that follows to calculate the newborn mortality rate and fetal mortality rate at Community Hospital for the year. In this exercise, deaths are included in the discharges. Round to two decimal places.

Community Hospital January–December 20XX Newborn Service	
Live births	307
Newborn discharges and deaths	306
Newborn deaths	3
Fetal deaths:	
Early	5
Intermediate	4
Late	2

Cancer Mortality Rate

The **cancer mortality rate** is the proportion of patients who die from cancer. The National Center for Health Statistics collects data on all cancer deaths occurring in the US and classifies them by sex, age, race, and cancer site so that mortality for a given time period can be determined for the entire country or selected areas (CDC 2018).

The formula for calculating the cancer mortality rate for a population is:

$$Cancer\ Mortality\ Rate = \frac{Number\ of\ cancer\ deaths\ during\ a\ period}{Number\ in\ population\ at\ risk}$$

Example 6.13: In 2017, 599,108 people died from cancer in the US. The estimated 2017 US population was 325,719,178 (NCHS 2018). Calculate the cancer mortality rate for the US in 2017. Report the answer as per 100,000 to the nearest tenth:

$$US\ Cancer\ Mortality\ Rate\ for\ 2017 = \frac{Number\ of\ cancer\ deaths\ in\ 2017}{US\ population\ in\ 2017}$$

$$US\ Cancer\ Mortality\ Rate\ for\ 2017 = \frac{599,108}{325,719,178} = 0.0018393$$

Reported as per 100,000 = 0.001839 × 100,000 = 183.93. Rounded to nearest tenth = 183.9.

Knowledge of healthcare statistics is an essential tool for cancer registrars. A **cancer registrar** is an individual who is responsible for maintaining a **cancer registry**. A cancer registry is a collection of information about the occurrence of cancer, the types of cancers that occur and their locations within the body, the extent of cancer at the time of diagnosis (disease stage), and the kinds of treatment that patients receive. Hospital cancer registries were developed as organized programs in hospitals to collect information about cancer patients. Their primary goal is to help improve treatment of cancer through various methods, including comparing different types of therapies used to treat cancer. The American College of Surgeons Commission on Cancer offers the opportunity for hospitals and treatment centers to become accredited. Accurate cancer data are vital to the fight against cancer, and cancer registrars are critical to capturing that data. Hospital and other cancer registry data are reported to population-based (central or regional) registries.

When calculating the cancer mortality rate in a facility, use the formula for case fatality rate presented earlier in the chapter. The disease in this case would be cancer or the type of cancer of interest.

Example 6.14: Community Hospital had five cases of prostate cancer patients who died last year. There was a total of 189 prostate cancer patients discharged in the same time period. Calculate the prostate cancer mortality rate for last year. Report the answer as a percentage to the nearest tenth of a percent.

$$Prostate\ Cancer\ Mortality\ Rate = \frac{Number\ of\ prostate\ cancer\ patients\ who\ died}{Number\ of\ cancer\ patients\ discharged}$$

$$Prostate\ Cancer\ Mortality\ Rate = \frac{5}{189} = 0.02645$$

Reported as a percentage: 0.02645 × 100 = 2.645%. Round to the nearest tenth of a percent: 2.6%.

Exercise 6.17

Use the information from Community Hospital's cancer registry in the table that follows. Prepare an Excel spreadsheet to calculate the mortality rates for each type of cancer and the total for this annual period. Deaths are included in the discharges. Round to the nearest hundredth of a percent.

Community Hospital Cancer Registry Annual Report Selected Cancers Reported 20XX			
Type of Cancer	No. of Discharges and Deaths	No. of Deaths	Cancer Mortality Rate
Breast	311	15	
Prostate	208	17	
Digestive system	102	13	
Lung and bronchus	162	12	
Urinary system	98	13	
Female reproductive	48	3	
Melanoma of the skin	21	14	
All other sites	215	52	
Total			

Exercise 6.18

Use the statistics from a multihospital system in the table that follows to calculate the cancer mortality rate for each hospital listed and for the entire healthcare system. In this exercise, the deaths are included in the discharges. Round to the nearest hundredth of a percent.

Community Healthcare System Annual Statistics, 20XX			
Hospital	No. of Cancer Discharges and Deaths	No. of Cancer Deaths	Cancer Mortality Rate
Urban Hospital	15,634	207	
Rural Hospital	6,203	154	
Suburban Hospital	2,073	58	
Total			

Exercise 6.19

Use the information in the table that follows. Prepare an Excel spreadsheet to calculate the mortality rates for University Hospital's cancer registry for each of the cancers reported and the total for this annual period. In this exercise, the deaths are included in the discharges. Round to two decimal places.

Type of Cancer	No. of Discharges and Deaths	No. of Deaths	Mortality Rate
Oral cavity and pharynx	24	1	
Digestive system	198	5	
Respiratory system	242	16	
Bone and joint	218	4	
Skin (excludes basal cell)	34	1	
Breast	190	12	
Female genital system	47	8	
Male genital system	228	25	
Urinary system	77	7	
Brain and other nervous system	42	19	
Endocrine system	28	1	
Lymphoma	47	6	
Myeloma	25	2	
Leukemia	15	4	
Total			

University Hospital
Cancer Registry Annual Report
Selected Cancers Reported
20XX

Chapter 6 Formulae for Calculation of Mortality Statistics

Statistic	Numerator	Denominator
Gross mortality rate (hospital mortality rate)	Number of inpatient deaths, including NBs, for a period	Number of discharges, including deaths and NB, for the same period
Net mortality rate (institutional mortality rate)	Number of inpatient deaths, including NBs, minus deaths < 48 hours for a period	Number of discharges, including deaths and NB, minus deaths < 48 hours for the same period
Postoperative mortality rate	Number of deaths within 10 days after surgery for a period	Number of patients operated on for the same period
Anesthesia mortality rate	Number of deaths caused by anesthesia agents for a period	Number of anesthetics administered for the same period
Maternal mortality rate	Number of maternal deaths for a period	Number of live births, for the same period
OB case fatality rate	Number of direct maternal deaths for a period	Number of OB discharges for the same period
Newborn mortality rate	Total number NB deaths for a period	Number of NB discharges, including deaths, for the same period

(*continued on next page*)

Statistic	Numerator	Denominator
Infant mortality rate	Number of infant deaths during a period	Number of live births during same period
Fetal mortality rate	Number of intermediate and late fetal deaths for a period	Number of live births plus number of intermediate and late fetal deaths for the same period
Cancer mortality rate	Number of deaths from cancer during a period	Number in population at risk during a period
Cancer case fatality rate	Number of deaths from cancer during a period	Number of discharges for cancer during a period

Chapter 6   Matching Quiz

Match the definitions with the terms.

Definitions:

a. The number of inpatient deaths that occurred during a given time period divided by the total number of inpatient discharges, including deaths, for the same time period

b. The ratio of deaths within 10 days after surgery to the total number of operations performed during a specified period of time

c. The death of a product of human conception that is fewer than 20 weeks of gestation and 500 grams or less in weight before its complete expulsion or extraction from the mother

d. An all-inclusive term that refers to both stillbirths and neonatal deaths

e. An inpatient who was born in a hospital at the beginning of the current inpatient hospitalization

f. Occurring after childbirth

g. A medical condition that arises during an inpatient hospitalization

h. A term referring to the incidence of death in a specific population

i. The number of newborns who died divided by the total number of newborns, both alive and dead

j. The total number of inpatient deaths minus the number of deaths that occurred less than 48 hours after admission for a given time period divided by the total number of inpatient discharges minus the number of deaths that occurred less than 48 hours after admission for the same time period

Terms:

1. _____ Complication

2. _____ Postpartum

3. _____ Newborn mortality rate

4. _____ Perinatal death

5. _____ Net mortality rate

6. _____ Gross mortality rate

7. _____ Newborn

8. _____ Postoperative mortality rate

9. _____ Mortality

10. _____ Early fetal death

Chapter 6   Review

Use the data reported for the past year in the table that follows to perform the calculations for questions 1 through 10. Round these to two decimal places.

Community Hospital Mortality Report Annual Statistics			
Discharges (includes deaths)		Deaths	
Total adults and children	13,954	Total adults and children	48
Total newborns	1,965	Total newborns	1
The following are included in the discharges:		The following are included in the deaths:	
OB delivered	1,971	Within 10 days postop	3
OB aborted	120	< 48 hours after admission	14
OB undelivered, prepartum	27	≥ 48 hours after admission	34
OB undelivered, postpartum	23	Anesthetic death	1
The following are included in the discharges:		Obstetrical deaths:	
Medicine service discharges	7,678	Undelivered, prepartum	1
Surgery service discharges	4,165	Aborted	1
Patients discharged with a primary diagnosis of cancer	565	Medicine service deaths	41
		Surgery service deaths	5
		Cancer deaths	53
		Fetal deaths:	
		Early	5
		Intermediate	4
		Late	3
Admissions			
Total adults and children	14,023	Total patients operated on	4,165
Total live births	1,964	Total anesthetics administered	4,165

1. What is the gross mortality rate?
    a. 0.030%
    b. 0.31%
    c. 3.10%
    d. 3.11%

2. What is the net mortality rate?
   a. 0.22%
   b. 2.20%
   c. 0.022%
   d. 22.00%

3. What is the postoperative mortality rate?
   a. 0.007%
   b. 0.07%
   c. 7.70%
   d. 77.02%

4. What is the anesthesia mortality rate?
   a. 0.002%
   b. 0.24%
   c. 0.02%
   d. 2.24%

5. What is the hospital maternal mortality rate?
   a. 0.009%
   b. 0.93%
   c. 0.09%
   d. 9.34%

6. What is the newborn mortality rate?
   a. 0.05%
   b. 0.50%
   c. 5.08%
   d. 5.10%

7. What is the fetal mortality rate?
   a. 0.03%
   b. 0.04%
   c. 0.36%
   d. 3.55%

8. What is the mortality rate for the medicine service?
   a. 0.05%
   b. 0.53%
   c. 5.33%
   d. 5.34%

9. What is the mortality rate for the surgery service?
   a. 0.12%
   b. 1.20%
   c. 12.00%
   d. 12.04%

10. What is the cancer mortality rate?
    a. 0.01%
    b. 0.09%
    c. 9.30%
    d. 9.38%

11. Which of the following statistics is also called the institutional mortality rate?
    a. Crude mortality rate
    b. Gross mortality rate
    c. Net mortality rate
    d. Postoperative mortality rate

12. Your hospital reported 287 deaths to cancer patients with 3,821 discharges of patients with a principal diagnosis of cancer. What is the cancer mortality rate?
    a. 0.75%
    b. 7.50%
    c. 7.51%
    d. 75.11%

Use the information in the table that follows to answer questions 13 through 15. In these exercises, the deaths are included in the discharges; this includes deaths occurring in less than 48 hours and postoperative deaths.

Community Hospital Annual Statistics, 20XX				
Service	**Discharges**	**Deaths**	**<48 hours**	**Postop**
Medicine	1,478	92	8	0
Surgery	1,385	25	10	2
Obstetrics	751	1	0	0
Newborn	753	1	1	0
Psychiatric	486	2	0	0
Rehabilitation	362	22	1	0
Total				
Additional Information				
Anesthetics administered		1,386		
Anesthetic deaths		1		
Patients operated on		1,385		
Total live births		753		
Fetal deaths:				
Early		5		
Intermediate		5		
Late		1		

13. What is the gross mortality rate for the rehabilitation service?
    a. 0.67%
    b. 0.68%
    c. 6.07%
    d. 6.08%

14. What is the total hospital net mortality rate?
    a. 0.24%
    b. 2.36%
    c. 2.37%
    d. 2.74%

15. What is the postoperative mortality rate?
    a. 0.14%
    b. 1.44%
    c. 14.10%
    d. 14.44%

7 | Hospital Autopsies and Autopsy Rates

Learning Objectives

At the conclusion of this chapter, you should be able to do the following:

- Identify alternate terms for autopsy
- Recognize a coroner's case and determine when it would be included in a hospital's autopsy rate
- Calculate the following autopsy rates: gross, net, adjusted hospital, newborn, and fetal
- Utilize software to complete spreadsheets

Key Terms

Adjusted hospital autopsy rate	Forensic autopsy	Medico-legal (ML) autopsy
Autopsy	Gross autopsy rate	Morgue
Autopsy rate	Home healthcare	Necropsy
Clinical autopsy	Hospital autopsy	Net autopsy rate
Coroner	Hospital autopsy rate	Newborn autopsy rate
Emergency department (ED)	Hospital inpatient autopsy	Postmortem examination
Fetal autopsy rate	Medical examiner	

An **autopsy** is the postmortem examination of the organs and tissues of a body to determine the cause of death or pathological conditions. The practice of autopsies has contributed to medical science by correlating changes in organs and tissues with the patient's symptoms. The practice of performing autopsies also supports the quality of care provided. An autopsy can be performed on the entire body or a particular body organ.

Another name for autopsy is **necropsy** or **postmortem** (after death) **examination**. Autopsies are classified as clinical or forensic. A **clinical autopsy** is one in which permission is granted by the next of kin and is primarily performed to confirm the cause of death or identify any other diseases that may have contributed to the death. Clinical autopsies are generally performed by either a hospital pathologist or a physician on the medical staff who has been delegated this responsibility. They are usually performed in the hospital **morgue**, but in the case of small hospitals that do not have a morgue, the body may be removed to an off-site lab or a funeral home for the autopsy. A morgue is a place where the bodies of persons who have died are kept until identified and claimed by relatives or released for burial. A **forensic autopsy** or **medico-legal (ML) autopsy** is an autopsy in which a legal representative has ordered an autopsy to be performed. It is performed with the aim of providing answers to questions about the identity, cause of death, time of death, circumstances of death, and the like, thus helping law enforcing agencies to solve a crime. Both examinations are similar, but the forensic autopsy must be carried out to preserve any evidence discovered during the examination (Kotabagi, 2011). Forensic autopsies are typically carried out by a coroner or medical examiner.

A **coroner** is the official (elected or appointed, physician or nonphysician) who is responsible for determining the cause, time, and manner of death in unattended, violent, or unexplained deaths, or in cases in which a law may have been broken. Coroners may also have other duties depending on their state. The **medical examiner** is usually an appointed official who is a physician, commonly holding a specialty in pathology or forensic medicine. Large metropolitan areas usually have a forensic pathologist who acts as the coroner and performs the postmortem examination. In smaller areas, the coroner may be a physician practicing in the community who is not trained as a pathologist.

Autopsy Rates

The rate of autopsy has declined substantially over the years. It is estimated that before 1972 the autopsy rate was 40 to 60 percent, but by 2007 the rate had decreased to 5 percent (Hoyer 2011). Autopsies more likely to occur when the physician is unable to determine the cause of death, such as in the cases of heart disease and cancer, or when there are external causes of the death. Autopsies are generally performed on patients under the age of 25. Disease conditions are usually the cause of death in older patients and are not ordinarily autopsied (Hoyer 2011).

Gross Autopsy Rate

The **autopsy rate** is the proportion of deaths in a healthcare organization that are followed by the performance of an autopsy. The **gross autopsy rate** is the ratio of all inpatient autopsies to all inpatient deaths during any given period. Outpatients are not included in this autopsy statistic. The gross autopsy rate is customarily reported as a percentage. Again, the concept of a rate applies here: the number of times something happened compared with the number of times it could have happened. Statistically speaking, every patient who dies could be autopsied. Typically, newborn autopsies are included in the gross autopsy rate but may be calculated separately as determined by the hospital's administration or medical staff committee.

The formula for calculating the gross autopsy rate is

$$Gross\ Autopsy\ Rate = \frac{Number\ of\ autopsies\ in\ inpatient\ deaths\ for\ a\ period}{Number\ of\ inpatient\ deaths\ for\ a\ period}$$

Example 7.1: During January, University Hospital discharged 1,027 patients. The hospital had 32 deaths (including newborns) and performed 11 autopsies. Calculate the gross autopsy rate. Round to nearest tenth of percent.

$$Gross\ Autopsy\ Rate = \frac{11}{32} = 0.34375$$

Convert the rate to a percentage: $0.3475 \times 100 = 34.375\%$.

Round to the nearest tenth: 34.4%.

Exercise 7.1

1. Calculate the gross autopsy rate based on the following statistics. In a one-month period, a 300-bed hospital with 20 bassinets reported 18 inpatient deaths. The medical staff performed 6 autopsies. Report the rate as a percentage rounded to the nearest tenth.

2. In January, Community Hospital had 185 discharges, 9 deaths, and 2 autopsies. What is the gross autopsy rate? Report the rate as a percentage rounded to the nearest tenth.

3. During the last semiannual period, University Hospital had 6,234 discharges, 18 deaths, and 15 autopsies. What is their gross autopsy rate? Report the rate as a percentage rounded to the nearest tenth.

Exercise 7.2

Use the information in the table that follows to calculate the gross mortality rate, the net mortality rate, and the gross autopsy rate for Community Hospital for the time period. Round to nearest tenth of percent.

Community Hospital Hospital Statistics July–December 20XX	
Total inpatient discharges (including deaths)	724
Total inpatient deaths	19
<48 hours—included in total inpatient deaths	3
Total autopsies	6

Net Autopsy Rate

The **net autopsy rate** is the ratio of the total number of inpatient autopsies performed by the hospital pathologist for a given time period to the total number of inpatient deaths minus not autopsied coroners' or medical examiners' cases for the same time period. The formula for net autopsy rate differs slightly from the formula for gross autopsy rate in that it excludes bodies that have been removed by the coroner for a forensic autopsy. Because the body has been removed from the hospital, it is not available for autopsy and therefore not considered in this rate.

The formula for calculating the net autopsy rate is:

$$Net\ Autopsy\ Rate = \frac{Total\ autopsies\ on\ inpatient\ deaths\ for\ a\ period}{[Total\ inpatient\ deaths\ for\ a\ period] - [Cases\ removed\ by\ coroner\ or\ medical\ examiner]}$$

Example 7.2: During April, Community Hospital had 14 patient deaths and performed 3 autopsies. One body was released to the county coroner for autopsy. Calculate both the gross and net autopsy rates. Round to nearest hundredth of percent

$$Gross\ Autopsy\ Rate = \frac{3}{14} = 0.21428$$

Convert to a percentage: 0.2142 × 100 = 21.428%.
Round to the nearest hundredth: 21.43%.

$$Net\ Autopsy\ Rate = \frac{3}{(14-1)} = 0.23076$$

Convert to a percentage: 0.23076 × 100 = 23.076%.
Round to the nearest hundredth: 23.08%.

The net autopsy rate will always be greater than or equal to the gross autopsy rate.

QUICK TIP

Exercise 7.3

During the past year, University Hospital had 18,251 discharges (including deaths), 267 inpatient deaths, and 170 autopsies. The bodies of 20 patients were released to the medical examiner for autopsy. Calculate the gross mortality, gross autopsy, and net autopsy rates for University Hospital. Round to nearest hundredth of a percent.

Exercise 7.4

Use the information in the table that follows to calculate the gross mortality, gross autopsy, and net autopsy rates for University Hospital. In this exercise, the deaths are included in the discharges. Round to the nearest hundredth of a percent.

Community Hospital Quarterly Statistics April–June 20XX	
Discharges (including deaths):	
Adults and children	1,080
Newborn	270
Deaths:	
Adults and children	33
Newborn	2
Inpatient autopsies	12
Coroner's cases (unavailable for autopsy)	3

Exercise 7.5

Use the information in the table that follows. Create an Excel spreadsheet to calculate the gross mortality, gross autopsy, and net autopsy rates for each month and the year for University Hospital. In this exercise, the deaths are included in the discharges. Round to the nearest hundredth of a percent.

University Hospital Annual Statistics 20XX							
Month	Discharges	Inpatient Deaths	Autopsies	Coroner's Cases	Gross Mortality Rate	Gross Autopsy Rate	Net Autopsy Rate
January	598	5	2	1			
February	587	6	2	2			
March	607	7	5	1			
April	624	5	1	0			
May	620	6	2	1			
June	599	7	3	2			
July	609	9	5	2			
August	575	5	2	0			
September	611	7	3	1			
October	578	8	4	1			
November	622	6	2	0			
December	572	7	2	2			
Total							

Hospital Autopsies

A **hospital inpatient autopsy** is a postmortem (after-death) examination performed on the body of a patient who died during an inpatient hospitalization by a hospital pathologist or a physician of the medical staff who has been delegated the responsibility. In contrast, a **hospital autopsy** is the examination performed on the body of a person who has at some time been a hospital patient by a hospital pathologist or a physician of the medical staff who has been delegated the responsibility. Former inpatients may include emergency department (ED) patients, outpatients, and home healthcare patients. The **hospital autopsy rate** is calculated as the total number of autopsies performed by a hospital pathologist for a given time period divided by the number of deaths of hospital patients (inpatients and outpatients) whose bodies were available for autopsy for the same time period

Normally, hospital autopsies are performed in hospitals. However, a small hospital or a specialty hospital (for example, obstetrical or psychiatric) may not have many deaths and thus may not be equipped with the necessary facilities to perform autopsies. In such cases, the autopsies are performed in another designated place. Hospital autopsies are typically only performed on inpatients who have died during their hospitalization. However, because of the educational value of autopsies, former inpatients who were not in the hospital at the time of death may be considered for hospital autopsies. These individuals may include **emergency department** (ED) patients, outpatients, and **home healthcare** or hospice deaths. ED patients are those who are admitted to the emergency department of a hospital for the diagnosis and treatment of a condition that requires immediate medical, dental, or allied health services in order to sustain life or to prevent critical consequences. Outpatients are those who receive ambulatory care services in a hospital-based clinic or department. Home healthcare patients are those who receive care within their own home provided by a home health agency. **Hospice patients** are those who are receiving an interdisciplinary program of palliative care and supportive services that addresses the physical, spiritual, social, and economic needs of terminally ill patients and their families. Fetal autopsies are not included in the hospital autopsy rate because a fetus is not considered a patient.

The essential components for a hospital autopsy are the following:

1. The autopsy must be performed by a staff pathologist or a designated physician.

2. There must be a consent from the patient's next of kin or legal representative to perform an autopsy, which is filed in the patient's health record.

3. The consent may be for a full body autopsy or a partial autopsy.

4. The autopsy report must be filed in the patient's health record. The tissue specimens must be filed in the hospital laboratory along with the autopsy report.

Examples of hospital autopsy cases include the following:

*   A patient dies in the hospital and is autopsied by the hospital's pathologist in the local morgue.

*   A patient dies in the hospital, and one of the hospital's physicians is designated to perform the autopsy in the absence of the staff pathologist.

*   A former patient is pronounced dead on arrival in the hospital's ED, and the staff pathologist performs the autopsy.

Adjusted Hospital Autopsy Rate

The **adjusted hospital autopsy rate** is the proportion of hospital autopsies performed following the deaths of patients whose bodies are available for autopsy. Although many hospitals calculate the net autopsy rate for various surveys and external reports, the adjusted hospital autopsy rate is a more accurate indication of the hospital's resources for physician education because it includes all autopsies.

The formula for calculating the adjusted hospital autopsy rate is:

$$Adjusted\ Hospital\ Autopsy\ Rate = \frac{Number\ of\ hospital\ autopsies}{Number\ of\ bodies\ that\ are\ available\ for\ autopsy}$$

Patients whose bodies are available for hospital autopsy are deceased patients who have, at some point, been a hospital patient. These patients include the following:

- Inpatient deaths when the bodies are not removed from the hospital by legal authorities such as the coroner or medical examiner.
- Other patients, including home healthcare patients, outpatients, and previous hospital patients who have died elsewhere and whose bodies have been made available for the performance of a hospital autopsy.

Example 7.3: Community Hospital had 260 discharges in June; 7 were deaths. The hospital pathologist performed 3 of the autopsies. During this period, 2 home healthcare patients and 1 outpatient died and were brought to the hospital for autopsy. Calculate the adjusted hospital autopsy rate. Express the rate as a percentage rounded to the nearest tenth.

To determine the adjusted hospital autopsy rate, add all the hospital autopsies performed to determine the numerator (3 inpatients + 2 home healthcare patients + 1 outpatient). The denominator contains all the patients whose bodies were available for autopsy. This includes the 7 inpatients, 2 home healthcare patients, and 1 outpatient who died in June (7 + 2 + 1).

$$Adjusted\ Hospital\ Autopsy\ Rate = \frac{(3+2+1)}{(7+2+1)} = \frac{6}{10} = 0.600$$

Convert to a percentage: 0.600 × 100 = 60.00%.

Round to the nearest tenth: 60.0%.

 In the previous formulas, outpatients, ED patients, and home healthcare patients were not included with the inpatients. When calculating the adjusted hospital autopsy rate, the outpatients, ED patients, and home healthcare patients would be included if their bodies were autopsied by the hospital pathologist.

Exercise 7.6

During the past quarter, Community Hospital had 22 inpatient deaths, 7 of whom were autopsied. Two of the 22 deaths were coroners' cases, but 1 was autopsied by the hospital pathologist (included in the 7). In addition, the following bodies were brought to the hospital for autopsy: 2 former patients who died in the ER, 1 former inpatient who died in a skilled nursing facility, 2 former inpatients who died at home, and 1 patient who died during a round of outpatient chemotherapy. What is the adjusted hospital autopsy rate? Express the rate as a percentage rounded to the nearest hundredth.

Exercise 7.7

Which of the following represents a hospital autopsy? Select all that apply:

a. A former inpatient died at home a month after discharge from the hospital, and his body was brought to the hospital for autopsy.

b. The coroner authorized the hospital pathologist to perform an autopsy on a patient who died in the ED after a car accident.

c. A patient who had been receiving radiation therapy on an outpatient basis at the hospital died at home; her body was brought to the hospital for autopsy.

d. A victim of gunshot wounds who died in the ED was autopsied by the medical examiner.

e. A cardiac patient died in the ED, and the hospital pathologist performed the autopsy.

f. The hospital pathologist designated a physician to cover for her while she was away. The physician performed an autopsy on a deceased hospital inpatient.

g. A late fetal death (stillbirth) was autopsied by the hospital pathologist.

Exercise 7.8

Use the information in the table that follows to calculate the gross mortality, gross autopsy, net autopsy, and adjusted hospital autopsy rates for University Hospital. In this exercise, the deaths are included in the discharges. Round to the nearest hundredth of a percent.

University Hospital Annual Statistics 20XX	
Discharges and (including deaths):	
Adults and children	14,892
Newborn	5,223
Deaths:	
Adults and children	362
Newborn	4
Deaths in the ED and OPD*	12
Autopsies:	
Inpatient	97
ED/OPD	12
Coroner's cases (unavailable for autopsy)	6

*ED = Emergency department; OPD = Outpatient department

Exercise 7.9

Use the information in the table that follows to calculate the adjusted hospital autopsy rate. Round to the nearest hundredth of a percent.

Community Hospital September 20XX Statistics	
Deaths	
Inpatient deaths	12
ED deaths	2
Home health death	1

(continued on next page)

Community Hospital September 20XX Statistics	
Autopsies	
Inpatient autopsies	3
ED autopsies	2
Home health autopsy	1
Coroner's case (unavailable for autopsy)	2

Exercise 7.10

During the first quarter of 20XX, Community Hospital had 24 inpatient deaths, 6 of whom were autopsied. Of the 24 deaths, 2 were coroners' cases—1 of whom was autopsied by the hospital pathologist (included in the 6 autopsies) and 1 was removed to be autopsied by the coroner. Additionally, these patients were also autopsied: 1 patient who died in the hospital's skilled nursing facility two days after discharge from the hospital, a patient who died in the ED after a motor vehicle accident, 1 outpatient who died in the physical therapy department after a fall, and a former patient who died at home while under the care of the hospital's hospice department. Calculate the adjusted hospital autopsy rate for Community Hospital for this quarter. Round to two decimal places.

Newborn Autopsy Rate

The **newborn autopsy rate** is number of autopsies performed on newborns who died during a given time period divided by the total number of newborns who died during the same time period. This is analogous to the formula used to calculate the hospital autopsy rate but limited to newborns only.

The formula for calculating the newborn autopsy rate is:

$$Newborn\ Autopsy\ Rate = \frac{Newborn\ autopsies\ for\ the\ period}{Total\ newborn\ deaths\ for\ the\ period}$$

Example 7.4: Community Hospital had 33 births during the month of June with 2 newborn deaths. One of the newborns died shortly after birth and was autopsied. Calculate the newborn autopsy rate. Round to the nearest tenth of a percent.

$$Newborn\ Autopsy\ Rate = \frac{1}{2} = 0.50,$$

Convert to a percentage : 50.0%

Example 7.5: Use the information in the table that follows to calculate the newborn mortality rate and the newborn autopsy rate for Community Hospital. In this exercise, the deaths are included in the discharges. Round to two decimal places.

Community Hospital Newborn Statistics January–June 20XX	
Births	210
Discharges and Deaths	208
Deaths	4
Autopsies	3

$$Newborn\ Mortality\ Rate = \frac{4}{208} = 0.01923$$

Convert to a percentage: $0.01923 \times 100 = 1.923\%$.

Round to two decimal places: 1.92%.

$$Newborn\ Autopsy\ Rate = \frac{3}{4} = 0.75000$$

Convert to a percentage: $0.75000 \times 100 = 75.000\%$.

Round to two decimal places: 75.00%.

Exercise 7.11

In November 20XX, the newborn unit at Community Hospital reported three stillbirths and two newborn deaths. Autopsies were performed on one of the newborns and two stillbirths. Calculate the newborn autopsy rate for November. Round to one decimal place.

Exercise 7.12

University Hospital reported the following semiannual statistics for January through June 20XX: 966 newborn discharges, and 5 of these were newborn deaths. There were 2 newborn autopsies. One newborn was born in a taxi on the way to the hospital, was admitted, and later died. It was autopsied. One newborn was born at home and brought to the hospital and admitted. It also died and was autopsied. Calculate University Hospital's newborn mortality rate and newborn autopsy rate. In this exercise, the deaths are included in the discharges. Round to two decimal places.

Fetal Autopsy Rate

The **fetal autopsy rate** is the proportion of hospital autopsies performed following the deaths of intermediate and late fetal deaths.

The formula for the fetal autopsy rate is:

$$Fetal\ Autopsy\ Rate = \frac{Autopsies\ performed\ on\ intermediate\ and\ late\ fetal\ deaths\ for\ the\ period}{Total\ intermediate\ and\ late\ fetal\ deaths\ for\ the\ period}$$

Example 7.6: University Hospital's newborn service reported 10 fetal deaths last quarter: 2 early, 6 intermediate, and 2 late. Of these, the 2 late fetal deaths and 1 intermediate fetal death were autopsied. Apply the formula above to calculate the fetal autopsy rate. Round to a tenth of a percent.

Number of intermediate and late fetal deaths = 6 intermediate + 2 late = 8

Number of autopsies performed on intermediate and late fetal deaths = 1 intermediate + 2 late = 3

$$Fetal\ Autopsy\ Rate = \frac{3}{8} = 0.375$$

Convert to a percentage: $0.375 \times 100 = 37.5\%$.

Round to a tenth of a percent: 37.5%.

Exercise 7.13

Use the information in the table that follows to calculate the newborn mortality, fetal mortality, newborn autopsy, and fetal autopsy rates for the newborn service at University Hospital. In this exercise, the newborn deaths are included in the newborn discharges. Round to two decimal places.

University Hospital Newborn Service Statistics July–December 20XX	
Births	687
Discharges and deaths	686
Newborn deaths	3
Newborn autopsies	2
Fetal deaths:	
Early	4
Intermediate	7
Late	3
Fetal death autopsies:	
Early	10
Intermediate	1
Late	2

Exercise 7.14

Community Healthcare System reported the statistics in the table that follows for its four facilities during its past semiannual period. Use an Excel spreadsheet to calculate the newborn mortality, fetal mortality, newborn autopsy, and fetal autopsy rates for each facility and for the system as a whole. In this exercise, the deaths are included in the discharges. Round to two decimal places.

Community Healthcare System Newborn Statistics January–June 20XX				
	Urban Hospital	Suburban Hospital	Rural Hospital	Specialty Hospital
Live births	252	247	176	201
Newborn discharges and deaths	250	245	173	200
Newborn deaths	2	2	2	12
Fetal deaths:				
Early	3	1	1	7
Intermediate	4	4	2	8
Late	3	1	1	3
Autopsies:				
Newborn	1	1	1	8
Fetal (late and intermediate)	2	1	2	8

Chapter 7 Formulae for Autopsy Rate Statistics

Rate	Numerator	Denominator
Gross autopsy rate	Total number of autopsies on inpatient deaths for a given period	Total number of inpatient deaths for the same period
Net autopsy rate	Total number of autopsies on inpatient deaths for a given period	Total number of inpatient deaths minus autopsied coroner or medical examiner cases for the same period
Adjusted hospital autopsy rate	Total number of hospital autopsies including ED, OP and home healthcare patients for a given period	Total number of deaths of hospital patients whose bodies are available for autopsy
NB autopsy rate	Total number of autopsies on newborn deaths for a given period	Total number of newborn deaths for the same period
Fetal autopsy rate	Total number of autopsies on intermediate and late fetal deaths for a given period	Total number of intermediate and late fetal deaths for the same period

Chapter 7   Matching Quiz

Match the definitions with the terms.

Definitions:

a. The place where the bodies of persons who have died are kept until identified and claimed by relatives or released for burial

b. The postmortem examination of the organs and tissues of a body to determine the cause of death or pathological conditions

c. A public officer whose principal duty is to inquire via an inquest into the cause of any death that there is reason to suppose is not due to natural causes

d. The total number of autopsies (inpatient and outpatients) performed by a hospital pathologist for a given time period divided by the number of deaths of hospital patients (inpatients and outpatients) whose bodies were available for autopsy for the same time period

e. The number of autopsies performed on newborns who died during a given period of time divided by the total number of newborns who died during the same period

f. A situation in which the required conditions have been met to allow an autopsy to be performed on a hospital patient who has died

g. A postmortem examination performed on the body of a patient who died during an inpatient hospitalization by a hospital pathologist or a physician of the medical staff who has been delegated the responsibility

h. The number of inpatient autopsies conducted during a given time period divided by the total number of inpatient deaths for the same time period

i. The proportion of hospital autopsies performed following the deaths of patients whose bodies are available for autopsy

j. The total number of autopsies on inpatient deaths for a given period divided by the total inpatient deaths minus the not autopsied coroners' or medical examiners' cases

Terms:

1. _____ Autopsy
2. _____ Hospital autopsy rate
3. _____ Morgue
4. _____ Newborn autopsy rate
5. _____ Medical examiner

6. _____ Hospital inpatient autopsy
7. _____ Adjusted hospital autopsy rate
8. _____ Gross autopsy rate
9. _____ Net autopsy rate
10. _____ Available for hospital autopsy

Chapter 7 Review

Use the statistics reported by Community Hospital in the table that follows to calculate the rates for questions 1 through 5. Calculate all rates to two decimal places.

Community Hospital Annual Statistics 20XX	
Inpatient discharges (including deaths):	
Adults and children	8,234
Newborn	820
Inpatient deaths (included in discharges):	
Adults and children	54
Newborn	3
Fetal deaths:	
Early	4
Intermediate	5
Late	3
Inpatient autopsies:	
Adults and children	12
Newborn	2
Coroner's cases:	
Unavailable for autopsy	4
Autopsy by hospital pathologist (included in inpatient autopsies)	1
Fetal death autopsies:	
Intermediate and late	4
Former hospital patient brought in for autopsy	2

1. What is the gross autopsy rate?
   a. 24.00%
   b. 24.56%
   c. 0.24%
   d. 2.45%

2. What is the net autopsy rate?
   a. 0.26%
   b. 2.64%
   c. 26.41%
   d. 26.42 %

3. What is the adjusted hospital autopsy rate?
   a. 29.90%
   b. 2.90%
   c. 29.09%
   d. 0.29%

4. What is the newborn autopsy rate?
   a. 0.66%
   b. 0.67%
   c. 6.67%
   d. 66.67%

5. What is the fetal autopsy rate?
   a. 0.50%
   b. 5.00%
   c. 50.00%
   d. 0.050%

Use the information reported by University Hospital for September 20XX in the table that follows to calculate the rates for questions 6 through 12. Round to two decimal places.

University Hospital September 20XX Statistics	
Discharges (including deaths):	
Total adults and children	1,432
Newborn	123
Total live births	120
Deaths (included in discharges):	
Adults and children	87
Newborn	3
Autopsies:	
Adults and children	23
Newborn	2
Hospital autopsied outpatients	7
Coroner's cases (unavailable for autopsy)	3

(*continued on next page*)

University Hospital September 20XX Statistics	
Fetal deaths:	
Early	0
Intermediate	5
Late	2
Fetal death autopsies:	
Intermediate and late	4

6. What is the gross mortality rate?
    a. 0.05%
    b. 0.57%
    c. 5.79%
    d. 57.87%

7. What is the gross autopsy rate?
    a. 0.27%
    b. 27.77%
    c. 27.78%
    d. 2.78%

8. What is the net autopsy rate?
    a. 0.28%
    b. 2.87%
    c. 2.88%
    d. 28.74%

9. What is the adjusted hospital autopsy rate?
    a. 34.04%
    b. 0.34%
    c. 3.40%
    d. 3.04%

10. What is the newborn autopsy rate?
    a. 0.66%
    b. 0.67%
    c. 6.67%
    d. 66.67%

11. What is the fetal mortality rate?
    a. 0.55%
    b. 5.51%
    c. 55.10%
    d. 0.06%

12. What is the fetal autopsy rate?
    a. 0.05%
    b. 0.57%
    c. 5.71%
    d. 57.14%

13. What is the principal difference between net autopsy rate and adjusted hospital autopsy rate?
    a. The net autopsy rate considers only inpatient deaths.
    b. Hospital autopsy rates include only those deaths in which the bodies are available for autopsy.
    c. Fetal deaths are not counted in hospital autopsy rates.
    d. Legal cases sometimes are excluded from deaths when computing net autopsy rates.

14. In which of the following rates are outpatients who were autopsied counted in an autopsy rate?
    a. Gross autopsy rate
    b. Net autopsy rate
    c. Adjusted hospital autopsy rate
    d. Newborn autopsy rate

15. Hospital autopsies include which of the following?
    a. Inpatients only
    b. Inpatients and outpatients who die in the hospital
    c. Inpatients, outpatients, and home healthcare patients
    d. Inpatients and any other patient who has at some time been a hospital patient

CHAPTER 8

Morbidity and Other Miscellaneous Rates

Learning Objectives

At the conclusion of this chapter, you should be able to do the following:

- Summarize calculations based on morbidity, mortality, infection, postoperative infection, complication, consultation, readmission
- Explain the difference between a surgical operation and surgical procedure
- Identify the attributes that constitute a clean surgery case

Key Terms

Cesarean section (C-section)
Cesarean section rate
Chronic
Clean surgical case
Complication
Complication rate
Concomitant

Consultation
Consultation rate
Delivery
Hospital-acquired infection (HAI)
Iatrogenic
Infection rate
Morbidity

Nosocomial infection
Nosocomial or hospital-acquired infection rate
Postoperative infection rate
Surgical site infection (SSI)
Surgical site infection (SSI) rate

Health statistics and data are important to facilities because they measure a variety of indicators. Data collected can provide comparisons with other facilities or information for improved quality of care. Data can help administrators see where additional services are needed and help them plan.

Morbidity Rates

The term **morbidity** refers to the state of being diseased or the number of sick persons including illness, injury, or deviation from normal health. Morbidity may be infectious or have other causes. For example, the presence of **concomitant** (taking place at the same time) or **chronic** (of long duration) conditions may constitute comorbidity. Moreover, morbidity may be pre-existing (arising prior to admission to the hospital) or **iatrogenic** (induced inadvertently by a physician or surgeon or by medical treatment or diagnostic procedures).

Infection Rate

Preventing morbidity due to infection is an important clinical and quality management function. Frequently, the healthcare facility establishes a committee whose primary function is to evaluate infections and determine their causes so that recurrence can be avoided. Typically called the infection control committee, or infection prevention committee, it is composed of representatives from medical staff, nursing, pharmacy, laboratory, housekeeping, and health information management (HIM). Charged with the duty of infection prevention, committee members establish procedures for the management and reporting of infections. Effective management of infections acquired in the hospital or **nosocomial infections** more commonly referred to as **hospital-acquired infections (HAIs)**, sometimes requires finding cases beyond the infections documented by physicians in the health record. The HIM practitioner can help identify such cases in the course of performing qualitative analysis and coding of health records.

In 1970, the Centers for Disease Control and Prevention (CDC) developed a voluntary reporting system, the National Nosocomial Infections Surveillance (NNIS) System, to monitor the incidence of HAIs. In 2008, the CDC's Division of Healthcare Quality Promotion developed the National Healthcare Safety Network (NHSN), which includes the previous work of the NNIS. "The NHSN is a secure, internet-based surveillance system that integrates former CDC surveillance systems, including the National Nosocomial Infections Surveillance System (NNIS), National Surveillance System for Healthcare Workers (NaSH), and the Dialysis Surveillance Network (DSN). It is the nation's most widely used healthcare-associated infection tracking system. NHSN allows healthcare facilities to track blood safety errors and important healthcare process measures such as healthcare personnel influenza status" (CDC 2019a).

As defined in chapter 2, *Mathematics Review,* the term *rate* refers to the number of times something happened (part) compared with the number of times it could have happened (base).

$$Rate = \frac{Part}{Base} = \frac{P}{B}$$

Each healthcare facility's medical staff must determine the criteria for inclusion of a patient in both the numerator (infection) and denominator (patients at risk of infection). The inclusion and exclusion criteria for rates that are reported to external entities such as the NHSN or Centers for Medicare and Medicaid Services (CMS) are defined at the national level to ensure comparability across facilities.

Most healthcare facilities differentiate between nosocomial infections or HAIs as well as exacerbation or recurrence of previous infections. For example, if an obstetrical patient develops a urinary tract infection, a physician must determine whether it was hospital-acquired or due to a recurrence of a previous urinary tract infection. Most infection prevention departments are interested in determining whether nosocomial infections are attributable to specific patient care units, specific operations, patients with specified diseases, the organized medical staff units, or individual physicians or hospital employees so that appropriate actions may be taken to reduce the risk of further infections.

The nosocomial or hospital-acquired infection rate is the number of HAIs in the hospital for a given time period divided by the total number of inpatient discharges (including deaths) for the same time period.

The formula for calculating the nosocomial infection rate is:

$$HAI\ Rate = \frac{Number\ of\ HAIs\ for\ the\ period}{Number\ of\ discharges,\ including\ deaths,\ for\ the\ period}$$

Example 8.1: In February, Community Hospital had 289 discharges and deaths. Twelve of these patients had HAIs. Calculate the nosocomial infection rate. Round to two decimal places.

$$HAI\ Rate = \frac{12}{289} = 0.04152$$

Convert to a percentage: $0.04152 \times 100 = 4.152\%$

Round to two decimal places: 4.15%

Infection rates may be calculated separately for specific source or location of infection, such as surgical wound infections, puerperal infections (infections that occur immediately after childbirth), and infections of the respiratory tract, urinary tract, bloodstream, and so on.

The general formula for calculating the **infection rate** at a facility is:

$$Infection\ Rate = \frac{Number\ of\ infections\ for\ the\ period}{Number\ of\ discharges,\ including\ deaths,\ for\ the\ period}$$

Example 8.2: In May, Community Hospital had 360 discharges, 4 of whom developed sepsis while in the hospital. Calculate the sepsis infection rate for the facility. Round to two decimal places.

$$Infection\ Rate = \frac{4}{360} = 0.0111$$

Convert to a percentage: $0.0111 \times 100 = 1.111\%$

Round to two decimal places: 1.11%

Exercise 8.1

Use the information in the table that follows to calculate the rates requested for Community Hospital. In this exercise, deaths are included in the discharges. Round to two decimal places.

Community Hospital Annual Statistics 20XX	
Discharges and deaths:	
Adults and children	2,190
Newborn	127
Deaths:	
Adults and children	13
Newborn	1
Nosocomial or hospital-acquired infections:	
Adults and children	18
Newborn	2

Exercise 8.2

Use the information in the table that follows, create an Excel spreadsheet to calculate the gross mortality and HAI rates for each service and in total. In this exercise, the deaths are included in the discharges. Round to two decimal places.

University Hospital Semiannual Statistics July–December 20XX			
Service	No. of Discharges (Includes Deaths)	No. of Deaths	No. of Nosocomial Infections
Medicine	2,469	201	52
Surgery	2,890	144	56
Obstetrics	785	2	6
Psychiatry	786	1	4

(*continued on next page*)

University Hospital Semiannual Statistics July–December 20XX			
Service	No. of Discharges (Includes Deaths)	No. of Deaths	No. of Nosocomial Infections
Rehabilitation	847	18	27
Pediatrics	945	3	3
Newborn	791	1	1
Total			

Postoperative Infection Rate

Another specific type of infection of great concern to hospitals is the **postoperative infection rate** or **surgical site infection (SSI) rate.** This is because a postoperative infection can contribute to the increased morbidity, mortality, and cost of care.

 The term SSI is used more often in practice at this time, but the term postoperative infection rate is included in this discussion since both may still be encountered in the field.

Postoperative infections or SSIs occur after surgery. The CDC estimates that SSIs account for 31 percent of all HAIs (CDC 2019b). Even though hospitals take care to avoid an infection after surgery, one still can occur.

Two terms previously defined in chapter 6, *Mortality Rates,* are revisited here since they are crucial in understanding the calculation of post-operative infection rates: need to be considered here:

- A **surgical procedure** is defined as any single, separate, systematic process upon or within the body that can be complete in itself; normally is performed by a physician, dentist, or other licensed practitioner; can be performed with or without instruments; and is performed to restore disunited or deficient parts, remove diseased or injured tissues, extract foreign matter, assist in obstetrical delivery, or aid in diagnosis (AHIMA 2017).

- A **surgical operation** is defined as one or more surgical procedures performed at one time for one patient via a common approach or for a common purpose (AHIMA 2017).
    - An example of a surgical operation including more than one surgical procedure is an abdominoperineal resection, which involves resection of both the abdomen and the peritoneum.
    - An example of two surgical operations and two surgical procedures is a tonsillectomy followed by a cholecystectomy. Even though the procedures were performed at one time for one patient, the approach to each procedure is different and the two procedures are not performed for a common purpose.

The CDC classifies wounds into four classes: clean, clean-contaminated, contaminated and dirty or infected (CDC 2019b). These are developed according to the likelihood and degree of wound contamination at the time of the operation.

A clean wound is one in which no inflammation is encountered and the respiratory, alimentary, genital, or uninfected urinary tracts are not entered. Many infection prevention departments report the number of postoperative infections relative to the type of surgery that was performed. For example, if a patient has no infection prior to a coronary artery bypass graft but develops one after surgery, then the infection prevention department would report this as a postoperative infection in a clean case.

A clean-contaminated case is one in which the respiratory, alimentary, genital, or urinary tract is entered. Specifically, operations involving the biliary tract, appendix, vagina, and oropharynx are included in this category. For instance, a patient who develops an infection after an abdominal hysterectomy would be reported as an infection in a clean-contaminated case.

A contaminated wound includes an open, fresh, accidental wound; an operation with a break in sterile technique or gross spillage from the gastrointestinal tract; and incisions in which acute, nonpurulent inflammation is encountered.

A dirty wound is one that involves old traumatic wounds or devitalized tissue, an existing clinical infection, or perforated viscera. Organisms were present before the procedure (CDC 2019b).

If you are assisting the infection prevention department with their statistics, be sure to determine how they are classifying postoperative infections.

The postoperative infection or SSI rate is the ratio of all infections in clean surgical cases to the number of surgical operations performed. A general definition of a **clean surgical case** is one in which no infection existed prior to surgery.

The formula for calculating the SSI rate is:

$$SSI\ Rate = \frac{Number\ of\ infections\ in\ clean\ surgical\ cases\ for\ period}{Number\ of\ surgical\ operations\ for\ period}$$

Example 8.3: During May, a hospital reported that 578 surgical operations were performed. The infection prevention committee reported three postoperative infections in clean surgical cases. Calculate the SSI rate for May. Round to two decimals.

$$SSI\ Rate = \frac{3}{578} = 0.00519$$

Convert to a percentage: $0.00519 \times 100 = 0.0519\%$

Round to two decimals: 0.52%

A postoperative infection may be difficult to determine because it is not always evident whether the patient entered the hospital with an infection or acquired one because of the surgical techniques used. Therefore, the medical staff should provide guidance to the HIM practitioner and the infection prevention department on what constitutes a clean surgical case and which infections should be considered postoperative infections.

Exercise 8.3

Use the information in the table that follows to calculate the postoperative infection and postoperative mortality rates for University Hospital during this semiannual period. Round to two decimal places.

University Hospital Surgery Service July–December 20XX	
Number of surgical operations	2,176
Number of patients operated on	2,170
Number of postoperative infections	14
Number of postoperative deaths	8

Exercise 8.4

Use the information in the table that follows, create an Excel spreadsheet to calculate the rates requested below. Round to two decimal places.

Community Hospital Semiannual Report January–June 20XX							
		Deaths		Infections		No. of Patients	No. of Surgical
Month	Live Discharges	Postop	Other	Postop	Nosocomial	Operated On	Operations
Jan	540	2	10	2	4	478	479
Feb	660	3	12	3	5	642	648
Mar	680	3	8	1	4	660	663

(*continued on next page*)

		Deaths		Infections		No. of Patients	No. of Surgical
Community Hospital **Semiannual Report** **January–June 20XX**							
Month	Live Discharges	Postop	Other	Postop	Nosocomial	Operated On	Operations
Apr	669	2	12	4	3	650	653
May	701	5	15	4	2	690	690
Jun	693	3	11	5	3	685	685
Total							

Calculate the following rates.

1. The month with the lowest SSI rate:

2. The SSI rate for the semiannual period:

3. The month with the highest postoperative mortality rate:

4. The postoperative mortality rate for the semiannual period:

5. The gross mortality rate for the surgical service during the semiannual period:

Exercise 8.5

Use the information in the table that follows to calculate the infection rates requested. In this exercise, the deaths are included in the discharges. Round to two decimal places.

Type of Infection	No. of Infections	Infection Rate
Community Hospital **Infection Prevention Committee Report on Infections** **January–March 20XX** **389 discharges**		
Central line-associated bloodstream infections	8	
Catheter-associated urinary tract infections	12	
Ventilator-associated pneumonia	4	
Surgical-site infections	6	
Cardiovascular system infections	2	
Gastrointestinal tract infections	3	
Skin and soft-tissue infections	1	

(continued on next page)

Community Hospital Infection Prevention Committee Report on Infections January–March 20XX 389 discharges		
Type of Infection	**No. of Infections**	**Infection Rate**
Ears, nose, and throat infections	9	
Central nervous system infections	7	
Systemic infections	5	

Complication Rate

In addition to infections, healthcare facilities are concerned with any other type of complication that results from or occurs during the course of care. A **complication** is a medical condition that arises during an inpatient hospitalization. According to the CMS, a complication is a condition that occurs during the patient's hospital stay that extends the length of stay by at least one day in 75 percent of cases (Casto 2018, 117).

Complications may be the result of the patient's disease process, social condition (for example, homeless) or related to the quality of care received by patients. The purpose of collecting a **complication rate** is to determine if changes in the treatment or practice in the facility can prevent them from occurring again.

Examples of complications include blood transfusion reactions, injuries sustained during cardiopulmonary resuscitation, reactions to medications given, vaccination reactions, and patient falls out of bed, just to name a few. Infections, of course, can be complications, but they are generally calculated separately. Any of these examples would change the way the patient was treated from the original reason for hospitalization.

Many facilities calculate these rates at usual intervals: monthly, quarterly, semiannually, or annually.

The general formula for calculating the complication rate is

$$Complication\ Rate = \frac{Number\ of\ patients\ with\ complications\ for\ period}{Number\ of\ discharges\ for\ period}$$

Example 8.4: From July through December, Community Hospital had 32 patients with complications and 2,394 discharges. Calculate the complication rate. Round to two decimals.

$$Complication\ Rate = \frac{32}{2,394} = 0.01336$$

Convert to a percentage: 0.01336 = 1.336%

Round to two decimals: 1.34%

Complication rates are typically calculated for specific types of complications. This is done so that interventions may be determined to prevent complications of that type. When calculating event-specific complication rates, recall that the rate is the number of events divided by the number of times the event could have occurred (part or base).

Example 8.5: In July, Community Hospital had 18 patients who had a blood transfusion. Of those, 2 developed an adverse reaction to the transfusion. Calculate the blood transfusion reaction rate. Round to two decimals.

In this example, the "part" is the number of patients with adverse blood reactions (2) and the base is the number of patients who had blood transfusions (18).

$$Blood\ Transfusion\ Reaction\ Rate = \frac{2}{18} = 0.11111$$

Convert to a percentage: 0.1111 × 100 = 11.111%

Round to two decimals: 11.11%

Exercise 8.6

Use the information for University Hospital in the table that follows, create an Excel spreadsheet to calculate the complication rate for each service and the total for this quarterly period. Round to two decimal places.

University Hospital Statistics January–March 20XX			
Service	Discharges and Deaths	Complications	Complication Rate
Medicine	2,742	197	
Surgery	2,075	208	
Obstetrics	492	7	
Newborn	490	3	
Total			

Exercise 8.7

Use the information in the table that follows, create an Excel spreadsheet to calculate the complication rates by physician and the total for this semiannual period for Community Hospital. Round to two decimal places.

Community Hospital Complication Rate by Physician January–June 20XX			
Physician No.	No. Discharges and Deaths	No. Complications	Complication Rate
102	298	2	
237	247	4	
391	110	3	
518	144	2	
637	206	3	
802	82	1	
900	100	3	
Total			

Cesarean Section Rate

Most hospitals determine the percentage of deliveries that are performed by cesarean section (commonly called C-section) as compared with spontaneous vaginal deliveries. A **cesarean section** is a surgical operation for delivering a child by cutting through the wall of the mother's abdomen. Hospitals determine the **cesarean section rate**, which is the ratio of all C-sections to the total number of deliveries, including C-sections, during a specified period of time. Much attention has been given to high C-section rates by specific physicians, hospitals, and areas of the country because of concerns about adverse effects to the mother and child. It may be necessary to report C-section rates to accrediting agencies or the American Medical Association (AMA) for such reasons as residency programs.

A **delivery** is defined as the process of delivering a liveborn infant or dead fetus (and placenta) by manual, instrumental, or surgical means.

 A pregnant mother who delivers has one delivery but may have multiple births. For example, a woman who delivers a liveborn infant is counted as one delivery and one live birth whereas a woman who delivers liveborn twins is counted as one delivery and two live births. A woman who delivers a stillbirth is counted as one delivery and one intermediate or late fetal death. This is also considered to be one delivery and one birth since a stillbirth is a birth but not a live birth.

The formula for calculating the C-section rate is

$$C-Section\ Rate = \frac{Number\ of\ C-section\ deliveries\ in\ period}{Total\ number\ of\ deliveries\ in\ period}$$

 The C-section rate is not based on the number of patients discharged but, rather, on the number of deliveries. A rate compares the number of actual occurrences with the total possible.

Example 8.6: Forty C-sections were performed in a month during which there were 350 deliveries. Calculate the C-section rate for the month. Round to two decimals.

$$C-Section\ Rate = \frac{40}{350} = 0.11428$$

Convert to a percentage: $0.11428 \times 100 = 11.428\%$

Round to two decimals: 11.43%

Exercise 8.8

Use the information in the table that follows to calculate the C-section rate and the vaginal delivery rate at University Hospital for the semiannual period. Round to two decimal places.

University Hospital Obstetrics Service Semiannual Statistics July–December 20XX	
Admissions	672
Discharges and Deaths:	
Delivered	504
Not delivered	147
Aborted	21
Vaginal deliveries	403
C-sections	101

Exercise 8.9

Use the information in the table that follows to calculate the C-section rate, the newborn mortality rate, and the fetal mortality rate at University Hospital for the month of July. Round to two decimal places.

University Hospital Newborn Service July 20XX	
Discharges (includes deaths)	130
Births:	
Single live births	125
Multiple live births	1 set of twins 1 set of triplets
Deliveries:	
Vaginal	110
C-section	20
Deaths:	
Newborn	1
Fetal:	
Early	4
Intermediate	2
Late	2

Consultation Rates

A **consultation** is the response by one healthcare professional to another healthcare professional's request to provide recommendations or opinions regarding the care of a particular patient or resident. A patient's attending physician may occasionally request that a consultant (another physician or healthcare practitioner) examine a patient and give an opinion as to his or her condition. Ordinarily the consultant is called in to help identify and treat a patient whose diagnosis is outside the expertise of the attending physician. For example, a patient who is being treated by an orthopedist for a fractured hip consults with a cardiologist when the patient has postoperative high blood pressure. Consultants are usually specialists in their specific field of medicine. The consultant has the opportunity to visit with the patient and review the health record and then prepare a consultation report that includes the findings of the examination and recommendations for treating the patient. The consultation report is made a part of the patient's health records.

The formula for calculating the **consultation rate** is

$$Consultation\ Rate = \frac{Number\ of\ patients\ receiving\ a\ consultation\ for\ period}{Number\ of\ patients\ discharged,\ including\ deaths,\ for\ period}$$

Example 8.7: During the month of May, Community Hospital's medicine unit had 103 discharges, 14 of whom were seen by a consultant. Calculate the consultation rate. Round to two decimals.

$$Consultation\ Rate = \frac{14}{103} = 0.13592$$

Convert to a percentage: $0.13592 \times 100 = 13.592\%$

Round to two decimals: 13.59%

Exercise 8.10

Use the information in the table that follows to calculate the consultation rate at Community Hospital for each service and the total for the semiannual period. Round to two decimal places.

	Community Hospital Semiannual Statistics July–December 20XX		
Service	**Discharges and Deaths**	**No. of Patients Receiving Consultations**	**Consultation Rate**
Medicine	3,240	962	
Surgery	3,745	827	
Obstetrics	690	35	
Psychiatric	155	10	
Total			

Exercise 8.11

Use the information in the table that follows, create an Excel spreadsheet to calculate the rates requested below for Community Hospital. In this exercise, the deaths are included in the discharges. Round to two decimal places.

	Community Hospital Surgery Service Annual Statistics, 20XX				
Month	**Disch Including Deaths**	**Deaths**	**Consults**	**Consultation Rate**	**Gross Morality Rate**
January	602	18	119		
February	675	12	107		
March	598	11	92		
April	555	14	74		
May	630	10	105		
June	592	6	96		
July	581	9	85		
August	593	7	72		
September	621	5	89		
October	610	12	56		
November	601	10	95		
December	581	14	82		
Total					

(*continued on next page*)

Calculate the following rates.

1. Consultation rate for each month:

2. Consultation rate for the year for the surgery service:

3. Gross mortality rate for each month:

4. Gross mortality rate for the year for the surgery service:

Exercise 8.12

Use the information in the table that follows, create an Excel spreadsheet to calculate the consultation rates by physician for Community Hospital. Round to two decimal places.

Community Hospital Consultation Rate by Physician January–June 20XX			
Physician No.	**No. of Discharges and Deaths**	**No. of Consultations**	**Consultation Rate**
102	298	12	
237	247	3	
391	110	7	
518	144	8	
637	206	5	
802	82	12	
900	100	10	
Total			

Example 8.8: Use the information in the table that follows to calculate the readmission rates for each month and the semiannual period for University Hospital. Round to two decimal places.

$$30 - day\ Readmission\ Rate = \frac{Number\ of\ patients\ readmitted\ within\ 30\ days\ of\ a\ discharge}{Number\ of\ patients\ discharged\ (excluding\ deaths)}$$

University Hospital Surgery Service Semiannual Statistics July–December 20XX		
Month	No. of Patients Discharged Alive	No. of Patients Readmitted within 30 Days of the Previous Discharge	Readmission Rate
July	673	38	$\frac{38}{673} = 0.05646$ Convert to percentage: 5.646% Round to two decimals: 5.65%
August	765	43	$\frac{43}{765} = 0.05620$ Convert to percentage: 5.620% Round to two decimals: 5.62%
September	789	49	$\frac{49}{789} = 0.06210$ Convert to percentage: 6.210% Round to two decimals: 6.21%
October	750	32	$\frac{32}{750} = 0.04266$ Convert to percentage: 4.266% Round to two decimals: 4.27%
November	769	36	$\frac{36}{769} = 0.04681$ Convert to percentage: 4.681% Round to two decimals: 4.68%
December	778	45	$\frac{45}{778} = 0.05784$ Convert to percentage: 5.784% Round to two decimals: 5.78%
Total	4,524	243	$\frac{243}{4,524} = 0.05371$ Convert to percentage: 5.371% Round to two decimals: 5.37%

Notice in the readmission rate example that patients who died in the hospital are excluded. This ensures that the rate follows the guideline that the denominator should only be those that could have the event occur (part or base). Since patients that died in the hospital could not be readmitted, they are excluded.

Exercise 8.13

Use the information in the table that follows, create an Excel spreadsheet to calculate the readmission rates requested for Community Hospital. Round to two decimal places.

MS-DRG	Title	No. Live Disch	No. Readmissions within 30 days of Previous Discharge	Readmission Rate
	Community Hospital **Semiannual Statistics, 20XX** **Readmission by Selected MS-DRGs**			
190	COPD with MCC	12	2	
191	COPD with CC	14	5	
192	COPD without CC/MCC	42	11	
193	Simple pneumonia & pleurisy with MCC	8	1	
194	Simple pneumonia & pleurisy with CC	15	4	
195	Simple pneumonia & pleurisy without CC/MCC	97	8	
280	Acute myocardial infarction discharged alive, with MCC	10	3	
281	Acute myocardial infarction discharged alive, with CC	8	2	
282	Acute myocardial infarction discharged alive, without CC/MCC	180	10	
291	Heart failure & shock with MCC	3	1	
292	Heart failure & shock with CC	6	1	
293	Heart failure & shock without CC/MCC	63	2	
469	Major joint replacement or reattachment, lower extremity with MCC	15	2	
470	Major joint replacement or reattachment, lower extremity without MCC	49	4	

Exercise 8.14

Use the information in the table that follows, create an Excel spreadsheet to calculate the rate of readmitted patients by physician at Community Hospital for each month and for this quarter. Round to two decimal places.

Physician	No. of Live Discharges	No. of Readmissions within 30 days of Previous Discharge	Readmission Rate
	Community Hospital **Semiannual Statistics, 20XX** **Readmissions by Physicians**		
102	298	8	
237	247	4	
391	110	3	

(continued on next page)

Community Hospital Semiannual Statistics, 20XX Readmissions by Physicians			
Physician	No. of Live Discharges	No. of Readmissions within 30 days of Previous Discharge	Readmission Rate
518	144	2	
637	206	12	
802	82	6	
900	100	5	
Total			

Exercise 8.15

Use the information in the table that follows to calculate the rates requested for the medicine service at Community Hospital. Round to two decimal places.

Community Hospital Medicine Service Selected Annual Statistics, 20XX	
Total hospital discharges: 9,845	
Medicine Service	Number
Discharges and deaths	5,967
Complications	236
Hospital-acquired infections	89
Deaths (included in discharges)	71

Calculate the following rates.

1. Percentage of total hospital patients in the medicine service:

2. Complication rate in the medicine service:

3. Hospital-acquired infection rate in the medicine service:

4. Gross mortality rate in the medicine service:

Chapter 8 – Formulae for Morbidity and Other Rates

Rate	Numerator	Denominator
Infection rate	Total number of infections for a period	Total number of discharges (including deaths) for the same period
Postoperative infection rate	Total number of infections in clean surgical cases for a period	Number of surgical operations for the same period
Complication rate	Total number of complications for a period	Total number of discharges (including deaths) for the same period
C-section rate	Total number of C-sections for a period	Total number of deliveries (including C-sections) in the same period
Consultation rate	Total number of patients receiving consultations for a period	Total number of discharges (including deaths) for the same period
Readmission rate	Number of patients readmitted within 30 days of the previous discharge	Total patients discharged (excluding deaths)

Chapter 8   Matching Quiz

Match the definitions with the terms.

Definitions:

a. The ratio of all infections to the number of discharges, including deaths
b. Disease of long duration
c. A medical condition that arises during an inpatient hospitalization
d. Accessory; taking place at the same time
e. The process of delivering a liveborn infant or dead fetus by manual, instrumental, or surgical means
f. An infection acquired by a patient while receiving care or services in a healthcare organization; also called a hospital-acquired infection
g. The state of being diseased
h. Induced inadvertently by a physician or surgeon or by medical treatment or diagnostic procedure
i. One or more surgical procedures performed at one time for one patient via a common approach or for a common purpose
j. A surgical case in which no infection existed prior to surgery

Terms:

1. _____ Morbidity
2. _____ Infection rate
3. _____ Delivery
4. _____ Complication
5. _____ Clean surgical case

6. _____ Concomitant
7. _____ Chronic
8. _____ Surgical operation
9. _____ Iatrogenic
10. _____ Nosocomial infection

Chapter 8   Review

Use the information in the table that follows to answer questions 1 through 4.

Discharges and deaths	
Adults and children	8,191
Newborn	809
Surgical procedures	2,376
Surgical operations	2,371
Patients receiving consultations	2,789
Hospital-acquired infections	27
Surgical site infections (included in total HAIs)	6

1. The hospital-acquired infection rate (including newborns) is _____.
    a. 0.03%
    b. 0.30%
    c. 3.00%
    d. 30.00%

2. The consultation rate (including newborns) is _____.
    a. 0.03%
    b. 0.30%
    c. 3.09%
    d. 30.99%

3. What is the SSI rate?
    a. 0.25%
    b. 0.025%
    c. 2.53%
    d. 25.30%

4. A hospital reported the following statistics for the past year: births, 1,702; deliveries, 1,708; C-sections, 360; and obstetrical discharges, 1,827. The C-section rate for that year is _____.
    a. 0.21%
    b. 2.10%
    c. 21.08%
    d. 20.77%

Use the information in the table that follows to answer questions 5 through 8.

Women's Hospital September 20XX	
Deliveries	284 Two sets of twins
Births	286
Obstetrical Discharges	287
First-time C-sections	5
Repeat C-sections	4

5. What is the C-section rate for September?

    a. 0.03%

    b. 0.31%

    c. 3.17%

    d. 31.69%

6. What is the percentage of multiple births?

    a. 0.14%

    b. 14.00%

    c. 13.98%

    d. 1.40%

7. What is the percentage of patients with multiple births?

    a. 0.07%

    b. 0.70%

    c. 7.04%

    d. 70.42%

8. A third-party review company reported the statistics in the table below. Calculate the rate of admissions approved for each month and for the quarter. Round to two decimal places.

	July	August	September
Number of admission claims reviewed	875	892	925
Number of claims approved for admission to the hospital	851	888	920

Use the information in the table that follows to answer questions 9 through 12.

Community Hospital Selected Semiannual Statistics, 20XX						
Month	No. of Patients Discharged Alive	No. of Deaths	No. of Patients Readmission within 30 days	No. of Hospital-acquired Infections	No. of Consultations	No. of Complications
Jan	187	5	7	9	12	3
Feb	207	6	10	7	10	8
Mar	315	8	8	5	15	5
Apr	327	6	6	4	9	7
May	288	5	5	6	11	6
Jun	292	4	9	8	14	4
Total						

9. The readmission rate for the entire semiannual period is _____.
   a. 0.27%
   b. 27.84%
   c. 0.02%
   d. 2.78%

10. What is the hospital-acquired infection rate for the entire semiannual period?
   a. 2.36%
   b. 23.63%
   c. 0.23%
   d. 0.02%

11. The consultation rate for the entire semiannual period is _____.
   a. 0.43%
   b. 0.04%
   c. 4.30%
   d. 43.03%

12. The complication rate for the entire semiannual period is _____.
   a. 0.20%
   b. 0.02%
   c. 20.00%
   d. 2.00%

Use the information in the table that follows to answer questions 13 through 15. In these questions, the discharges include the deaths.

Community Hospital Selected Semiannual Statistics, 20XX						
Month	No. of Surgical Operations	No. of Post-op Infections	No. of Deliveries	No. of C-sections	No. of Discharges and Deaths	No. of Deaths
Jul	127	3	142	4	238	8
Aug	132	2	137	8	264	7
Sept	147	4	130	3	288	8
Oct	140	6	138	9	292	9
Nov	137	3	140	5	246	7
Dec	110	2	152	6	220	3
Total						

13. What is the SSI rate for this semiannual period?
   a. 0.25%
   b. 2.52%
   c. 0.02%
   d. 25.22%

14. What is the C-section rate for this semiannual period?

    a. 4.17%

    b. 40.17%

    c. 0.41%

    d. 0.04%

15. What is the gross mortality rate for this semiannual period?

    a. 0.27%

    b. 0.02%

    c. 27.13%

    d. 2.71%

Statistics Computed within the Health Information Management Department

Learning Objectives

At the conclusion of this chapter, you should be able to do the following:

- Relate the following terms: full-time equivalent employee, budget, fiscal year, variance and variance analysis, payback period
- Explain the use of various statistics to operations in a health information management (HIM) department in terms of unit labor cost, productivity, staffing levels, and budgets
- Differentiate between operational and capital budgets
- Develop the appropriate statistics to use in the management of an HIM department

Key Terms

Budget	Full-time equivalent employee (FTE)	Release of information (ROI)
Capital budget	Operational budget	Unit labor cost
Electronic signature	Payback period	Variance
Fiscal year	Productivity	Variance analysis

Statistics computed for use within the health information management (HIM) department usually relate to labor costs, productivity, and staffing and often are used in determining whether the department may be able to hire a new employee, set benchmarks for productivity, determine absentee rates, and so on. The following sections provide examples of common, everyday computations made by HIM staff members.

Health Information Statistics

Health information professionals can improve processes and procedures by keeping track of common statistics such as employee compensation, unit labor costs, staffing and productivity, and department budgets and verifying statistical reports generated by the HIM department and others. The HIM professional is at the center of all this data and should use the data to help make informed decisions.

Employee Compensation and Unit Labor Costs

One example of where health information managers must make effective decisions is regarding employee compensation and **unit labor cost**.

Unit labor cost is determined by dividing total annual compensation by total annual productivity. For example, coding workload in an HIM department is commonly measured in number of records coded. To determine the unit labor cost, divide the total annual compensation by the total annual productivity, as shown below:

$$Unit\ Labor\ Cost = \frac{Total\ annual\ compensation}{Total\ annual\ productivity}$$

The annual compensation for an individual employee is calculated by multiplying the number of hours worked per year (2,080 for a full-time employee) by the hourly wage and then multiplying that number by the benefits received. Then, add the amount of the benefits to the base salary. A sample calculation follows:

$$(2,080\ hours \times \$15\ per\ hour) \times 30\%\ benefits = \$31,200 \times .30 = \$9,360 + \$31,200 = \$40,560$$

 A quicker way to compute this is to multiply by 1.3 (if 30 percent benefits).

To determine the annual productivity, multiply the amount of work completed (for example, lines transcribed, number of records coded, and such) per day by the number of workdays in the year (5 workdays per week × 52 weeks per year = 260 workdays). Note that this calculation includes any vacation time or sick leave that an employee may take. This is necessary since the amount budgeted for the salary includes paid time off.

Example 9.1: Two full-time coding professionals in the HIM department each code 20 records per day. One employee earns $15.00 per hour and is paid an annual salary of $31,200; the other employee earns $15.65 per hour and is paid an annual salary of $32,552. What is the unit labor cost for these two professionals?

First, determine the annual productivity, by multiplying the number of records coded by the two employees (20 per day per coding professional or 40 per day) by the number of workdays in the year (5 workdays per week × 52 weeks per year = 260 workdays). Note that this calculation does not include any allowance for paid time off.

$$2(260\ workdays \times 20\ records) = 10,400\ records\ coded\ per\ year$$

Next, determine unit cost, by adding the two salaries ($31,200 + $32,552 = $63,752).

Finally, divide by the total number of records coded by the two employees in one year (10,400).

$$Unit\ Labor\ Cost = \frac{\$63,732}{10,400} = \$6.13\ per\ record$$

Example 9.2: If an analyst is compensated at $14.50 per hour and analyzes six records per hour, what is the unit labor cost?

First, determine the employee's annual productivity, by multiplying six records per hour by 2,080 worked hours per year.

$$Total\ Productivity = \frac{6\ records}{hour} \times \frac{2,080\ hours}{year} = 12,480\ records\ per\ year$$

Next, determine the employee's annual salary, as follows:

$$Total\ compensation = \frac{\$14.50}{hour} \times \frac{2,080\ hours}{year} = \$30,160\ per\ year$$

$$Unit\ Labor\ Cost = \frac{30,160}{12,480} = \$2.416 = \$2.42\ per\ record$$

Exercise 9.1

Complete the exercises that follow.

1. Accurate Transcription Company hires transcriptionist A, a full-time employee earning $15.00 per hour and an annual salary of $31,200. She transcribes 1,200 lines per day for a total of 312,000 lines per year. What is the unit transcription labor cost for transcriptionist A (or how much does a line cost when transcribed by transcriptionist A)?

2. The same transcription company hires transcriptionist B, a full-time employee earning $14.00 per hour and an annual salary of $29,120. He transcribes 900 lines per day for a total of 234,000 lines per year. What is the unit transcription labor cost for transcriptionist B?

3. University Hospital has eight full-time transcriptionists. Five of them produce 1,000 lines each per day. Of these five, one earns $14.00 per hour, three earn $14.80 per hour, and one earns $16.00 per hour.

   Two other transcriptionists in the department produce 1,100 lines per day. Of these two, one earns $14.25 per hour and the other earns $17.00 per hour. Finally, the eighth transcriptionist produces 1,200 lines per day and earns $14.00 per hour. Use an Excel spreadsheet to calculate the unit labor cost for each employee and answer the questions below.

   a. What is the difference in cost per line between the employee who produces 1,000 lines per day and makes $14.00 per hour and the employee who produces 1,200 lines per day and makes $14.00 per hour?

   b. What general observations can you make about the unit labor cost and the two employees just mentioned?

   c. What is the difference in cost per line between the employee who produces 1,000 lines per day and makes $16.00 per hour and the employee who produces 1,100 lines per day and makes $14.25 per hour?

   d. What is the total unit cost for transcription?

4. The HIM department at Community Hospital has three full-time coding professionals. One is considered the lead coding professional and his salary is $20.35 per hour. One coding professional is a new graduate who makes $15.50 per hour, and the third coding professional is an experienced employee who earns $18.90 per hour. The lead coding professional codes four records per hour; the new coding professional codes three records per hour, and the experienced coding professional codes six records per hour.

   a. Using a 7.5-hour productive day, what is the unit cost per coding professional?

   b. What is the total unit cost for all three coding professionals?

Some employers consider 7.5 hours a productive workday, thinking in terms of an 8-hour day minus breaks the employee may take. The salary cost is still based on an 8-hour paid workday.

QUICK
TIP

5. University Hospital employs ten full-time coding professionals. Use the information in the table that follows to determine the individual salary per year, the unit cost of coding for each employee, and the total unit cost for the coding department. Use 7.5 hours per day as a productive workday. Use an Excel spreadsheet to calculate the unit cost for each coding professional. Round unit cost to whole cents.

Coding Professional	Salary	Records Coded per Hour	Salary per Year	Unit Cost
A	$15.00	4	$31,200	
B	$15.45	5	$32,136	
C	$15.10	4	$31,408	
D	$16.79	6	$34,923	
E	$18.22	6	$37,898	
F	$22.65	6	$47,112	
G	$16.03	6	$33,342	
H	$16.85	6	$35,048	
I	$21.76	8	$45,261	
J	$17.34	6	$36,067	
Total			$364,395	

Unit Cost for Release of Information

The Health Insurance Portability and Accountability Act (HIPAA), commonly referred to as the Privacy Rule, allows a facility to charge a reasonable, cost-based fee for any requests for **release of information (ROI)**. ROI is the process of disclosing patient information from the medical record to another party. Federal, state and local regulations exist to govern the release of a patient's medical record information. Time studies would need to be performed in order to validate the cost. Some activities involved could be the following:

- Looking up the patient in the master patient index
- Keeping track of the time it takes to review and log the request
- Determining the location of the health record, either paper or electronic
- Determining whether other departments have portions of the medical record and have possibly made a disclosure
- Retrieving the record if it is a paper record or locating the record online and printing any scanned documents
- Preparing an invoice for the patient
- Updating the release of the information log

The HIM department also may consider nonlabor expenses such as those listed in example 9.3. However, the facility's chief financial officer (CFO) is usually consulted to determine whether other nonlabor costs can be applied.

Another aspect that will need consideration is that some health information departments are copying records onto a CD or thumb drive and giving them directly to a patient. This may affect the cost of the ROI. Health information exchanges (HIEs) may also affect the time it takes to answer an ROI request. The health information director should calculate the time needed to transfer the information rather than copy the information.

Example 9.3: Calculate the cost per request based on the statistics in the table that follows.

Community Hospital Health Information Department Release of Information Costs Average Requests per Month = 410	
Item	**Cost per Request**
Postage: $510 per month	$\dfrac{\$510}{410} = \$1.24$
Service contract (includes copier): $250 per month	$\dfrac{\$250}{410} = \$0.61$
Equipment (includes copies): $125 per month	$\dfrac{\$125}{410} = \$0.30$
Supplies (includes toner, printer cartridges, paper): $90 per month	$\dfrac{\$90}{410} = \$0.22$
Wages: $14.00 per hour = monthly salary of $2,427 ($14.00 × 2,080 hours = $29,120 annual salary, $\dfrac{\$29,120}{12 \text{ months}} = 2,426,66 = \$2,427$ per month	$\dfrac{\$2,427}{410} = \$5.92$
Total	**$8.30**

Exercise 9.2

Use the information in the table that follows, create an Excel spreadsheet to calculate the cost breakdown per item and the monthly cost for the ROI services at Community Hospital. Round wages to whole numbers.

Community Hospital Health Information Department Release of Information Costs Average Requests per Month = 540	
Item	**Cost per Month**
Postage	$675
Service contract (includes copier)	$250
Equipment (includes copies)	$125
Supplies (includes toner, printer cartridges, paper)	$95
Wages	$15.00 per hour
Monthly cost	**$**

Exercise 9.3

Use the information in the table that follows to complete the following exercises. Round annual wages to whole numbers.

Community Hospital Health Information Department Release of Information Costs Average Requests per Month = 550	
Item	**Cost per Month**
Postage	$790
Service contract (includes copier)	$265
Equipment (includes copies)	$150
Supplies (includes toner, printer cartridges, paper)	$95
Wages	$13.00 per hour

1. Calculate the cost breakdown for each item.

2. What is the monthly cost for the ROI services?

3. On average, the ROI section brings in $1,800 per month. What is the difference between cost and income?

4. An ROI contract company has approached the director of HIM with a proposal to take over the ROI function for free, and they would then charge the third parties for the copies. What are the advantages and disadvantages of this proposal?

5. The HIM department at Community Hospital had 100,000 active records. During January through June 20XX, they received 6,382 requests for records.

   a. What is the request rate for this six-month period? Round to two decimal places.

   b. Of the 6,382 requests, 3,375 were located within the 25-minute time frame, which was set as one of the department's quality indicators. What is the rate of compliance in answering these requests for records? Round to two decimal places.

Other Labor Unit Costs

The HIM department also processes patient record (chart) requests, which consumes a great deal of staff time. Responsibilities in maintaining records include the following:

- *Scanning of records*: Some facilities choose to scan the paper record to make it available online. These facilities may have an electronic document management system to help manage all their documents for a patient. This technology allows users to do the following:
  - Scan documents
  - Move documents from other systems to the electronic health record (EHR)
  - Enter information online
  - Handle the **electronic signature** of records, which is any representation of a signature in digital form, including an image of a handwritten signature
  - Allow text-editable deficiencies, which are those that a physician or other healthcare practitioner can enter through the computer or mobile device to make changes to a specific document
  - Index documents as they are entered into the computer system
  - Access information from a variety of locations
  - And more

  The main calculations for this function are productivity and quality. These are regularly computed and used for staffing issues and benchmarking. New technologies will continue to evolve, and managers in health information departments will continue to determine the costs and benefits of these new systems.

- *Provider-patient email*: As patients become more comfortable with emailing their physicians through patient portals, and as healthcare insurers begin to reimburse physicians for their time used to email patients, this will become an everyday issue for healthcare organizations. Email and text messages are considered healthcare business records and thus are subject to the same rules and regulations as any other health record. Facilities will usually make all email messages sent or received part of the patient's medical record. Email can be used to schedule appointments, refill prescriptions, transfer department results, or request that information be sent to other providers. Organizations may decide to keep track of the time spent responding to emails, gathering information before the email is answered, and deciding what can be answered via email (Pendergrass 2016).

- *Loose papers*: Often these are copies of health records sent from other healthcare facilities or prenatal records coming from obstetricians that must be included in the EHR. The number of pieces of paper received in the HIM department for filing is a significant factor in determining staffing levels. Loose papers may be measured in inches or by individual pieces, which is a more accurate measure. Because of the time involved in tracking this information, departments may choose to sample this activity for a one-week period several times a year.

- *Performance improvement activities*: HIM managers will often keep track of the activity in the department to determine if they are meeting their performance improvement targets. For example, the coding supervisor may monitor the number of days it takes the coding professionals to code a discharged record. The HIM department may be responsible for resubmitting claims that have been denied.

Example 9.4:

Your physician clinic's CFO has determined that it costs the clinic $3.50 per telephone call for the receptionist to schedule an appointment with a physician in the clinic, compared with $1.50 per online request to schedule an appointment.

1. What would the per-appointment cost savings be if, during one day at the clinic, 250 patient appointments were arranged by online request rather than by telephone?

   First calculate the cost of each method:

   Telephone appointment: $3.50 × 250 = $875.00.

   Email appointment $1.50 × 250 = $375.00.

   Calculate the cost savings:

   Cost Savings: $875.00 − $375.00 = $500.00.

2. What percentage of savings does this represent? Round to two decimals.

% Cost Savings: savings/total cost = 500/875 = 0.57142.

Convert to a percentage: $0.5714 \times 100 = 57.142\%$.

Round to two decimals: 57.14%.

Exercise 9.4

Complete the following exercises.

1. The HIM department at Community Hospital completed a time study, and the data are listed in the table below. Use an Excel spreadsheet to determine the number of hours worked in each activity. Hint: Create separate columns for hours per week (h/w) and number of weeks.

Community Hospital Health Information Department Time Allocation Report September 20XX		
Service/Division	Number of Hours	Hours Worked
Inpatient records:		
Medicine	450 h/w × 4 weeks	
Surgery	460 h/w × 4 weeks	
Pediatrics	12 h/w × 4 weeks	
Psychiatry	10 h/w × 4 weeks	
Obstetrics	60 h/w × 4 weeks	
Newborn	48 h/w × 4 weeks	
Subtotal inpatient records		
ED records:		
Supervisory	5 h/w × 4 weeks	
Correspondence	7 h/w × 4 weeks	
Clerical/processing	28 h/w × 4 weeks	
Subtotal ED records		
General clinic:		
Supervisory	5 h/w × 4 weeks	
Transcription	0.10 h/record × 370 records	
Clerical/Processing	6 h/w × 4 weeks	
Subtotal general clinic		
Outpatient/ambulatory surgery		

(continued on next page)

Community Hospital Health Information Department Time Allocation Report September 20XX		
Service/Division	**Number of Hours**	**Hours Worked**
Clerical/primary:	16 h/w × 4 weeks	
Filing	3 h/w × 4 weeks	
Admissions	3 h/w × 4 weeks	
Combining records	1 h/w × 4 weeks	
Tumor registry	1 h/w × 4 weeks	
Correspondence	3 h/w × 4 weeks	
Record completion	12 h/w × 4 weeks	
Supervisory	10 h/w × 4 weeks	
Transcription	0.10 h/record × 720 records	
Coding	0.15 h/record × 1,000 records	
Subtotal outpatient/ambulatory surgery		
Total hours worked		

2. What percentage of the total hours is spent in each category of inpatient records? Round to two decimal places.

Exercise 9.5

1. The information services department has requested data about the electronic signature system being used in your facility. They would like to know the locations where physicians are accessing the system. Review the information in the table that follows to determine the percentage of use from each site using an Excel spreadsheet. Round to two decimal places.

Community Hospital Electronic Signature System 500 Physicians on Staff; 489 Using the System		
Site	**No. of Physicians Using the System at This Site**	**% of Physicians Using the System at This Site**
Medicine, 2 West	54	
Medicine, 2 East	62	
Pediatrics, 3 West	42	
Obstetrics, 1 West	12	
Physician's lounge	87	
HIM department	65	
Personal mobile device	92	
Physician home	75	

2. What is the percentage of physicians not using the electronic signature system? Round to one decimal place.

Exercise 9.6

1. Review the report that follows and use an Excel spreadsheet to calculate the unapproved abbreviations for each physician. Round to two decimal places.

	Community Hospital Health Information Services Unapproved Abbreviations List November 20XX		
Physician No.	No. of Discharges	No. of Unapproved Abbreviations	Rate of Unapproved Abbreviations
102	298	34	
237	247	21	
391	110	26	
518	144	22	
637	206	4	
802	82	21	
900	100	12	
Total			

2. Review the report that follows and use an Excel spreadsheet to calculate the rate of deficiency for each physician. Round to two decimal places.

	Community Hospital Health Information Services Physician Documentation Deficiencies January 20XX		
Physician No.	No. of Admissions	No. of H&Ps Not Completed within 24 hours of Admission	Rate of Deficiency
102	189	5	
237	234	4	
391	98	8	
518	122	5	
637	178	3	
802	92	7	
900	99	2	
Total			

Productivity

Productivity is defined as a unit of performance defined by management in quantitative standards. Productivity allows organizations to measure how well the labor is converted into a product or service.

Most HIM departments have productivity standards for different areas in the department. For example, in the coding section, a productivity standard may be that employees should code four inpatient records per hour. In a 7.5-hour workday (considering breaks the employee will take), 30 inpatient records would be coded per day. But how does the HIM manager or supervisor know how many records should be coded in a day? Several factors influence this decision. Some things the supervisor should consider are as follows:

- Does the coding professional do anything in addition to coding, such as abstracting, answering the phone, or querying the physician for additional information about the diagnoses and procedures?
- What kinds of records is the coding professional coding? Are they long or short lengths of stay? Are they complex or relatively simple cases to code?

Two simple formulas that accurately calculate labor productivity have been suggested (Miller and Waterstraat 2004):

$$Completed\ work = Total\ work\ output - Defective\ work$$

and

$$Labor\ Productivity = \frac{Completed\ work}{Time\ to\ produce\ total\ work\ output}$$

Determining the total work output and the hours worked is clear; however, determining the defective work involves auditing the work for any errors. The manager could perform a review of all the work performed or the manager could perform a review of a fixed percentage of the work chosen through a random sample. The last suggestion is the most efficient. This method requires the manager to select a fixed percentage of an employee's total work for review. The manager also has a predetermined quality standard in mind and then reviews the work and classifies it as completed work or defective work. Additional work could be reviewed if more information is needed to determine the type of defect or until all the work has been reviewed (Miller and Waterstraat 2004).

Example 9.5. Use the information in the table that follows, create an Excel spreadsheet to calculate the inpatient coding productivity for one month.

Coding Professional	Work Output (All Records Coded)	Total Hours Worked	Average Work Output per Hour	Completed Work Percentage	Completed Work Output (Records Coded Accurately)	Completed Work per Hours Worked
A	500	140		91%		
B	475	140		96%		
C	300	80		80%		
D	375	80		64%		

Work Output: number of work units as recorded by the employee or the process
Total Hours Worked: number of hours worked by the employee to produce work, which does not include time for meals, breaks, and meetings
Average Work Output per Hour: work output divided by total hours worked
Completed Work Percentage: percentage of completed work from audit
Completed Work Output: work output multiplied by completed work percentage
Completed Work per Hours Worked: completed work output divided by total hours worked

Excel formula version:

	A	B	C	D	E	F	G
1	Coding Professional	Work Output (All Records Coded)	Total Hours Worked	Average Work Output per Hour	Completed Work Percentage	Completed Work Output (Records Coded Accurately)	Completed Work per Hours Worked
2	A	500	140	= B2/C2	0.91	= B2*E2	= F2/C2
3	B	475	140	= B3/C3	0.96	= B3*E3	= F3/C3
4	C	300	80	= B4/C4	0.8	= B4*E4	= F4/C4
5	D	375	80	= B5/C5	0.64	= B5*E5	= F5/C5
6	Department Summary	=SUM(B2:B5)	=SUM(C2:C5)	=F6/C6		=SUM(F2:F5)	=F6/C6
7							

Excel calculated version:

	A	B	C	D	E	F	G
1	Coding Professional	Work Output (All Records Coded)	Total Hours Worked	Average Work Output per Hour	Completed Work Percentage	Completed Work Output (Records Coded Accurately)	Completed Work per Hours Worked
2	A	500	140	3.57	91%	455	3.25
3	B	475	140	3.39	96%	456	3.26
4	C	300	80	3.75	80%	240	3.00
5	D	375	80	4.69	61%	240	3.00
6	Department Summary	1,650	440	3.16		1,391	3.16
7							

Example 9.5 shows the calculation for determining inpatient coding productivity for one month. Notice that coding professional D's average work output is 4.69 records per hour ($\frac{work\ output}{total\ hours\ worked} = \frac{375}{80} = 4.69$). However, after auditing the work, it was determined that 240 of those records were coded accurately (completed work output). Coding professional D's completed work is really 3.00 ($\frac{240}{80} = 3.00$) per hour.

Staffing Levels

Healthcare organizations use a variety of methods to determine appropriate staffing levels. For example, many outpatient facilities use patient encounters per **full-time equivalent employee (FTE)** per month. A patient encounter is any personal contact between a patient and a physician or other person authorized to furnish healthcare services for the diagnosis or treatment of the patient. These may include laboratory services, x-ray services, physical therapy, and other ancillary services.

The staffing level may be determined by dividing the number of patient encounters by the expected productivity for each FTE. An FTE is the total number of workers, including part-time, in an area as the equivalent of full-time positions. The number of FTEs does not always equal the actual number of employees because two or more part-time employees might equal one FTE.

$$Required\ Number\ of\ FTEs = \frac{Number\ of\ encounters}{Expected\ productivity}$$

Example 9.6: Community Physician Clinic, a large clinic with 85 providers, experiences 1,500 patient encounters per day. A coding professional is expected to code 150 records per day. Determine the number of coding professionals needed.

$$Required\ Number\ of\ FTEs = \frac{Number\ of\ encounters}{Productivity\ Rate} = \frac{1,500}{150}$$

$$= 10\ coding\ professionals$$

Hospital HIM departments often use discharges as their method to determine inpatient staffing levels.

 When computing FTEs, the manager does not ordinarily round up or down to a whole number. For example, the administration may only want to approve a person working 50 percent time (0.5 FTE) if a full-time employee is not needed to perform the work.

Example 9.7: At Community Hospital, the new HIM director wants to determine the number of employees needed in a coding section. She knows that the average number of inpatient records coded is six per hour. The hospital discharges an average of 65 patients per day. How many FTEs are required for inpatient coding? Assume that the FTEs work 7.5 hours per day and round to two decimals.

First, calculate the number of records each FTE can code per day:

$$(6\ records\ per\ hour) \times (7.5\ hours\ per\ day) = 45\ records$$

Next, divide the number of discharges per day by the number of records coded per FTE:

$$Required\ Number\ of\ FTEs = \frac{Number\ of\ encounters}{Productivity\ Rate} = \frac{65}{45} = 1.444$$

Round to two decimals: 1.44 FTEs or one full-time employee and one 44% part-time employee.

A 44% part-time employee would work 40 hours/week × 0.44 = 17.6 hours per week.

Another way to determine the number of employees needed is to calculate how many minutes and hours it would take to perform all the work, then divide by the number of productive hours.

Example 9.8: An HIM director would like to know how many FTEs are needed to analyze the weekly discharges in her facility. There are 350 discharges per week. It takes one employee 15 minutes to code and analyze one record. Using a productive week as 37.5 (7.5 × 5 days) hours, the director determines that she will need 2.3 employees to analyze the week's discharges.

$$15\ minutes \times 350\ records = 5,250\ minutes$$

$$\frac{5,250\ minutes}{60\ minutes\ (in\ one\ hour)} = 87.5\ hours$$

$$\frac{87.5\ hours}{37.5\ productive\ hours} = 2.3\ FTE$$

Exercise 9.7

1. Community Physician's Clinic is a large clinic with 85 physicians. They treat about 9,000 patients each week. Coding professionals are expected to code 100 clinical records each day. How many FTEs are needed to code these records? (Assume a five-day work week and 7.5 hours as a productive day.)

2. Community Physician's Clinic is merging with the Medical Center Physician's Clinic. They will be adding 24 physicians who treat 65,104 patients per year. The coding supervisor at Community Physician's Clinic will be responsible for adding credentialed coding professionals to her current staff. The coding professionals will be expected to code 100 clinical records per day. How many more FTEs will be needed to code these records?

3. Accurate Transcription Company is taking on your hospital as a new client for a one-month trial period. You report that the average number of transcribed lines per month is 142,500. The daily production standard they require is 950 lines per day per transcriptionist. With 20 workdays in the month, calculate the number of FTEs needed for this volume.

4. The supervisor over the coding division in the HIM department at Community Hospital reviewed the productivity logs of four newly hired coding professionals after their first month. Use the information in the table that follows, create an Excel spreadsheet to determine which employee will require additional assistance in order to meet the standard of 20 medical records coded per day.

Community Hospital Coding Productivity Report Coding Standard: 20 Medical Records per Day				
Coding Professional	Week 1	Week 2	Week 3	Week 4
1	90	105	98	107
2	100	105	105	95
3	75	80	85	105
4	80	95	115	110

5. Use the information in the table that follows, create an Excel spreadsheet to calculate the labor productivity for the following coding professionals. Round to two decimal places.

Inpatient coding productivity calculation for September, 20XX						
Coding Professional	Work Output (All Records Coded)	Total Hours Worked	Average Work Output per Hour	Completed Work Percentage	Completed Work Output (Records Coded Accurately)	Completed Work per Hours Worked
1	400	150	2.67	93.75%	375	
2	405	150	2.70	98.77%	400	
3	345	140	1.75	99.13%	342	
4	400	140	2.86	95.00%	380	

Exercise 9.8

1. Community Hospital wants to make the transition to an electronic data management system. The process will involve scanning 7,500 inpatient records, 3,000 outpatient records, and 2,500 emergency department (ED) records into the new system. The hospital estimates that there are 30 pages per inpatient record, 4 pages per outpatient record, and 4 pages per ED record. Assuming one scanning clerk can scan 7,500 pages per day, how many days will it take to complete the transition?

2. Use the scenario in the question above to answer this question. The HIM department would like to complete this project in 10 days. How many FTEs will the HIM department manager need to hire to complete this in the desired time frame? Round to one decimal place.

3. Use the information in the table that follows to create an Excel spreadsheet to answer the following questions. Each employee worked 7.5 hours per day during the 21 workdays in September. Round all answers to two decimal places. Hint: create a calculated column in the spreadsheet for each of the statistics in a-e below.

   a. What percentage of the total number of records did each employee code during the month?

   b. How many records is each coding professional coding each workday?

   c. How many records is each coding professional coding per hour? (Use a 7.5-hour workday.)

   d. How many minutes does it take each coding professional to code one record?

   e. What percentage of records is not passing the quality screens for each coding professional?

Community Hospital Health Information Management Department Coding Section—Productive and Quality Audit Reports September 20XX		
Coding Professional	**No. of Records Coded**	**No. of Records Not Passing Quality Screens**
A	450	4
B	510	4
C	385	11

Exercise 9.9

1. An HIM manager must determine the number of FTEs needed to code 750 discharges per week. It takes 20 minutes to code each record. Each coding professional works 37.5 productive hours per week. How many FTEs will the HIM manager need? Round to one decimal place.

2. The coding department at Community Physician's Clinic developed the following report for the denials committee at the clinic. The billing report shows the following information. Create an Excel spreadsheet to calculate the percentage of denials for each third-party payer category and the total. Round to two decimal places.

Community Physician's Clinic Coding Department Denials–October 20XX			
Payment Source	**Number of Claims Sent**	**Number of Denials**	**Percentage of Denials**
Medicare	460	43	
Medicaid	345	35	
Tricare/military	182	14	
Commercial payers	1,307	83	
Worker's compensation	6	1	
Total			

3. Use the information from number 2 to determine how many hours it will take to reconcile these denials if each denial takes 1.5 hours to review and resubmit the bill?

4. The coding manager would like the denials listed in number 2 reconciled within one month (20 workdays). How many FTEs will the coding manager need?

5. The coding manager at Community Physician's Clinic submitted the following report to administration to explain the charge-lag time experienced. Their goal is to bill the insurance companies within three days of seeing the patient.

Community Physician's Clinic Charge-Lag Report October 20XX Total Claims = 2,300	
Reason not billed within three days of encounter:	
Physician not completed with documentation	120
Physician documentation completed, but record not coded	18
Business office hold	32

Use the following formula to calculate the percentage of non-billed claims for each category. Round to two decimal places.

$$\frac{Reason\ claim\ not\ billed}{Total\ number\ of\ claims}$$

Charge-Lag Time Reason Attributed to:	Percentage of Non-Billed Claims
Physician	
Coding professional	
Business office	

Budgets

If you are responsible for supervising a group of employees, you will most likely also be responsible for budgeting. Usually, health information departments are involved with expense and capital budgets.

A **budget** is a plan that converts the organization's goals and objectives into targets for revenue and spending. Planning for the budget begins several months before the facility's **fiscal year** begins. A fiscal year is any consecutive 12-month period an organization uses as its accounting period. During the planning process, the HIM supervisor uses skills learned in statistics to help approximate the department's expenses for the coming year. Departmental expenses may include employee wages and benefits, supplies, travel and education, membership dues, subscriptions, postage, copying, and equipment maintenance contracts.

The HIM department may also generate some revenue for the department, for example, if it is responsible for the ROI activity or provides transcription or coding services for hospital physicians.

 A fiscal year is a consecutive 12-month period used by an organization as its accounting period. The fiscal year does not have to be a calendar year but must be a period of 12 consecutive months. For example, the US government's fiscal year begins October 1 and ends September 30.

QUICK
TIP

Operational Budget

An **operational budget** is a type of budget that allocates and controls resources to meet an organization's goals and objectives for the fiscal year. During the year, usually each month, a department director receives budget reports showing amounts budgeted and actual amounts spent. This report generally alerts the department director as to whether he or she is over or under budget. Any differences between the budgeted amount and the amount actually spent are called variances A budget variance is a disagreement between two figures. The variance can be used as a device to monitor the department's activities. Budgets also may be available on the organization's intranet for viewing at any time. This is an easy way for the manager to stay aware of his or her department's budget. An intranet is a private network that works like the internet but can only be accessed by certain individuals, such as employees of a company.

> *The term variance has multiple meanings depending on the context. In the budget context, variance is the difference between a value and a target. In the descriptive statistics context, variance is a measure of the spread or dispersion of a set of data points (see chapter 10).*

The department director should check the budget report at least monthly to determine whether any adjustments must be made in order to stay within the budget. Often the director may be required to explain budget variances if the department is over or under budget. This assessment of a department's financial transactions to identify differences between the budget amount and the actual amount of a line item is called a variance analysis.

To determine the percent variance, subtract the budgeted amount from the actual amount and then divide the difference by the budgeted amount.

Example 9.9: Determine the percent budget variance for each of the departments listed in the table that follows. Round to one decimal place.

Item	Budgeted Amount	Actual Amount	Variance
Supplies	$3,000	$4,000	($1,000)
Training	$1,000	$2,000	($1,000)

Use the information in the preceding table to determine the variance for supplies is $1,000, or 33.3 percent, over budget.

$$Percent\ Variance\ for\ Supplies = \frac{Variance\ amount}{Budget\ amount} = \frac{-1,000}{3,000} = -0.3333$$

Convert to a percentage: $-0.3333 \times 100 = -33.33\%$.
Round to one decimal place: -33.3%.

$$Percent\ Variance\ for\ Training = \frac{Variance\ amount}{Budget\ amount} = \frac{-1,000}{2,000} = -0.5000$$

Convert to a percentage: $0.5000 \times 100 = -50.00\%$.
Round to one decimal place: -50.0%.

The variances computed above are examples of unfavorable variances; that is, the amounts spent were more than the amounts budgeted.

Favorable variances occur when the amounts spent are less than or equal to the amounts budgeted, as shown in the table that follows.

Item	Budgeted Amount	Actual Amount	Variance
Supplies	$10,000	$8,000	$2,000
Education/training	$3,500	$2,000	$1,500

$$Percent\ Variance\ for\ Supplies = \frac{Variance\ amount}{Budget\ amount} = \frac{2,000}{10,000} = 0.2000$$

Convert to a percentage: $0.2000 \times 100 = 20.00\%$.
Round to one decimal place: 20.0%.

$$Percent\ Variance\ for\ Training = \frac{Variance\ amount}{Budget\ amount} = \frac{1,500}{3,500} = 0.4285$$

Convert to a percentage: $0.4285 \times 100 = 42.85\%$.
Round to one decimal place: 42.9%.

Capital Budget

A **capital budget** is allocation of resources for long-term investments and projects. It accounts for the major assets the facility will purchase during the fiscal year; for example, equipment for the HIM department or a new CT machine. Capital budget items usually are "high-dollar" purchases. Each facility defines what "high-dollar" means. For example, one facility may consider any assets purchased at a cost of more than $500 to be part of the capital budget.

Moreover, items included in a capital budget usually have a "life" of more than one year; that is, each item's usefulness should last longer than a year. Health information professionals are usually involved in assisting the department director in a cost justification for the capital budget. This is very important because only a certain amount of dollars can be allocated to the facility's departments and supervisors who wish to have their projects approved. The department director may ask the supervisor to calculate the **payback period** of the project. The payback period is a financial method used to evaluate the value of a capital expenditure by calculating the time frame that must pass before inflow of cash from a project equals or exceeds outflow of cash. The formula is as follows:

$$Payback\ Period = \frac{Total\ cost\ of\ the\ project}{Annual\ incremental\ cash\ flow}$$

The annual incremental cash flow refers to the savings that a department realizes from the project. For example, if the HIM department needs a new copy machine, the department director may ask the department supervisor to determine, first, how much a new copy machine costs, and then, what kind of savings would be realized from the purchase of a new machine. The supervisor would investigate the cost from different vendors and then calculate an estimate of the savings. Savings considerations might include the time not spent recopying pages, fixing the copy machine, or releasing papers trapped in the machine, as well as the cost of additional paper.

> **Example 9.10:** A new copy machine costs $3,000, and the department will realize a savings of $1,000 per year. Calculate the payback period for the new copy machine. Round to one decimal place.
>
> $$Payback\ Period = \frac{3,000}{1,000} = 3.0\ years$$

Exercise 9.10

Complete the following exercises.

1. In deciding whether to purchase or lease new scanning equipment, the HIM supervisor at Community Hospital calculates the payback period. The hospital's required payback period is three years. If the equipment costs $32,000 and generates $4,500 per year in savings, what would be the payback period for this equipment? Should the department purchase this equipment?

2. The coding section in the HIM department shows its first-quarter budget analysis as having a budgeted cost of operation of $72,000. However, the actual cost of operation was $76,000. Calculate the budget variance. Round to one decimal place.

3. Administration at Community Hospital System (which includes an inpatient hospital, skilled nursing facility, durable equipment company, mental health facility, and outpatient counseling center) will begin a conversion project from the current EHR to another that will allow all the facilities access to one EHR. The estimated cost of the new EHR is $2,750,000. The savings with the new system is estimated to be $575,000 per year. What is the payback period? Round to two decimal places.

4. The HIM department shows the following monthly report. Create an Excel spreadsheet to calculate the percentage of variance for each line item and the total. Round to two decimal places.

Community Hospital HIM Department Budget Variance Annual Report, 20XX			
Line Item	**Budgeted Amount**	**Actual Amount**	**Percentage of Variance**
Service contracts	$2,000	$2,500	
Education/conferences	$4,500	$2,400	
Travel	$2,000	$1,750	
Dues/memberships	$720	$545	
Subscriptions/books	$600	$250	
Supplies	$600	$725	
Total			

5. Your HIM manager has been approved to add $25,000 to the salary budget to pay the coding professionals overtime to catch up on coding records so the claims may be billed. Coding professional A earns $15.75 per hour, coding professional B earns $16.00 per hour, coding professional C earns $18.40 per hour, and coding professional D earns $17.29 per hour. How many total hours of overtime can be worked if each coding professional works an equal amount of overtime earning time and a half? Round to two decimal places.

Chapter 9 Matching Quiz

Match the definitions with the terms.

Definitions:

a. The amount of work minus any defective units

b. A plan that converts the organization's goals and objectives into targets for revenue and spending

c. Any representation of a signature in digital form, including an image of a handwritten signature

d. The total number of workers, including part-time, in an area as the equivalent of full-time positions

e. Any consecutive 12-month period an organization uses as its accounting period

f. A financial method used to evaluate the value of a capital expenditure by calculating the time frames that must pass before inflow of cash from a project equals or exceeds outflow of cash

g. A type of financial plan that allocates and controls resources to meet an organization's goals and objectives for the fiscal year

h. The difference between a budget and actual value

Terms:

1. _____ Budget

2. _____ Full-time equivalents

3. _____ Payback period

4. _____ Variance

5. _____ Completed work

6. _____ Electronic signature

7. _____ Fiscal year

8. _____ Operational budget

Chapter 9   Review

Complete the following exercises.

1. A coding supervisor must determine the number of FTEs needed to code 600 discharges per week. If it takes an average of 20 minutes to code each record and each coding professional works 7.5 productive hours per day, how many FTEs will the coding supervisor need? Round to one decimal place.

2. The HIM department at Community Hospital will experience a 15 percent increase in the number of discharges coded per day as the result of opening an orthopedic clinic in the facility. The 15 percent increase is projected to be 50 additional records per day. The standard time to code this type of record is 15 minutes. Compute the number of FTEs required to handle this increased volume in coding based on a 7.5-hour productive day. Round to one digit after the decimal.

3. The HIM coding supervisor agrees to pay a new graduate $15.00 per hour. This is a full-time coding position at 2,080 hours per year. The cost for a full-time employee's fringe benefits is 25 percent of the employee's salary. How much must the supervisor budget for the employee's salary and fringe benefits?

4. The same supervisor in the scenario above agreed to increase the salary of the employee to $16.00 per hour once she passed her RHIT certification exam. Three months after beginning her employment, the employee passed her RHIT certification exam. What will the new budget be for salary and fringe benefits?

5. The forms used to query physicians in your coding area cost $50.00 per 250 forms for the first 500 and $40 for every 100 thereafter. If you need to order 850 forms, what is the total cost to be budgeted?

6. You currently lease scanning equipment at a cost of $2,750 per quarter and two copy machines at $150 each per month plus $0.01 per page copied. You estimate you will copy a total of 30,000 pages a year per copier. What will you need to budget annually for this leased equipment?

7. Use an Excel spreadsheet to determine the variance and percent of variance for each item listed in the HIM department budget shown in the table that follows. Round to two decimal points.

Community Hospital Health Information Department Fiscal Year 20XX			
Item	Budget Amount	Actual Amount	Variance/% of Variance
Supplies	$1,500	$1,495	
Outside temp service	$10,500	$8,500	
Travel	$2,500	$2,575	
Conference fees	$750	$800	
Postage	$2,000	$1,035	
Subscriptions	$325	$320	
Maintenance contracts	$6,000	$3,525	

8. All patients who present to the emergency department with a suspected acute myocardial infarction (AMI) are expected to receive an electrocardiogram (ECG) within 10 minutes of their arrival. Of the 45 patients who had a suspected AMI during the last quarter, 33 had an ECG within the specified time frame. What was the rate of compliance? Round to two decimal places.

9. Last month, the ROI specialist received 580 requests for information. He was able to answer 307 within the specified time frame of three working days. What is the rate of compliance in answering requests within the specified time frame? Round to two decimal places.

10. Create an Excel spreadsheet of the hospital charges for the patients listed in the table that follows based on an average charge of $1,500 per day.

Community Hospital		
Patient Number	**LOS**	**Estimated Charges**
126745	4	
853275	6	
903629	2	
956825	7	
957032	10	
903412	8	
934818	11	
563498	9	
985476	5	
894532	3	

11. Last year, Community Hospital had 32,687 discharges. Of these, 1,789 were readmissions. What is the hospital's readmission rate? Round to two decimal places.

12. In September, the hospital had three coding professionals who coded 1,500 inpatient records, and 22 of the records failed the quality screens.

    a. What is the average number of records coded by each coding professional?

    b. What was the average number of records coded each working day (Monday through Friday at 21 workdays) in September? Round to two decimal places.

    c. What percentage of records passed the quality screens? Round to two decimal places.

13. At Community Hospital, each full-time employee is required to work 2,080 hours annually. The table that follows shows the amount of time that five employees were absent from work over the past year. Create an Excel spreadsheet to answer the questions that follow. Round all answers to two decimal places. Hint: add columns to the spreadsheet for each calculation in a and b; add a total row for part c.

Community Hospital Health Information Management Department Coding Section Absentee Report Annual Statistics 20XX		
Employee Name	**Vacation Hours Used**	**Sick Leave Hours Used**
A	40	6
B	22	16
C	36	8
D	80	32
E	16	40

    a. What is the total absentee rate for each employee?

    b. What is the sick leave rate for each employee?

    c. What is the total sick leave rate for this group of employees for the year?

14. The coding department of Community Physician's Clinic is interested in purchasing a software program that will edit claims before they are sent to the billing office. The license fee for the software is $60,000 per year. The software is expected to reduce the number of errors on claims and thus reduce the number of denials returned to the clinic. Currently, the department codes 47,600 provider visits per month and 500 claims are returned each month for recoding. The facility pays two FTEs in the billing office $14.00 per hour each plus 25 percent in benefits to refile the returned claims. The software company promises that its software will reduce the number of returned claims by 90 percent.

    a. What is the rate of claims that are currently being returned for recoding each month? Round to two decimal places.

    b. How many claims are estimated to be returned after the installation of the software?

    c. If the clinic eliminated the two FTEs that handle the returned claims, what savings would it realize after installation of the software?

    d. What is the payback period?

CHAPTER 10

Descriptive Statistics in Healthcare

Learning Objectives

At the conclusion of this chapter, you should be able to do the following:

- Explain how and why percentiles are used
- Compute the percentile from an ungrouped distribution
- Prepare statistics measuring central tendency such as mean, median or mode
- Prepare statistics measuring variation such as range, variance, standard deviation, and correlation

Key Terms

Decile
Descriptive statistics
Frequency distribution
Measures of central tendency
Median
Mode

Normal distribution
Outlier
Percentile
Quartile
Range
Skewness

Standard deviation (SD)
Variability
Variable
Variance

Descriptive statistics describe data in ways that are manageable and easily understood. They describe the attributes of a population or sample. They also summarize data, and we can easily get a sense of the data. The following sections discuss the basic concepts of rank, quartile, decile, percentile, measures of central tendency (mean, median, and mode), measures of variation (range, variance, and standard deviation [SD]), and correlation.

Concepts in Descriptive Statistics

Health information professionals use descriptive statistics in many aspects of their day-to-day work. For example, they determine the number of patients in certain payment categories and review the top 10 surgical procedures for medical staff committee reports. The concepts covered in this chapter will help health information professionals summarize large amounts of data using the appropriate statistics.

Frequency Distribution

Before studying measures in descriptive statistics, it would be useful to briefly cover two concepts: variables and frequency distribution. A **variable** is a characteristic that can have different values. For example, a person may be HIV negative or positive. The variable is HIV status and the values are negative and positive. Third-party payers, race, length of stay (LOS), and services are examples of variables. Within each variable, there is more than one possible value. For example, third-party payers include numerous insurance companies. The variable is "third-party payer" while the values are the names of the organizations paying for services.

Because it is difficult to draw conclusions from data in raw form, they are often summarized into frequency distributions. A **frequency distribution** shows the values that a variable can take, and the number of observations associated with each value. In the previous example, a facility conducting HIV testing may be interested in the number or frequency of HIV negative and positive individuals using their services. This information is valuable when seeking funding.

For example, table 10.1 provides the frequency distribution in which types of third-party payers are identified, along with the number of patients discharged by Community Hospital associated with each payer during the month of June.

Table 10.1. Example of a frequency distribution of number of patients discharged by third-party payer

Community Hospital Patients Discharged by Payer June 20XX	
Third-Party Payer	**No. of Patients**
Medicare	98
Medicaid	56
Tri-Care	23
Blue Cross	85
Mutual of Omaha	67
Other Private Payer	76
Total	**405**

Rank

Rank denotes a value's position in a group relative to other values organized in order of magnitude. For example, a rank of 50 means that a value or score is 50th from the beginning (or end) of a series. The number of scores in a sequence is important in determining the significance of a rank. If there are only 60 scores, a rank of 50th is interpreted much differently than if there are 1,000 scores. For this reason, it may be more useful to express data as percentiles.

In ranked data, the position of the observation is more important than the number associated with it. For example, it is possible to list the major causes of death in the US, along with the number of lives that each cause claimed. If the causes of death were ordered starting with the one that resulted in the greatest number of deaths and ending with the one that caused the fewest, and these were assigned consecutive integers, the data are said to be ranked.

Table 10.2 shows a report listing the top 10 leading causes of death in the US for the latest data available (2016). Note that stroke would be ranked fifth regardless of whether it caused 154,595 (one less than chronic lower respiratory disease) or 116,103 (one more than Alzheimer's disease) deaths.

Percentile

Percentiles separate the scores into 100 equal parts. If a person scores at the 54th percentile, their score is greater than or equal to 54 percent of all the scores in the group. This is called a percentile rank.

How and Why Percentiles Are Used

Percentiles help people understand their score relative to all scores from a group. If a student is told that she received a score of 34 on a test and she did not know how many points were possible, the 34 has no meaning to her. However, if she

Table 10.2. Top 10 leading causes of death in the US in 2016

Rank	Causes of Death	Total Deaths
1	Heart disease	635,260
2	Cancer	598,038
4	Accidents (unintentional injuries)	161,374
	Chronic lower respiratory diseases	154,596
5	Stroke (cerebrovascular diseases)	142,142
6	Alzheimer's disease	116,103
7	Diabetes mellitus	80,058
8	Influenza and pneumonia	51,537
9	Nephritis, nephritic syndrome, and nephrosis	50,046
10	Intentional self-harm (suicide)	44,965

Source: CDC n.d.

is told that the score was in the 95th percentile, this would give a better understanding of the score compared with her peers; that is, only 5 percent of the class received a higher score.

To find the score that falls within a given percentile in a group of data arranged in order of magnitude, do the following:

1. Multiply the desired percentile's percentage by the total number of scores in the given group of scores (N). For example, the 38th percentile's percentage would be 38 percent. Likewise, the 90th percentile's percentage would be 90 percent.
2. This number indicates the rank of the score in the group that represents the desired percentile.

Example 10.1: The following numbers represent lengths of newborns in inches:

12, 12, 12, 13, 13, 15, 15, 16, 17, 18, 19, 20, 21, 21, 22, 22, 23, 23, 24, 25. Find the 60th percentile.

$N = 20$

To find the 60th percentile:

1. Multiply 60 percent or 0.60 by 20 (N) = 12.
2. Count up to the 12th score.
3. The 60th percentile is 20.

This means that 40 percent of the newborns were over 20 inches in length at birth and 60 percent were under 30 inches in this sample.

On the other hand, if you want to know in what percentile a score is, take that score and divide the number of scores that are equal to and less than your score by the total number of scores, and then multiply by 100.

Example 10.2: Find the percentile of newborns that are 17 inches in length, in the example above.

1. Determine the rank of the value 17. Seventeen is the 9th value and, therefore, has rank 9.
2. Take 9 (17 is the 9th score) divided by 20 (the N) × 100.

$$\left(\frac{9}{20}\right) \times 100 = 45\text{th percentile}$$

Seventeen falls in the 45th percentile. This means that 45 percent of the newborns were 17 inches or less in length at birth and 55 percent (100 percent − 45 percent) were over 17 inches in length at birth.

Example 10.3: Dr. Davis, a new endocrinologist at the Community Physician's Clinic, acquired 20 new diabetic patients during his first month of practice. Their A1C results, a measure of blood glucose levels, are listed in the spreadsheet that follows. Dr. Davis would like to offer a weight-loss clinic to the patients who are above the 40th percentile of the results. Create an Excel spreadsheet that will identify which patients should be included.

	A	B
1	**New patients seen by Dr. Davis**	
2	**October 20XX**	
3	**Patient Number**	**AIC result**
4	893245	5.7
5	879554	5.8
6	766509	6.2
7	752354	6.1
8	918756	6.8
9	457656	11.5
10	235423	10.7
11	561115	6.7
12	872208	6.8
13	544565	9.2
14	876745	8.4
15	929827	7.2
16	648382	6.9
17	980053	5.5
18	768997	5.7
19	741452	6.7
20	861942	10.4
21	146349	8.5
22	749961	9.6
23	656511	6.0
24		

1. Sort patients by A1C value. Hint: Select the patient number and AIC results columns when sorting (cells A3:B23).

	A	B
1	**New patients seen by Dr. Davis**	
2	**October 20XX**	
3	**Patient Number**	**AIC result**
4	980053	5.5
5	893245	5.7
6	768997	5.7
7	879554	5.8
8	656111	6.0
9	752354	6.1
10	766509	6.2
11	561115	6.7
12	741452	6.7
13	918756	6.8
14	872208	6.8
15	648382	6.9
16	929827	7.2
17	876745	8.4
18	146349	8.5
19	544565	9.2
20	749961	9.6
21	861942	10.4
22	235423	10.7
23	457656	11.5
24		

2. Determine the total number of observations: $N = 20$.
3. Determine the rank of the value representing the 40th percentile: $0.40 \times 20 = 8$.
4. Find the 8th ranked score by counting: 6.7 (patients 561115 and 741452).
5. All patients with an A1C above 6.7 qualify.

Quartile

In addition to determining the percentile or rank of the score in a group, it can be helpful to divide data into parts to better understand the relationship among scores. Data organized in order of magnitude can be divided into four equal parts, or **quartiles**. The first quartile corresponds to the 25th percentile and includes the first 25 percent of the data, the second quartile corresponds to the 50th percentile and includes 50 percent of the data, and so on. The 50th percentile is also referred to as the median of the distribution.

QUICK TIP *Quartiles may be denoted by Q_1, Q_2, Q_3.*

Example 10.4: The following birth weights, in pounds, were recorded: 7.8, 5.6, 8.9, 9.10, 5.7, 4.8, 8.1, 9.2, 9.1, 9.4, and 7.6. Calculate the quartiles.

1. Write the data in increasing order: 4.8, 5.6, 5.7, 7.6, 7.8, **8.1**, 8.9, 9.1, 9.2, 9.4, 9.10.
2. Find the second quartile—the point that divides the series of values into two equal subsets. There are 11 values (n = 11), so the 6th value will divide the series into two subsets of 5 values. The 6th value is 8.1. Therefore, the second quartile is 8.1.
   Q_2 or the median = 8.1
3. The lower half of the data is 4.8, 5.6, **5.7**, 7.6, 7.8.
   Q_1 = 5.7 (the middle value)
4. The upper half of the data is 8.9, 9.1, **9.2**, 9.4, 9.10.
   Q_3 = 9.2 (the middle value)

Decile

In similar fashion, **deciles** represent data divided into 10 equal parts. The first decile corresponds to the 10th percentile and includes the first 10 percent of the scores, the second decile corresponds to the 20th percentile and includes the second 10 percent of the data, and so on.

Example 10.5: Community Physician's Clinic recorded the wait times for 20 patients. The wait times were (in minutes) as follows: 13, 3, 5, 12, 16, 7, 24, 6, 18, 14, 17, 4, 11, 8, 9, 15, 23, 10, 22, 19. Determine the 4th and 9th decile of the wait times.

1. Place the times in order:
   3, 4, 5, 6, 7, 8, 9, 10, 11, 12, 13, 14, 15, 16, 17, 18, 19, 22, 23, 24.
2. Determine which values represent the deciles by multiplying the number of values times 0.10 (10 percent):
   10 percent of 20 = 2—every two values is a decile.
3. The fourth decile is the 8th value (every 2 × 4 = 8) which is 10.
4. The ninth decile is the 18th value (every 2 × 9 = 18) which is 22.

Exercise 10.1

1. A pediatrician at the Community Physician's Clinic told a mother that her six-month-old child is in the 54th percentile in weight. This means that her child's weight is greater than or equal to 54 percent of all six-month-old children. True or false?
2. Use the information in the table that follows to create an Excel spreadsheet to determine the percentile for a score of 86.

Test Scores Out of 100 Points	
95	97
99	74
84	91
65	94
54	89
35	88
86	56
77	96
76	27
100	75
92	93

3. Use the information from University Hospital in the table that follows to create an Excel spreadsheet to answer the questions that follow.

University Hospital C-sections by Physician January–December 20XX	
Physician Number	**Number of C-sections**
101	3
202	7
303	27
305	33
401	5
407	8
508	1
518	12
629	9
710	2
911	4
912	18
933	22
944	15
975	20

   a. Which percentile is Dr. 975?
   b. Find the 60th percentile.

4. Dr. Sullivan, a new physician at Community Physician's Clinic, has acquired 20 new patients in the first month of his practice. Create an Excel spreadsheet to determine the quartiles of the distribution of the patients' weights.

New Patients Seen by Dr. Sullivan October 20XX	
Patient Number	**Weight**
892345	196
877654	207
764309	155
753254	185
912356	186
455656	192
232323	147
567815	209
875408	242
543465	307
872345	245
925627	232
647382	222

(*continued on next page*)

New Patients Seen by Dr. Sullivan October 20XX	
Patient Number	**Weight**
980753	150
765497	189
743952	195
867342	180
142849	175
745261	172
654811	165

Measures of Central Tendency

In summarizing data, it is often useful to have a single number that is representative of the typical value of a collection of data or specific population. Such numbers are customarily referred to as **measures of central tendency**. A common measure of central tendency is average or mean, which is the sum of a set of numbers divided by the number of data points. One of the most common examples of a mean or average in a healthcare facility involves average length of stay, or ALOS (average number of days from admission to discharge that patients stay in the hospital). The ALOS was discussed in detail in chapter 5, *Length of Stay*, and is discussed briefly in this chapter.

Three measures of central tendency are frequently used: mean, median, and mode. Each measure has advantages and disadvantages in describing a typical value.

Mean

The **mean** is a measure of central tendency that is determined by calculating the arithmetic average of the observations. It is common to use the term average to designate mean. It is computed by dividing the sum of all the scores (Σ) by the total number of scores (*N*). If a sample is used to estimate the mean, then the N is replaced by a lowercase n to denote a sample mean. The symbol $\bar{X}$ (pronounced "ex bar") is used to represent the mean in this formula:

$$\bar{X} = \frac{X_1 + X_2 + X_3 + \cdots + X_N}{N} = \frac{\sum X}{N}$$

Where $X_1, X_2, X_3 \ldots X_N$ are the observed values of the data.

Example 10.6: Seven hospital inpatients have the following lengths of stay: 2, 3, 4, 3, 5, 1, and 3 days. Determine the mean LOS for these patients. Round to one decimal place.

$$\bar{X} = \frac{2+3+4+3+5+1+3}{7} = \frac{21}{7} = 3.0 \; days$$

You may hear individuals refer to the average or mean as, "The average age is 10 to 20." This is the wrong use of this statistic. In this example, they are referring to a range of ages, which may be the desired expression in some instances. However, the average is only one value.
QUICK TIP

The mean is the most common measure of central tendency. One of its advantages is that it is easy to compute. It is used as the basis for a large proportion of statistical tests. One disadvantage of the mean is that it is sensitive to **outliers**, extreme statistical values that fall outside the normal range, and may distort its representation of the central tendency of a set of numbers.

Example 10.7: Determine the average weight for the following six women in a group who weighed 110, 115, 120, 122, 125, and 227 pounds. Round to one decimal place.

$$\bar{X} = \frac{110+115+120+122+125+227}{6} = \frac{819}{6} = 136.5 \; pounds$$

Notice that the mean weight for the women in example 10.7 is 136.5 pounds. This value is larger than all but one of the reported weights. The mean is influenced by the large outlier value of 227 pounds. In this situation, the median is a better measure of the central tendency of the distribution of the data.

Median

The **median** is the midpoint (center) of the distribution of values, or the point above and below which 50 percent of the values fall. Notice that this is also the definition of the second quartile. The median value is obtained by arranging the numerical observations in ascending or descending order and then determining the middle value. This may be the middle observation (if there is an odd number of values) or a point halfway between the two middle values (if there is an even number of values).

To arrive at the median in an even-numbered distribution, add the two middle values together and divide by two. When the two middle values are the same, the median is that value.

The median, second quartile, and 50th percentile are all terms used to describe the middle value in a set of data.

Example 10.8: Determine the median of the LOS values from example 10.6.

1. Sort the values in ascending order:
   1
   2
   3
   3 ← median (midpoint)
   3
   4
   5

2. There are 7 values, and the middle observation is the 4th value.
3. The median is 3.

Example 10.9: Determine the median weight of the women from example 10.7:

110
115
120

$\leftarrow$ median $\left(120 + 122 = \dfrac{242}{2} = 121\right)$

122
125
227

The median is 121. Since there is an even number of observations (6), the median is the average of the middle two values.

The advantage to using the median as a measure of central tendency is that it is unaffected by outliers. The value of 121 pounds is much more representative of the fact that five out of the six women weigh 125 pounds or less than the mean value of 136.5, as seen in the previous example.

The median is also often used in calculating LOS in long-term care. As discussed in chapter 5, a long-stay patient's discharge days are allocated to the period in which he or she is discharged. Sometimes this can give a distorted average, especially on a monthly (rather than annual) basis because of patients with extremely long lengths of stay.

Example 10.10: In March, a long-term care facility discharged 130 patients with a total LOS of 1,267 days. The LOS for one of the patients was 365 days. The ALOS for all 130 patients was 9.8 days ($\frac{1,267}{130} = 9.75$). If the stay of the one patient is removed from the total LOS, the ALOS becomes 6.99 or 7.0 days ($1,267 - 365 = \frac{902}{129} = 6.99$). Should one patient or a few patients in a population affect the average to this degree? Is the statistical computation meaningful for decision-making purposes? In this situation, the facility has two options:

- First, a notation can be made on the report that either the ALOS of 9.8 includes one patient who stayed 365 days or the ALOS of 7.0 excludes one patient who stayed 365 days. Both calculations can be made. Appropriate notes should be attached to the report to indicate the difference.

- Second, the computation using the median rather than the mean can be used. The individual LOSs would be arranged in numerical order from highest to lowest or vice versa.

Example 10.11. The list in table 10.3 includes the LOSs of 15 discharged patients. Create an Excel spreadsheet to calculate the mean and median LOS and age for this set of patients. Round to one decimal place. Which statistic is a better choice for the two distributions?

The median is the better choice because the two patients with long stays (21 and 28 days) cause the mean to over estimate the typical LOS.

Table 10.3.   LOSs of 15 discharged patients

Name	Age	Clinical Service	Admission Date	Length of Stay
Bertram	32	Medicine	6/01	4
Williams	22	Medicine	5/28	8
Capney	47	Medicine	6/01	4
Darcy	27	Medicine	5/08	28
Ediger	62	Surgery	6/01	4
Fitzroy	53	Medicine	5/31	5
Guilford	21	Obstetrics	6/03	2
Hansen	30	Obstetrics	6/01	4
Isaacs	76	Medicine	6/03	2
Jamison	35	Surgery	5/15	21
Kapowski	20	Obstetrics	6/03	2
Lawrence	50	Medicine	5/31	5
Bennett	41	Obstetrics	6/02	3
Oswald	14	Obstetrics	6/04	1
Petersen	48	Surgery	5/27	9
Total				**102**

Excel formula version:

	A	B	C	D	E
1	Name	Age	Clinical Service	Admission Date	Length of Stay
2	Bertram	32	Medicine	1-Jun	4
3	Williams	22	Medicine	28-May	8
4	Capney	47	Medicine	1-Jun	4
5	Darcy	27	Medicine	8-May	28
6	Ediger	62	Surgery	1-Jun	4
7	Fitzroy	53	Medicine	31-May	5
8	Guilford	21	Obstetrics	3-Jun	2
9	Hansen	30	Obstetrics	1-Jun	4
10	Isaacs	76	Medicine	3-Jun	2
11	Jamison	35	Surgery	15-May	21
12	Kapowski	20	Obstetrics	3-Jun	2
13	Lawrence	50	Medicine	31-May	5
14	Bennett	41	Obstetrics	2-Jun	3
15	Oswald	14	Obstetrics	4-Jun	1
16	Pertersen	48	Surgery	27-May	9
17	**Total**				102
18					
19	Mean	=AVERAGE(B2:B16)			=AVERAGE(E2:E16)
20	Median	=MEDIAN(B2:B16)			=MEDIAN(E2:E16)
21					

Excel calculated version:

	A	B	C	D	E
1	Name	Age	Clinical Service	Admission Date	Length of Stay
2	Bertram	32	Medicine	1-Jun	4
3	Williams	22	Medicine	28-May	8
4	Capney	47	Medicine	1-Jun	4
5	Darcy	27	Medicine	8-May	28
6	Ediger	62	Surgery	1-Jun	4
7	Fitzroy	53	Medicine	31-May	5
8	Guilford	21	Obstetrics	3-Jun	2
9	Hansen	30	Obstetrics	1-Jun	4
10	Isaacs	76	Medicine	3-Jun	2
11	Jamison	35	Surgery	15-May	21
12	Kapowski	20	Obstetrics	3-Jun	2
13	Lawrence	50	Medicine	31-May	5
14	Bennett	41	Obstetrics	2-Jun	3
15	Oswald	14	Obstetrics	4-Jun	1
16	Pertersen	48	Surgery	27-May	9
17	**Total**				102
18					
19	Mean	38.53			6.80
20	Median	35.00			4.00
21					

Mode

Mode is the third measure of central tendency presented in this text and is defined as the value that occurs most frequently in the data. In this sense, it is the value that is most typical. Its advantage is that it is the simplest of the measures of central tendency because it does not require any calculations. The example in table 10.3 shows that the mode is 4 because 4 is the most frequent value in the set.

While the mode is simple to use, there are disadvantages to using it. In the case of a small number of values, each value could occur only once and there would be no mode. Or, two values may be more common than others and you could have two or more modes.

The mode does not have to be numerical. If you ask every person in your class what his or her favorite food is and tally the answers, you will most likely find a mode or most frequently reported value.

QUICK
TIP

Example 10.12: Add another patient's LOS of 35 to example 10.6 and calculate the mean. median and mode with this additional value. The values are (1 2 3 3 3 4 5 35).

$$\bar{X} = \frac{2+3+4+3+5+1+3+35}{8} = \frac{56}{8} = 7.0 \ days$$

The median would be calculated as follows:

1
2
3
3
$\leftarrow$ median $\left(3+3 = \frac{6}{2} = 3\right)$
3
4
5
35

The median is 3, and the mode remains at 3.

This example shows that the median and the mode are not influenced by extreme values.

The mode is rarely used as a sole descriptive measure of central tendency because it may not be unique; there may be two or more modes. These are called bimodal (two modes) or multimodal (several modes) distributions.

Example 10.13: The following represents a collection of values of LOSs:

1
1
1
2
2
3
3
3
4
5
5
5
7
9

In this group of patients, the modes for the LOSs are 1, 3, and 5. The mode is the score that occurs most frequently; in this example, it occurred three times in 1, 3, and 5.

The choice of a measure of central tendency depends on the number of values and the nature of their distribution. Occasionally, the mean, median, and mode are identical. For statistical analyses, however, the mean is preferable, whenever possible, because it includes information from all observations. However, if the series of values contains a few that are unusually high or low, the median may represent the series better than the mean. The mode is often used in samples where the most typical value is preferred and when the data are non-numeric or categories.

Exercise 10.2

Complete the following exercises.

1. Fourteen patients have the following LOSs: 2, 6, 6, 4, 7, 18, 5, 5, 3, 8, 6, 7, 9, and 4. Calculate the mean, median, and mode. Round the mean to two decimal places.
2. A student's 10 scores on 10-point class quizzes include a 5, an 8, a 3, five 9s, a 7, and a 10. The student claims that her average grade on quizzes is 9 because most of her scores are 9s. Is this correct? Explain. Round the mean to one decimal place.
3. Fourteen patients have the following LOSs: 3, 4, 5, 2, 5, 17, 5, 3, 2, 6, 5, 4, 7, and 2. Calculate the mean, median, and mode. Round the mean to one decimal place.
4. An HIM supervisor timed his staff for 8 hours during the workday to determine the average number of inpatient records coded in 1 hour. Use the findings in the table that follows to create an Excel spreadsheet to calculate the mean, median, and mode records for each coding professional. Also, calculate the overall mean, median, and mode records for the coding section. Round to one decimal place.

Community Hospital HIM Department Number of Records Coded							
Coding Professional A		Coding Professional B		Coding Professional C		Coding Professional D	
Hour 1	3	Hour 1	3	Hour 1	5	Hour 1	4
Hour 2	4	Hour 2	4	Hour 2	6	Hour 2	4
Hour 3	6	Hour 3	6	Hour 3	3	Hour 3	3
Hour 4	3	Hour 4	1	Hour 4	5	Hour 4	4
Hour 5	2	Hour 5	4	Hour 5	4	Hour 5	5
Hour 6	5	Hour 6	6	Hour 6	4	Hour 6	6
Hour 7	4	Hour 7	3	Hour 7	2	Hour 7	2
Hour 8	4	Hour 8	4	Hour 8	5	Hour 8	1

5. The quality manager at Community Physician's Clinic is investigating a complaint that the wait times are too long at the clinic. She wishes to use the median to determine the wait times. Calculate the median and mean of the following wait times. Round the mean to one decimal place.

(In minutes): 12, 17, 11, 10, 9, 22, 18, 20, 8, 7, 6, 12, 12, 13

Measures of Variation

Measures of central tendency are not the only statistics used to summarize frequency distributions. A facility also may want to consider the spread of the distribution, also called the measure of variation. The measure of variation shows how widely the observations are spread out around the measure of central tendency. The mean gives a measure of central tendency of a list of numbers but tells nothing about the spread of the numbers in the list.

Example 10.14: Review the following three groups:

Group A	3	5	6	3	3
Group B	4	4	4	4	4
Group C	10	1	0	0	9

Each of these groups has a mean of $4(\frac{20}{5})$, and yet the amount of dispersion or variation within the groups is different. The measures of spread increase with greater variation in the values in the frequency distribution. The spread is equal to 0 when there is no variation; for example, when all the values in a frequency distribution are the same, as shown in group B.

Variability

Variability refers to the difference between each score and every other score in a frequency distribution. For example, if there are 100 scores, you would have to compute the difference between the first score and each of the 99 other scores, and then compute the difference between the second score and each of the 98 remaining scores, and so on. There would be 4,950 differences in all. A more feasible approach, which serves the purpose equally well, is to define statistics that summarize the differences of the various values in the data set.

Range

The **range** is the simplest measure of spread. It represents the difference between the largest and smallest values in a frequency distribution. In reviewing the three groups in the previous section on variability, the largest number in group A is 6 and the smallest is 3, a difference of 3. In group B, the difference is 0, and in group C, the difference is 10. Therefore, the range for group A is 3, the range for group B is 0, and the range for group C is 10.

Range has the advantage of being easy to compute, but it is far from optimal as a measure of variability because it is obviously affected by extreme values that are very different from other values in the data.

Exercise 10.3

Complete the following exercises.

1. Fourteen patients have the following LOSs: 3, 4, 5, 7, 19, 3, 2, 3, 1, 5, 3, 4, 7, and 2. What is the range of this distribution of numbers?

2. Find the range in the following sets:
   a. 2, 3, 7, 20, 6, 8
   b. 0, 1, 8, 20, 4, 7.65
   c. 85, 91, 132, 76, 35, 47

3. The range in a frequency distribution is 20. If the lowest value is 2, what is the highest value?

4. The range in a frequency distribution is 45. If the highest value is 109, what is the lowest value?

5. A group of women seen at a diabetes clinic weighed 140, 125, 210, 245, 202, 199, 173, and 197 pounds. What is the range?

Because the range is determined by two extremes only, a preferable measure of variability would include the distribution of all the values, not just those at the extremes. More informative measures of variation are variance and SD.

Variance

The **variance** of a frequency distribution is the square of the standard deviation or the average of the squared deviation from the mean. The symbol s^2 is used to show the variance of a sample. The formula for calculating the variance is as follows:

$$s^2 = \frac{(X_1 - \bar{X})^2 + (X_2 - \bar{X})^2 + (X_3 - \bar{X})^2 + \cdots (X_n - \bar{X})^2}{n-1}$$

Or, you could use the notation of

$$s^2 = \frac{\sum (X_i - \bar{X})^2}{n-1}$$

To calculate the variance, first determine the mean. Then, the squared deviations from the mean are calculated by subtracting the mean from each value in the distribution. The difference between the two values is squared $(X - \bar{X})^2$. The squared differences are summed and divided by $n - 1$. The definitions of the symbols used in the calculation of the sample variance are:

s^2 = variance

Σ = sum

X = value of a measure or observation

$\bar{X}$ = mean

n = number of values or observations in the sample

$n - 1$ is used in the denominator instead of n to adjust for the fact that the mean of the sample is used as an estimate of the mean of the underlying population.

The more the values in a distribution are different from one another, the greater the variance and SD. In Example 10.14, the variance in group B equals 0 because all the values are the same. Measures of variation equal 0 when there is no variation.

Example 10.15: Calculate the variance of a sample of 14 patients with the following LOSs: 2, 3, 3, 1, 4, 18, 3, 2, 1, 5, 4, 3, 6, and 1.

First, calculate the mean LOS:

$$\frac{56}{14} = 4 \text{ days}$$

Next, substitute the data values and sample mean into the formula for sample variance. The order of this computation is as follows:

1. Subtract the mean from each LOS score (enter result in column 3).
2. Square each result (enter result in column 4).
3. Add columns 3 and 4.
4. Divide column 4 by $(n - 1)$.

The variance is computed as follows:

$$s^2 = \frac{(2-4)^2 + (3-4)^2 + (3-4)^2 + (1-4)^2 + (4-4)^2 \text{ and so on}}{(14-1)} = \frac{240}{13} = 18.46$$

Column 1	Column 2	Column 3	Column 4
Patient	Length of Stay	LOS – Mean (4) $(X - \bar{X})$	(LOS – Mean)^2 $(X - \bar{X})^2$
1	2	–2	4
2	3	–1	1
3	3	–1	1
4	1	–3	9
5	4	0	0
6	18	14	196
7	3	–1	1
8	2	–2	4

(*continued on next page*)

Column 1	Column 2	Column 3	Column 4
Patient	Length of Stay	LOS – Mean (4) $(X - \bar{X})$	(LOS – Mean)² $(X - \bar{X})^2$
9	1	–3	9
10	5	1	1
11	4	0	0
12	3	–1	1
13	6	2	4
14	1	–3	9
Total	56	0	240

In this example, the size of the variance is influenced by the one LOS of 18 days. The more the values in a distribution are different from each other, the greater the variance.

 The sum of the deviations from the mean is always equal to zero. Therefore, by squaring the differences from the mean, the negative and positive deviations do not cancel each other out. When they are squared, negative as well as positive values become positive.

QUICK
TIP

Standard Deviation

The **SD** is a measure of variability that describes the deviation from the mean of a frequency distribution in the original units of measurement. It is computed as the square root of the variance. As such, it can be more easily interpreted as a measure of variation since it is measured in the same units as the data. For example, in example 10.15, the units associated with the variance is squared days. That is not a unit of analysis that is easily interpreted. Instead, in practice, the SD = 4.3 days (the square root of 18.46) is reported. If the SD is small, there is less dispersion around the mean. If the SD is large, there is greater dispersion around the mean.

The formula for calculating SD is

$$SD = s = \sqrt{s^2} = \sqrt{\frac{\sum(X_i - \bar{X})^2}{n-1}}$$

 The square root of a number is that number whose square is the number. The square of a number is that number multiplied by itself. For example, the square root of 9 is 3 (3 × 3 = 9).

QUICK
TIP

Exercise 10.4

The following sample report from a cancer registry shows the weights for 20 males with adenocarcinoma of the rectum. Create an Excel spreadsheet to calculate the mean, variance, and SD of the values. Round to one decimal place.

Patient	Weight lbs. (X)
1	142
2	148
3	151
4	155

(continued on next page)

Patient	Weight lbs. (X)
5	155
6	158
7	164
8	165
9	170
10	173
11	175
12	175
13	175
14	183
15	185
16	186
17	189
18	193
19	198
20	200

Normal Distribution and Other Curves

To understand the concept of distributions and variation, it is helpful to learn about what mathematicians call normal distribution of data. A **normal distribution** of data means that most of the values in a set of data are close to the "average" and relatively few values tend to one extreme or the other, creating a bell-shaped distribution curve as presented in figure 10.1.

The SD is a statistic that tells how closely all the observations are clustered around the mean in a set of data. When the examples are closely gathered and the bell-shaped curve is steep, the SD is small. When the examples are spread apart and the bell-shaped curve is relatively flat, the SD is relatively large.

Therefore, normal distribution means that if the variable of a particular characteristic for every member of the population were measured, the frequency distribution would display a normal or bell-shaped pattern, with most of the measurements near the center of the frequency. It also would be possible to accurately describe the population, with respect to a variable, by calculating the mean and SD of the values.

The normal distribution has some useful properties:

1. Approximately 2/3 (actually 68.2 percent) of the data is within one SD of the mean.
2. 95.4 percent of the data is within two SDs of the mean.
3. 99.7 percent of the data is within three SDs of the mean.

Example 10.16: Continuing with the LOS data used in example 10.15, the mean is 4 and the variance is 18.46. Thus, the SD is 4.3 (the square root of 18.46 = 4.30). If the LOS data followed a normal distribution, what range should contain 95.4 percent of the data?

Based on the properties of the normal distribution, 95.4 percent of the data should be in the range of the mean minus 2 SD and the mean plus 2 SD.

±2 SD includes values ranging from −4.6 to 12.6 (to get these figures, add 2 SD to the mean of 4, so ±2 SD = 4 − 8.6 to 4 + 8.6 = −4.6 to 12.6).

Not all distributions are symmetrical or have a bell-shaped curve. Some curves are skewed; that is, their numbers do not fall in the middle but, rather, on one end of the curve. **Skewness** is the horizontal stretching of a frequency distribution to one side or the other so that one tail is longer than the other. The direction of skewness is on the side of the long tail. Thus, if the longer tail is on the right, the curve is skewed to the right. If the longer tail is on the left, the curve is skewed to the left. (See figures 10.2 and 10.3.)

An example of skewness may occur in LOSs when one or more of a group of patients has an unusually long LOS. An unusually long LOS would raise the mean and thus result in a positive skewness.

Although less common than the normal, positive, and negative skewed curves, you may come across other types of curves in the graphical representation of data. Some examples of the other types of curves include a bimodal distribution, multimodal distribution, a J-shaped curve, and a reverse J-shaped curve, which are shown in figures 10.4 to 10.7.

Figure 10.1. Example of normal distribution

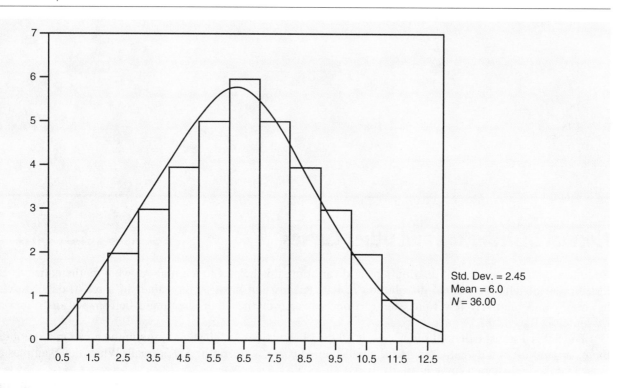

Std. Dev. = 2.45
Mean = 6.0
N = 36.00

Figure 10.2. Example of a curve skewed to the right (positive skew)

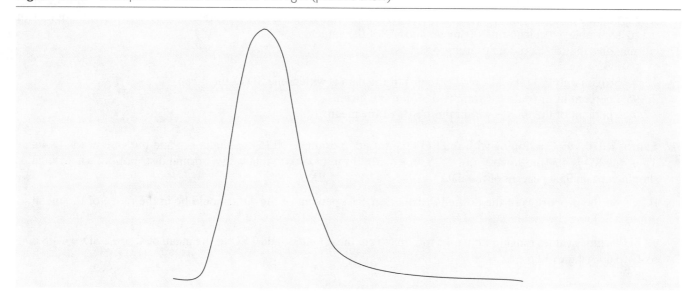

Figure 10.3. Example of a curve skewed to the left (negative skew)

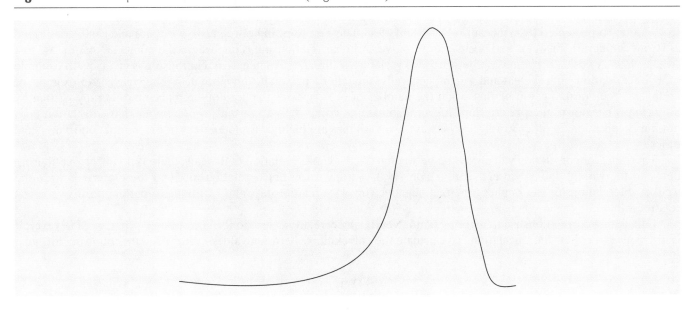

Figure 10.4. Bimodal

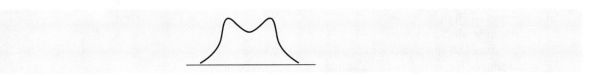

Figure 10.5. Multimodal

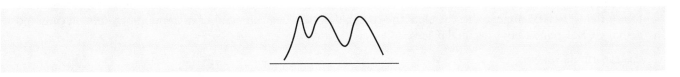

Figure 10.6. J-shaped

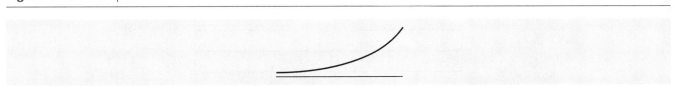

Figure 10.7. Reverse J-shaped

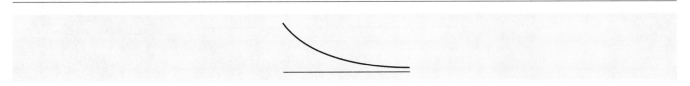

Correlation

Correlation (represented by r) measures the extent of a linear relationship between two variables and can be described as strong, moderate, or weak, and positive or negative. A linear relationship is one where the points lie on or close to a straight line. A positive relationship between two variables is direct, and a negative relationship is inverse. An example of a direct relationship is height and weight; generally, the taller a person is, the more he or she weighs. An example of an inverse relationship could be that when the number of prescriptions for hormone replacement therapy written by physicians goes down, the prescriptions for antidepressants go up. It is important to remember that correlation does not imply causation; in other words, just because two variables are highly correlated does not mean that one causes the other.

The value for correlation will always be between –1 and +1. A correlation of 0 means there is no linear relationship between the variables. The closer r is to –1 or +1, the stronger the linear relationship, and the closer r is to 0, the weaker the relationship. –1 implies a perfect negative (inverse) relationship, and +1 implies a perfect positive (direct) relationship.

Calculating correlations is intensive by hand. Nearly all correlations are done via computer programs. However, it is instructive to review the calculation. To calculate the correlation r between values x and y, use the following formula:

$$r = \frac{\Sigma xy - \dfrac{\Sigma x \Sigma y}{n}}{\sqrt{\left(\Sigma x^2 - \dfrac{(\Sigma x)^2}{n}\right)\left(\Sigma y^2 - \dfrac{(\Sigma y)^2}{n}\right)}}$$

Where:

Σx is the sum of all the x values.
Σy is the sum of all the y values.
Σxy is the sum of all the x values multiplied by the y values.
Σx^2 is the sum of the squares of all x values.
Σy^2 is the sum of the squares of all y values.
n is the number of subjects in the group.

Example 10.17: In this example, x = the number of phone calls per week to make an appointment to see a new psychologist; y = the number of actual visits to the psychologist plus any walk-ins. Create an Excel spreadsheet to use the CORREL function to calculate the correlation between the number of appointment phone calls and actual visits. Round to two decimal places.

Excel formula version:

	A	B
1	x (phone calls per week)	y (visits)
2	5	1
3	6	4
4	9	8
5	11	9
6	14	14
7	15	16
8	21	18
9		
10	=CORREL(A2:A8,B2:B8)	

Excel calculated version:

	A	B	C
1	x (phone calls per week)	y (visits)	
2	5	1	
3	6	4	
4	9	8	
5	11	9	
6	14	14	
7	15	16	
8	21	18	
9			
10	0.97		

In this example, $r = 0.97$ is a very strong positive correlation. Although causation cannot be implied, it can still be said that there is a strong positive linear relationship between the number of appointments made and the number of actual visits made with the psychologist. This means that appointments increase as phone calls increase.

Calculations for variance, SD, and correlation are not usually part of the health information technician's day-to-day activities; however, it is important to be familiar with these concepts. For example, you may pick up a journal article, listen to a speaker who is discussing these calculations, or be asked to validate the data. An understanding of them may be necessary in order to communicate this information with others.

Chapter 10   Matching Quiz

Match the definitions with the terms.

Definitions:

a. Horizontal stretching of a frequency distribution to one side or the other so that one tail is longer than the other

b. Midpoint (center) of the distribution of values, or the point above and below which 50 percent of the values fall

c. Describes a population

d. The difference between each score and every other score in a frequency distribution

e. An extreme statistical value that falls outside the normal range

f. A measure of central tendency that is determined by calculating the arithmetic average of the observations in a frequency distribution

g. The fourth equal part of a distribution

h. Distance or extent between possible extremes

i. A characteristic or property that may take on different values

j. A measure of central tendency that consists of the most frequent observation in a frequency distribution

Terms:

1. _____ Median

2. _____ Mean

3. _____ Mode

4. _____ Range

5. _____ Variability

6. _____ Descriptive statistics

7. _____ Quartile

8. _____ Variable

9. _____ Outlier

10. _____ Skewness

Chapter 10   Review

1. Your medical terminology instructor listed the following grades for the class out of a 75-point test:

    34, 36, 41, 43, 44, 49, 50, 55, 57, 60, 64, 66, 67, 67, 67, 68, 68, 69, 70, 73

    a. Find the 90th percentile.

    b. Your score was 64; what is your percentile?

2. Create an Excel spreadsheet using the list of number of discharges each day in September. Calculate the mean, median, mode, and range. Round the mean and median to one decimal point.

University Hospital Number of Discharge Days June 20XX					
Day	**No. of Discharges**	**Day**	**No. of Discharges**	**Day**	**No. of Discharges**
1	33	11	63	21	54
2	21	12	70	22	57
3	42	13	62	23	22
4	40	14	70	24	27
5	43	15	44	25	43
6	50	16	40	26	44
7	61	17	28	27	61
8	56	18	43	28	63
9	62	19	51	29	67
10	53	20	35	30	56

3. Use the information in the table that follows, create an Excel spreadsheet to calculate the ALOS, median LOS, and range for Community Nursing Center. The discharge date is June 2, 2019. Round the ALOS to one decimal place.

Community Nursing Center Discharge Report June 2, 2019		
Patients	**Admission Date**	**LOS**
1	January 2, 2019	
2	January 10, 2019	
3	February 8, 2019	
4	February 10, 2019	
5	February 26, 2019	

(continued on next page)

Community Nursing Center Discharge Report June 2, 2019		
Patients	**Admission Date**	**LOS**
6	March 1, 2019	
7	March 6, 2019	
8	March 12, 2019	
9	March 15, 2019	
10	April 1, 2019	
11	April 15, 2019	
12	May 3, 2019	
13	May 5, 2019	
14	May 6, 2019	
15	May 18, 2019	

4. The following table shows the LOSs for a sample of 11 discharged patients. Use the data in the table to calculate the mean, median, and mode, and then answer questions d and e. Round to one decimal place.

   a. Mean

   b. Median

   c. Mode

   d. What value is affecting the mean and SD of this distribution?

   e. Which is the best measure of central tendency for this data set?

Patient	Length of Stay
1	1
2	3
3	5
4	3
5	2
6	29
7	3
8	4
9	2
10	1
11	2

5. When two variables are correlated, it means that one is the cause of the other. True or false?

6. Dr. Anderson, a new pediatrician at Community Physician's Clinic, wants to study his new patient's growth charts to determine if they are within the guidelines for weight for age. His last 10 six-month-old male infants showed weights of 13.2, 14.6, 15.8, 16.5, 18.5, 12.1, 15.4, 16.1, 18.0, 13.2. What is the mean, median, and range of infant weights he is seeing? Round to one decimal place.

7. Dr. Anderson wants to follow the guidelines that recommend six-month-old infants should weigh 16.5 pounds. In what percentile is the 12.1-pound infant? Use the values presented in number 6.

8. A coding supervisor recorded the following salaries for the seven coding professionals in her HIM department section as \$15.25, \$16.72, \$17.23, \$15.34, \$15.93, \$17.05, and \$16.21. Find the first and third quartile (Q_1 and Q_3).

9. Last month, 10 patients between the ages of 11 and 13 were seen in their pediatrician's clinic. Their heights were recorded as 51, 57, 60, 51, 52, 49, 53, 57, 61, and 50 inches. Determine the mean, median, and mode. Round to one decimal place.

10. Community Physician's Clinic is examining the number of patients who make appointments by email and if they actually keep the appointment date and time. They collected the following information for the past month:

Week 1	Number of Appointments Made by Email	Number of Appointments Kept
1	10	9
2	8	8
3	6	6
4	12	11

Use an Excel spreadsheet to determine if there is a correlation between these variables. Round to two decimal places.

11. Use the information in the previous table to complete this sentence: The administrator of the clinic wants to have everyone make appointments by email instead of by telephone. However, the HIM professional tells him _____.

   a. This is a causal relationship and proves that patients who make appointments by email are more likely to keep the appointment.

   b. This is not a causal relationship; there is only a positive relationship between making the appointment by email and keeping the appointment.

   c. This is just a somewhat good correlation and may not be positive.

   d. This is a poor correlation and does not necessarily mean that appointments will be kept in the future.

12. A graph with a bell-shaped curve is referred to as having a _____.

   a. Normal distribution

   b. Bimodal distribution

   c. Left skewed distribution

   d. Right skewed distribution

13. When a distribution is skewed to the right, this means it_____.

   a. Has a positive skew

   b. Has a negative skew

   c. Has no skew

   d. Is multiskewed

14. Use the information in the table that follows, create an Excel spreadsheet to determine the mean and median age and range of ages of the patients discharged. Round the mean to one decimal place.

LOSs of 15 discharged patients				
Name	Age	Clinical Service	Admission Date	LOS
Bertram	32	Medicine	6/01	4
Williams	22	Medicine	5/28	8
Capney	47	Medicine	6/01	4
Darcy	27	Medicine	5/08	28
Ediger	62	Surgery	6/01	4
Fitzroy	53	Medicine	5/31	5
Guilford	21	Obstetrics	6/03	2
Hansen	30	Obstetrics	6/01	4
Isaacs	76	Medicine	6/03	2
Jamison	35	Surgery	5/15	21
Kapowski	20	Obstetrics	6/03	2
Lawrence	50	Medicine	5/31	5
Bennett	41	Obstetrics	6/02	3
Oswald	14	Obstetrics	6/04	1
Petersen	48	Surgery	5/27	9
Total				102

15. Decide whether the following statements are likely to have a positive or negative correlation:

   1. Positive correlation
   2. Negative correlation

   a. _____ People who suffer from depression have higher rates of suicide than those who do not.

   b. _____ The more absences you have in class, the more your grades will decrease.

   c. _____ The more you exercise your muscles, the stronger they become.

   d. _____ The more iron that an anemic patient takes, the less tired he will be.

   e. _____ As your attendance to your studies decreases, your achievement drops.

Presentation of Data

Learning Objectives

At the conclusion of this chapter, you should be able to do the following:

- Explain, differentiate, and apply the following terms: nominal, ordinal, interval, and ratio, and discrete and continuous data
- Distinguish between tables and the following graphs: bar graphs, pie charts, line graphs, histograms, frequency polygons, pictograms, and scatter diagrams, and choose the appropriate graph to use
- Create tables and graphs to display statistical information
- Prepare the basic elements of a report

Key Terms

Bar chart
Bar graph
Categorical data
Continuous data
Discrete data
Frequency polygon
Histogram

Interval data
Line graph
Nominal data
Ordinal data
Pictogram
Pie chart
Pie graph

Ratio data
Run chart
Scales of measurement
Scatter diagram
Table

Types of Data

A set of raw data may not provide an end user (such as an administrator, a physician, or a health information management [HIM] professional) with information that can be easily interpreted. As a result, additional data manipulation is needed. Descriptive statistics are the most common type of statistics that the HIM professional will encounter or be responsible for producing. Descriptive statistics describe populations, which can refer to patients, medical services, nursing units, or hospital departments. As mentioned in chapter 10, *Descriptive Statistics in Healthcare,* these statistics provide an overview of the general features of a set of data. The statistics can assume a number of different forms, the most common being tables and graphs. However, before choosing the appropriate method for displaying a set of data, it is important to determine whether the data are categorical or numerical.

Categorical Data

Categorical data are data that are collected and then sorted or divided into groups. There are two types or **scales of measurement** of categorical data: nominal and ordinal.

Nominal Data

A **nominal data** point is the lowest level of measurement. The word *nominal* means "pertaining to a name." In the nominal scale, observations are organized into categories in which there is no recognition of sequential order. Examples of nominal data include true or false, male or female, types of insurance carriers, or patient occupations. Often, numbers are used to represent categories. For example, male may be listed as 1 and female as 2; or persons may be grouped according to blood type, where 1 represents type A; 2, type B; 3, type AB; and 4, type O. The sequence of the values is not important. The numbers simply serve as labels for some piece of information and are used for convenience only.

Averages cannot be computed on nominal-level data. Nominal items may have numbers assigned to them and may appear to be a numeric values; however, they are not. For example, an average blood type of 2.3 for a given population is meaningless. Instead of calculating the mean for nominal data, the proportion (or "how many") that falls into each category is reported.

> **Example 11.1:** The following types of healthcare payment categories are an example of nominal data. Notice that the payment categories are represented by numbers, but the value of "Self-pay" is not necessarily higher than "Medicare." The numbers are simply category labels and therefore nominal data.
>
> **Payment Categories**
>
> 1   Medicare
>
> 2   Medicaid
>
> 3   Blue Cross
>
> 4   Other Commercial Insurance
>
> 5   Self-pay
>
> 6   Other

Ordinal Data

Ordinal data are types of data where the values are in ordered categories. The word *ordinal* means "to put something in order." On the ordinal scale, only the order of the numbers is meaningful, not the value of numbers themselves. This is because the intervals or distances between categories are not necessarily equal. For example, head injuries may be classified according to level of severity, where 4 is fatal; 3, severe; 2, moderate; and 1, minor.

A natural order exists among the groupings, with the largest number representing the most serious level of injury. However, the order could be reversed; there is no hard-and-fast rule. There is no reason why 1 could not represent the fatal injury and 4, the minor injury. In addition, the distance between a fatal and a severe injury may not necessarily be the same as the distance between a moderate and a minor injury.

> **Example 11.2:** The following list shows how this works in a classification of brain injury:
>
> 1   Minor
>
> 2   Moderate
>
> 3   Severe
>
> 4   Fatal

Another good example of ordinal data is the Likert scale used in many surveys: 1 = strongly disagree; 2 = disagree; 3 = neither agree nor disagree; 4 = agree; 5 = strongly agree. In this example, there is a natural order to the values 1 through 5; however, 1 could just as easily be "strongly agree" and 5, "strongly disagree."

Numeric Data

There are two scales of measurement for numeric data: ratio and interval. Within the two scales of measurement for numeric data, there are two types: discrete data and continuous data.

The categories in categorical data may be represented by number, but they are not considered numeric variables for the purposes of summarizing or analyzing. For example, severity levels 1 to 4 are represented by numbers, but it would not be appropriate to average them because they are labels for categories. Patients at severity level 4 are not twice as severely ill than those at level 2. This is a common mistake made in the field of healthcare statistics.

Interval Data

Interval data is a type of data that represents observations that can be measured on an evenly distributed scale beginning at a point other than true zero. The data include units of equal size, such as intelligence quotient (IQ) results. There is no true zero point. The most important characteristic is that the intervals between values are equal. An example of interval scale is time. Time is measured in terms of 24 hours in a day. The time between each hour is the same. For example, there are 60 minutes between 1:00 a.m. and 2:00 a.m. and between 5:00 p.m. and 6:00 p.m.

Example 11.3: Temperature is another example of interval data. The difference between 70 degrees and 71 degrees Fahrenheit is the equivalent to the difference between 75 and 76 degrees. Temperature has no zero point. The temperature could be 0 degrees, but that does not mean there is no temperature—only that it is really cold.

Ratio Data

Ratio data or scale is the highest level of measurement. On the ratio scale, there is a defined unit of measure, a real zero point, and the intervals between successive values are equal. Ratio data may be displayed by units of equal size placed on a scale starting with zero and thus can be manipulated mathematically, such as 0, 5, 10, 15, and 20. The concepts of "twice as much" or "half as much" have meaning in ratio data.

Example 11.4: An example of the ratio scale is age. The difference between two consecutive years would be the same (the difference between age 1 and 3 is two years; the difference between age 55 and 57 is two years, and so on). There is a "zero point" in that zero would mean an absence of age or birth; and someone who is 100 years old is twice as old as someone who is 50 years old.

Exercise 11.1

Community Hospital Discharges by Gender Annual Statistics, 20XX	
Male patients	1,203
Female patients	1,235

1. What example of scales of measurement is depicted in the table above?

2. Is it accurate to state that a temperature of 80 degrees Fahrenheit is twice as hot as 40 degrees Fahrenheit?

3. If a physician's office saw 50 patients yesterday and 100 patients today, is it correct to state that twice as many patients were seen today as yesterday?

4. Your health information instructor reported that on the last test given, 5 students received an A, 10 received a B, 3 received a C, 1 received a D, and no one received an F. What example of scales of measurement was given?

5. A physician's clinic conducted a survey to determine the level of patient satisfaction with various departments in the clinic. What type of scale is the following survey item?

> The information clerk at the clinic gave me the correct directions to find the department I was looking for. Please answer this question on a scale from 1 to 5 where 1 = strongly disagree and 5 = strongly agree.

Discrete Data

Discrete data are typically whole numbers; that is, they can have only a finite number of specified values. The number of children in a family is an example of discrete data. A family can have two or three children but cannot have 2.25 or 3.5 children. The numbers represent actual measurable quantities or counts rather than labels or categories.

Other examples of discrete data include the number of motor vehicle accidents in a particular community, the number of times a woman has given birth, the number of new cases of cancer in your state within the past five years, and the number of beds available in your hospital.

In discrete data, a natural order exists among the possible data values. In the example of the number of times a woman has given birth, a larger number indicates that she has had more children; the difference between one and two births is the same as the difference between four and five; and the number of births is restricted to whole numbers (a woman cannot give birth 2.3 times).

Continuous Data

Continuous data represent measurable quantities but are not restricted to certain specified values. A variable that is continuous can take on a fractional value. For example, a patient's temperature may be 102.6° Fahrenheit. Another example is height. One could say that someone is approximately 6 feet tall, refine it to 5 feet 10 inches, and refine it still further to 5 feet 10.5 inches. Age is yet another example. A person may have been 20 years old on your last birthday, but now the person would be 20 plus some part of another year.

The only limiting factor for a continuous observation is the degree of accuracy with which it can be measured. For analysis, continuous data often are converted to a range that acts as a category. For example, age can be categorized in ranges (0 to 20, 21 to 40, and so on).

Data Display

Data display is critical to data analysis because it reveals patterns and behaviors. When preparing a statistical report, the user must define its objectives and scope:

- What information is needed?
- What information do you want your audience to know?
- What information is available?
- Are the data collected routinely by the facility, or must additional data be collected?

If the purpose requires frequencies, percentages, or relationships among variables, the data may be presented in the form of a table or a graph. Basically, statistical tables are used for summarizing data; they simply list values into rows and columns and do not easily capture the audience's attention. On the other hand, graphs and charts can present data for quick visualization of relationships.

Tables

A **table** is an orderly arrangement of values that groups data into rows and columns. Almost any type of quantitative information can be grouped into tables. Columns allow you to read data up and down, and rows allow you to read data across. The columns and rows should be labeled. Many word-processing, spreadsheet, and database software programs help in the creation of tables. In table 11.1, variables arranged in columns across the page identify the individual patient name, age, clinical service, and length of stay. Each row represents one patient.

Table 11.1. Community Medical Center analysis showing patients discharged

Community Hospital Discharges 12/1/20XX			
Name	**Age**	**Clinical Service**	**Length of Stay**
Smith	5	Surgical	1
Valdez	22	Obstetrical	1
Chu	26	Obstetrical	2
MacDuff	18	Obstetrical	3
Johnson	10	Surgical	7
O'Brien	80	Surgical	8
Lewandowski	35	Surgical	11
Jones	52	Medical	15
Shultz	69	Medical	37
Martini	49	Medical	42

Source: Community Medical Center.

There are a number of advantages to using tables, including the following:

- More information can be presented.
- Exact values can be included to retain precision.
- Supportive details can be provided.
- Less work and fewer costs are required in the preparation.

The essential components of a table include the following:

- **Table number:** Use table numbers in a professional report to identify the table referenced in the body of the report.
- **Title:** The title must explain as simply as possible what is contained in the table. The title should answer these questions:
  - What are the data? For example, are these percentages or frequencies?
  - Who? Whom is the table about? For instance, are these male or female patients, a certain service, or a type of disease?
  - Where? For example, is this your hospital, the US, or your state?
  - When? What is the time period?
- **Headnote:** A headnote is a short explanatory note that applies to the values in the table, just under the title. Use a smaller print for this value. For example, if you were reporting data that were in the millions, you could place this in the headnote as "In Millions" unless you include it in the title.
- **Caption:** This refers to the headings of the columns. They should be brief and self-explanatory.
- **Stubs:** The categories (the left-hand column of a table).
- **Body or Cells:** The information formed by intersecting columns and rows. Data are entered into the cells.
- **Source footnote:** Located at the bottom of a table. This may include the source for any factual data or contain explanatory notes.

Table 11.2 illustrates the essential components of a table. Table 11.3 shows a sample table with the completed components.

Table 11.2.   Essential components of a table

Title (Headnote)			
	Caption	**Caption**	**Caption**
Stub	Cell	Cell	Cell
Stub	Cell	Cell	Cell
Stub	Cell	Cell	Cell

Source footnote:

Table 11.3.   Lung cancer by age and gender at Community Hospital, 20XX

Community Hospital Lung Cancer by Age and Gender Annual Statistics, 20XX		
Age, years	**Male**	**Female**
≤ 30	1	0
31–40	2	1
41–50	2	1
51–60	10	10
61–70	42	44
71+	29	27
Total	86	83

Although these rules are important in the construction of tables, it is more important to use good judgment. Check the table to ensure it is logical and self-explanatory. Remember to present the data in a format that illustrates a specific idea.

When reviewing a table, ask the following questions to be sure it is complete:
Are headings specific and understandable for every column and row?
QUICK TIP   *Are sources identified, if appropriate?*
Do totals add up in columns and rows? Is the table easy to read?

Frequency Distribution Tables

As discussed in chapter 10, a frequency distribution shows the values that a variable can take, and the number of observations associated with each value. A variable is a characteristic or property that may take on different values. For example, third-party payers, discharge service, and admission day are examples of variables. An example of a frequency table for the number of patients admitted on each day of the week is presented in table 11.4.

A frequency distribution table also may show the proportion; that is, the proportion of patients admitted on any of the days. To determine this, the value is divided by the total. The sum of the proportions should always equal 1.00.

Table 11.4. Report illustrating sample frequency distribution table

Sample Frequency Distribution for Admission Day June 20XX	
Day of the Week	**No. of Patients Admitted**
Sunday	20
Monday	29
Tuesday	28
Wednesday	12
Thursday	13
Friday	22
Saturday	8
Total	**132**

Example 11.5: The Utilization Resource Committee is interested in knowing the admission days for patients in your hospital. To construct a frequency distribution, you would list the days of the week and then enter the observations or number of patients admitted on the corresponding day of the week. Table 11.4 illustrates what this would look like. Create an Excel spreadsheet to add a column representing the proportion of patients admitted on each day of the week.

Excel—formula version

	A	B	C
1	Sample Frequency Distribution for Admission Day		
2	June 20XX		
3	Day of the Week	No. of Patients Admitted	Proportion of Patients Admitted
4	Sunday	20	=B4/B$11
5	Monday	29	=B5/B$11
6	Tuesday	28	=B6/B$11
7	Wednesday	12	=B7/B$11
8	Thursday	13	=B8/B$11
9	Friday	22	=B9/B$11
10	Saturday	8	=B10/B$11
11	**Total**	**132**	**=B11/B$11**

Excel—calculated version

	A	B	C
1	Sample Frequency Distribution for Admission Day		
2	June 20XX		
3	Day of the Week	No. of Patents Admitted	Proportion of admitted patients
4	Sunday	20	0.15
5	Monday	29	0.22
6	Tuesday	28	0.21
7	Wednesday	12	0.09
8	Thursday	13	0.10
9	Friday	22	0.17
10	Saturday	8	0.06
11	**Total**	**132**	**1.00**
12			

Table 11.5 shows a frequency distribution table of the prevalence of asthma nationally in 2017. The table includes the prevalence number in thousands as well as the percentage of people in that demographic category with asthma. Notice in the age group breakout that the number of people with asthma is the highest in the 35 to 64 years group, but the percentage with current asthma is highest in the 5 to 14 years group. This is because the population is larger in the 35 to 64 years group than the 5 to 14 years group. Standardizing by the size of the population allows the user to compare the rates as well as the total number.

Table 11.5.   Report illustrating frequency distribution

National Current Asthma Prevalence (2017)		
Characteristic*	**Number with Current Asthma (in thousands)**	**Percent with Current Asthma**
Total	25,191	7.9
Child (Age <18 years)	6,182	8.4
Adult (Age 18+ years)	19,009	7.7
All Age Groups		
0–4 years	869	4.4
5–14 years	4,010	9.7
15–19 years	2,020	9.4
20–24 years	1,498	7.3
25–34 years	3,311	7.6
35–64 years	10,036	8.1
65+ years	3,447	7

*Numbers within selected characteristics may not sum to total due to rounding
Source: CDC 2019a.

Table 11.6. Report illustrating frequency distribution

	Males				**Females**			
2014 Surgeon General's Report								
Smoking-Attributable Mortality by Gender, United States, 1965–2014								
Disease	**1965–1999**	**2000–2004**	**2005–2009**	**2010–2014**	**1965–1999**	**2000–2004**	**2005–2009**	**2010–2014**
Total cancers	3,091,600	522,360	501,500	501,500	1,053,700	281,880	317,000	317,000
Total cardiovascular and metabolic diseases	3,853,200	395,700	478,000	478,000	1,685,800	246,790	325,000	325,000
Total pulmonary diseases	1,440,700	268,980	291,000	291,000	715,800	247,720	274,500	274,500
Perinatal conditions	54,200	2,230	2,910	2,910	40,200	1,660	2,160	2,160
Residential fires	41,930	2,080	1,680	1,680	33,280	1,600	1,420	1,420
Total secondhand smoke	853,690	156,940	117,630	117,630	490,310	90,060	88,790	88,790

Source: HHS 2014.

Table 11.6 shows a frequency distribution table of deaths attributed to smoking by gender in the US from 1965 to 2013.

To display discrete or continuous data in the form of a frequency distribution table, the range of values of the observations must be broken down into a series of distinct groups that do not overlap. For example, when arranging a frequency distribution table by patient age, age ranges should not be listed as 1 to 10, 10 to 20, 20 to 30, 30 to 40, and so on because a patient could be placed in two categories if he were age 20: the 10-to-20 age range and the 20-to-30 age range. Thus, age ranges should be listed as 1 to 10, 11 to 20, 21 to 30, 31 to 40, and so on.

Notice the years in table 11.6. They do not overlap each other; 1965 to 1999, then the next group is 2000 to 2004, and so on.

Summarizing the data involves setting up categories and counting the number of cases that fall into each category, thereby creating a frequency distribution. Following are some general rules for choosing the classes or categories into which the data are to be grouped and the range of each:

- Use between 5 and 15 categories. However, the choice depends mostly on the number of values to be grouped.
- Define all categories. Choose categories that cover the smallest and largest values and do not produce gaps between categories.
- The categories should be mutually exclusive where each observation is grouped into one—and only one—category. Avoid successive classes that overlap or have common values.
- Whenever possible, make the classes cover equal ranges (or intervals) of values. These ranges also should be made up of numbers that are easy to work with.
- A table should be able to stand alone; meaning, the audience should be able to review the table and understand it without supporting information.

Example 11.6: The table that follows lists the patients seen last month at Community Hospital with their age and cholesterol reading. Use an Excel spreadsheet to create a table using common age categories and these ranges for cholesterol.

		Community Hospital Cholesterol Readings, October 20XX Desirable ≤ 199 Borderline High 200–239 High ≥ 240						
Age	**Cholesterol**	**Age**	**Cholesterol**	**Age**	**Cholesterol**	**Age**	**Cholesterol**
14	118	44	138	38	165	56	185
80	139	47	204	18	142	20	200
42	187	48	236	62	139	45	241
37	201	25	186	37	202	63	175
23	107	56	201	32	207	70	188
24	109	47	198	17	157	42	239
67	132	20	210	55	238	55	175
55	235	43	248	13	134	61	168
52	185	50	137	44	239	53	173
52	192	34	188	64	165	41	238
47	144	38	245	70	172	60	180
42	158	75	175	44	245	30	207
37	160	55	207	65	187	62	185
33	155	69	192	51	248	49	207
39	221	31	196	43	240	39	147
34	244	51	147	51	188	53	155
75	186	63	200	50	203	46	246
81	160	18	137	20	145	43	222
79	154	37	245	72	175	26	147
67	154	43	256	39	200	46	201
50	192	44	188	19	145	60	152
53	188	52	200	63	145	35	150
26	137	51	147	36	176	53	215
24	140	19	132	33	185	60	165
22	138	73	147	16	137	63	168

Note: This example will introduce functionality in Excel not previously used in this text.

Step 1: Create the cholesterol categories. This may be completed using a number of different methods in Excel. We will use the simplest method here. It is multistep, but much easier to follow than some of the other methods.

a. Copy the data so that there is one column for age and one for cholesterol.

b. Sort the table by cholesterol value.

c. Create a column called "Cholesterol Category" in column C.

d. Copy the term "Desirable <= 199" for each row with cholesterol <= 199.

e. Copy the term "Borderline High 200–239" for each row with cholesterol between 200 and 239.

f. Copy the term "High ≥ 240" for each row with cholesterol greater than or equal to 240.

Step 2: Create the age categories.

a. Sort the data by age value.

b. Label column D as "Age Category."

c. Ages range from 13 to 81; suggest using 10-year age categories.

d. Copy the term "10–19 years old" into column D where the age is between 10 and 19.

e. Copy the term "20–29 years old" into column D where the age is between 20 and 29.

f. Continue this process through the category 80–89 years old.

Step 3: Create the frequency table using a pivot table.

a. The first few rows of the table should look like this:

	A	B	C	D
1	Age	Cholesterol	Cholesterol Category	Age Category
2	13	134	Desirable <=199	10–19 years old
3	14	118	Desirable <=199	10–19 years old
4	16	137	Desirable <=199	10–19 years old
5	17	157	Desirable <=199	10–19 years old
6	18	137	Desirable <=199	10–19 years old
7	18	142	Desirable <=199	10–19 years old
8	19	132	Desirable <=199	10–19 years old
9	19	145	Desirable <=199	10–19 years old
10	20	145	Desirable <=199	20–29 years old
11	20	200	Borderline High 200–239	20–29 years old
12	20	210	Borderline High 200–239	20–29 years old

b. Click on one cell in columns A to D. Note: do not double click.

c. Click on "Insert" from the Excel menu.

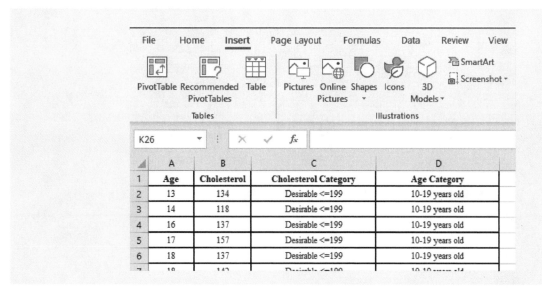

d. Click on "Pivot Table." The following window should appear. Ensure the table range includes all the cells populated with data.

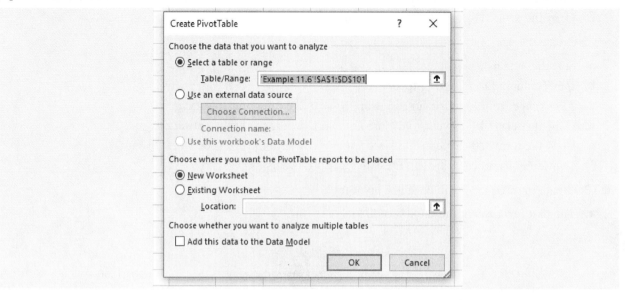

e. Click "OK."

f. Drag Cholesterol Category to the "Columns" window and Age Category to the "Rows" window; drag Age to the "Values" window. The PivotTable Fields window should look like this:

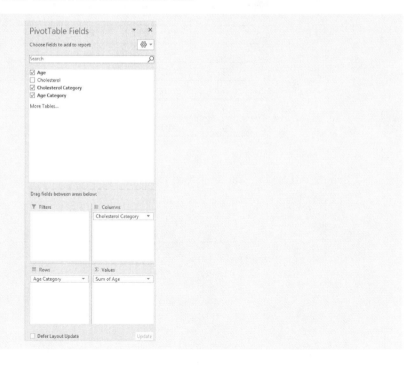

g. Since the values in the table should be counts of subjects, change the "Sum of Age" in the "Values" window to "Count of Age" by doing the following:

Click on "Sum of Age" and select "value field settings," select "Count" from the "Value Field Setting" window and then click "OK."

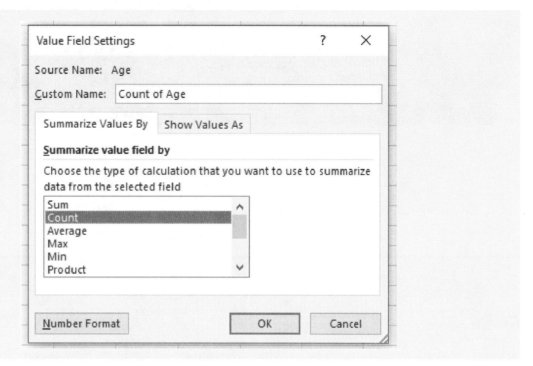

The resulting table is below:

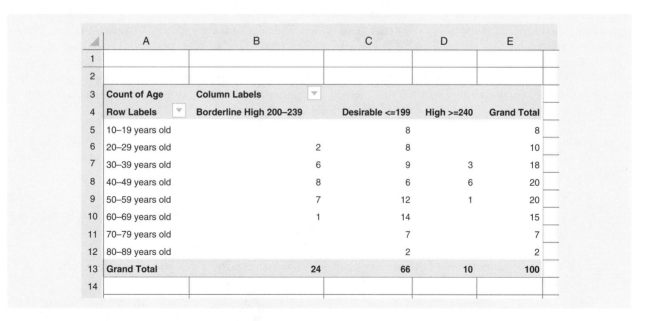

	A	B	C	D	E
1					
2					
3	**Count of Age**	**Column Labels**			
4	**Row Labels**	**Borderline High 200–239**	**Desirable <=199**	**High >=240**	**Grand Total**
5	10–19 years old		8		8
6	20–29 years old	2	8		10
7	30–39 years old	6	9	3	18
8	40–49 years old	8	6	6	20
9	50–59 years old	7	12	1	20
10	60–69 years old	1	14		15
11	70–79 years old		7		7
12	80–89 years old		2		2
13	**Grand Total**	24	66	10	100
14					

Pivot tables are a very powerful function in Excel that allows data to be summarized very easily. There are many tutorials and videos online that can be used to learn more about this method.

QUICK
TIP

Exercise 11.2

The table that follows shows a frequency distribution of patients with colon cancer treated at Community Hospital. Use an Excel spreadsheet to calculate the proportion of patients in each category. Round to two decimal places.

Community Hospital Ages of Patients with Colon Cancer Annual Statistics, 20X		
Age	**No. of Patients**	**Proportion**
≤ 30	3	
31–40	12	
41–50	18	
51–60	60	
61–70	65	
71+	48	

Graphs

Graphs of various types are the best means for presenting data for quick visualization of relationships. They often supply a lesser degree of detail than tables. However, data presented in a graph can be helpful in displaying statistics in a concise manner. There are advantages to using graphs. They grab the audience's attention. They are not meant to entertain the audience but rather present an easy-to-understand version of the data. The visual perception is more immediate when looking at the data rather than reading it. It is easier to see trends and comparisons with graphs.

Graphs should be easy to read, simple in content, and correctly labeled. The presentation of data in the form of a graph is an excellent way to convey the message you want to get across. Instead of presenting an entire statistical report in a table to a group, such as the medical staff or administration, you can create a graph to depict certain data. Many computer software programs are available that convert data into graphic form automatically and attractively.

When creating graphs, follow these general guidelines:

- The title must relate to what the graph is displaying. Follow the same general guidelines for the title in graphs as given in tables, including what the data are, what the graph is about, to whom it refers, and the time period.
- When several variables are included on the same graph (for example, males and females), each should be identified by using a legend or key.
- Categories should be natural; that is, the vertical axis should always start with zero. The scale of values for the x-axis reads from the lowest value on the left to the highest on the right. The scale of values for the y-axis extends from the lowest value at the bottom of the graph to the highest at the top.
- Scale captions are placed on both axes to identify the values clearly. These are simply titles placed on each axis to identify the values.
- Graphs should emphasize the horizontal. It is easier for the eye to read along the horizontal axis from left to right. Also, graphs should be greater in length than in height. A useful guideline is to follow the three-quarter-high rule, which states that the graph's height (y-axis) should be three-fourths of its length (x-axis).
- The exact reference to an outside source should be given.

Many software programs give users the opportunity to create three-dimensional graphs; however, it is recommended to not use these in presentations because they may be difficult to read.

QUICK
TIP

Bar Graphs

Bar graph, also called **bar chart** is graphic technique used to display frequency distributions of nominal or ordinal data that fall into categories. They are appropriate for displaying categorical data. The simplest bar graph is a one-variable bar graph. In this type of graph, the various categories of observations are presented along a horizontal axis, called the x-axis. (See figures 11.2 and 11.3.) The vertical axis, called the y-axis, displays the frequency of the data. Data representing frequencies, proportions, or percentages of categories are often displayed by using bar graphs. A grouped bar chart is used to display information from tables containing two or three variables. Figures 11.1, 11.2, and 11.3 show examples of one-, two-, and three-variable bar graphs, respectively.

Figure 11.1.   Example of a one-variable bar graph

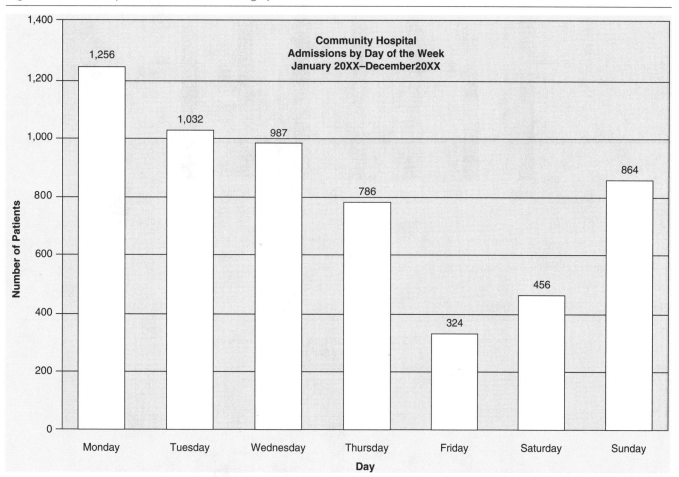

Source: Administrator's annual report.

Figure 11.2. Example of a two-variable bar graph

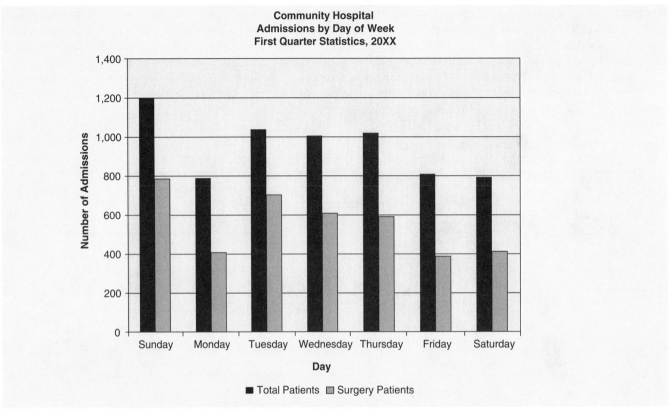

Source: Administrator's First Quarter Statistics 1/1/20XX to 3/31/20XX.

Figure 11.3. Example of a three-variable bar graph

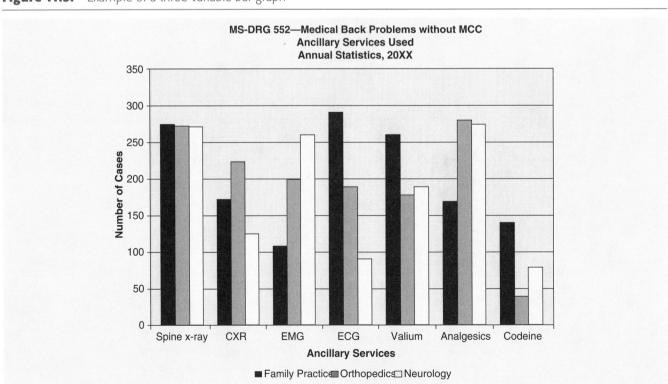

Source: Administrator's Annual Statistics 20XX.

Example 11.7: Use an Excel spreadsheet to create a bar chart to represent the number of patients in each age group from the data used in exercise 11.2.

Age	No. of Patients
≤ 30	3
31–40	12
41–50	18
51–60	60
61–70	65
71+	48

Step 1: Highlight the data table in Excel by selecting the cells and row and column titles.
Step 2: Click in "Insert" on the Excel menu and select the bar chart icon:

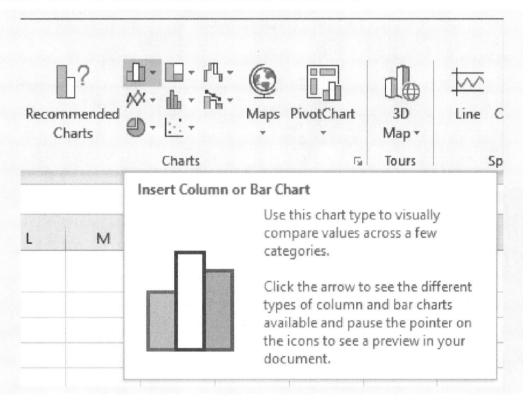

Step 3: Select the first choice. Notice that Excel shows you a preview of the chart:

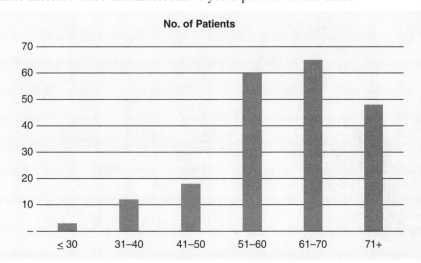

Step 4: Label the axes. While the chart is selected, "Add Chart Element" will be displayed on the menu bar. Click on that icon and there will be options to add labels and a chart title:

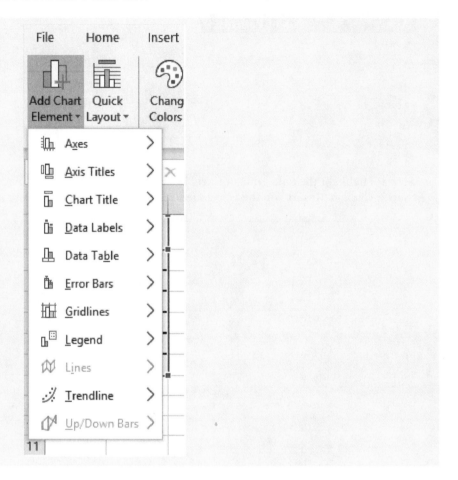

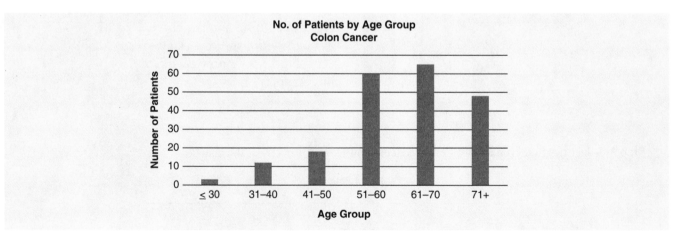

Pie Charts

A **pie chart**, also called a **pie graph**, is a method of displaying data as component parts of a whole. It is an easily understood chart in which the sizes of the slices of the pie show the proportional contribution of each part. Pie charts are best to use when you want to show each category's percentage of the total. They do not show changes over time. A circle is divided into sections such as wedges or slices. These represent percentages of the total (100 percent). To make a pie chart, include all the categories that make up a whole. Pie chart wedges may be shaded or colored to help differentiate the sections. In addition, they can be cut out of the pie to help emphasize a percentage. Computer software programs are extremely useful when creating pie graphs. See figures 11.4 and 11.5 for examples of pie charts.

Figure 11.4.   Pie graph showing nosocomial (hospital-acquired infections) by major service category

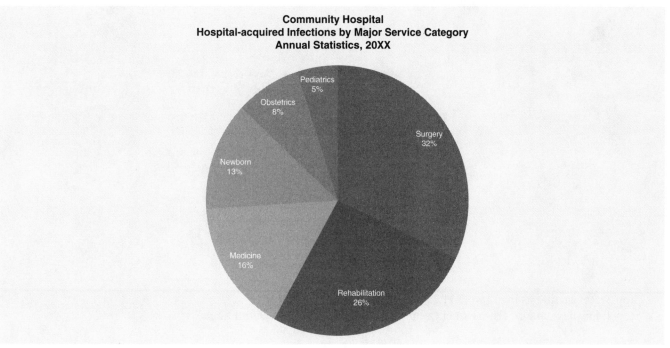

Source: ©AHIMA.

Figure 11.5.   Pie graph showing brain injury patients admitted from other facilities

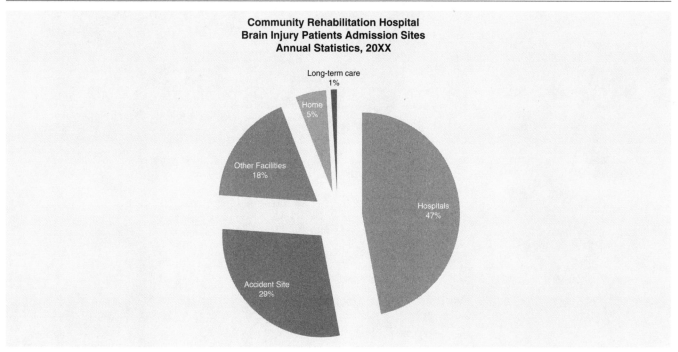

Source: ©AHIMA.

Example 11.8: Use Excel to create a pie chart to represent the number of patients in each age group from the data used in exercise 11.2.

Step 1: Highlight the data table in Excel by selecting the cells and row and column titles.
Step 2: Click on "Insert" from the Excel menu and select the pie chart icon:

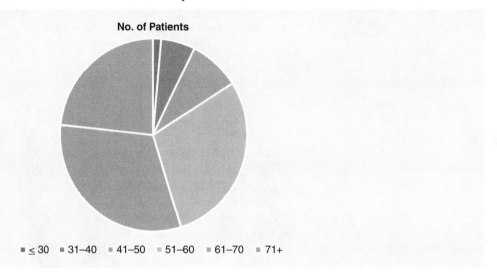

Step 3: Revise title as in example 11.7.
Step 4: Display data labels—right click on the pie and select "Add Data Labels":

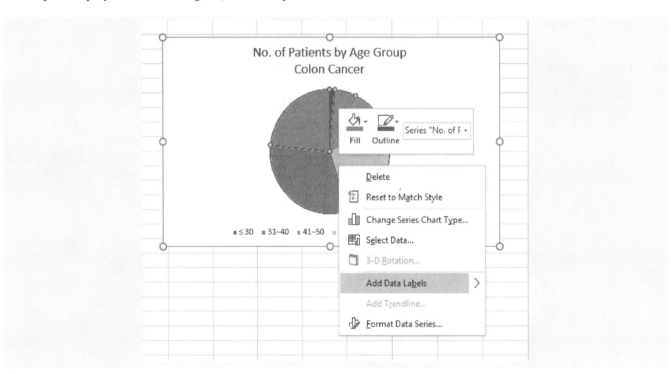

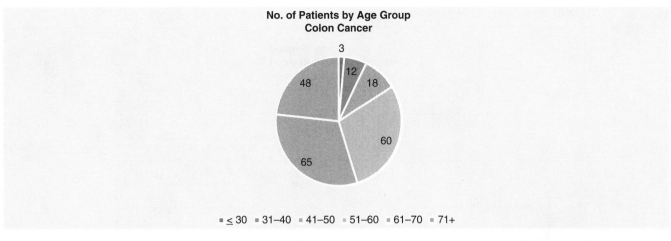

Which graph is more effective in presenting the age distribution of the colon cancer patients? The answer depends on the question to be answered by the graph. If the analyst wishes to know which age group includes the most patients, then either graph may work. If the analyst wants to determine what proportion of the patients are 61 years old or older, then the pie chart allows them to quickly determine that just over half of the patients are 61 or older. If the analyst would like to determine if the age distribution is skewed for colon cancer, then the bar chart shows the left skew much better than the pie chart.

Line Graphs

A **line graph** is often used to show data over time (for example, days, weeks, months, or years). The x-axis shows the time period, and the y-axis shows the values of the variables. A line graph consists of a line connecting a series of points. Line graphs also allow for several variables to be plotted. Line graphs are also referred to as **run charts** in the quality management field. The x-axis depicts the units of time from left to right, and the y-axis measures the values of the variable being shown. Refer to figures 11.6 and 11.7 for examples of line graphs.

Figure 11.6.   Example of a one-variable line graph

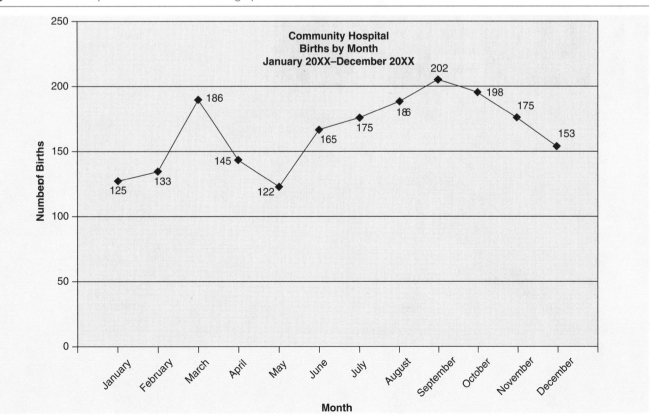

Source: Administrator's annual report.

Figure 11.7. Example of a two-variable line graph

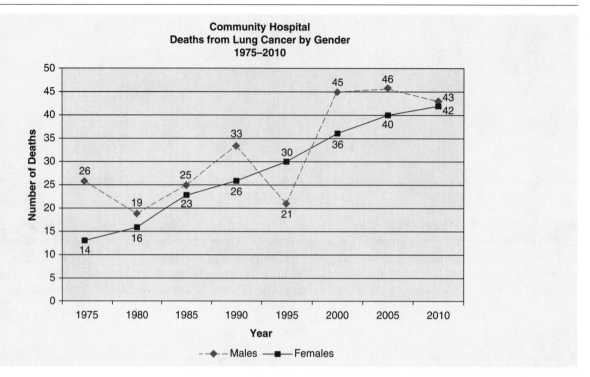

Source: ©AHIMA.

Example 11.9: University Hospital reported the following incidence of lung and bronchus cancer patients treated at the hospital during the past 10 years. Use Excel to construct a line graph of the data for males.

University Hospital Cancer Registry Data Lung and Bronchus Cancer by Year and Gender		
Year	**Male**	**Female**
2006	172	48
2007	175	47
2008	169	49
2009	165	50
2010	168	54
2011	121	93
2012	123	101
2013	130	118
2014	121	121
2015	112	123

Step 1: Select the data column of data for male patients.
Step 2: Click on "Insert" on the Excel menu and select the line chart.

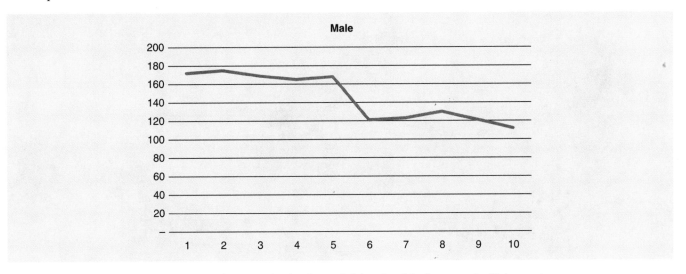

Step 3: Replace the sequence numbers on the horizontal (x) axis with the years in Column A.

a. Right click on the chart.

b. Click on "Select Data."

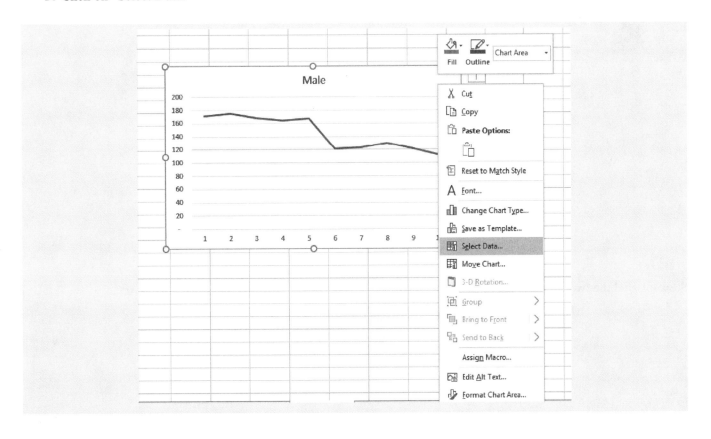

c. Click on "Edit" under the "Horizontal (Category) Axis Labels."

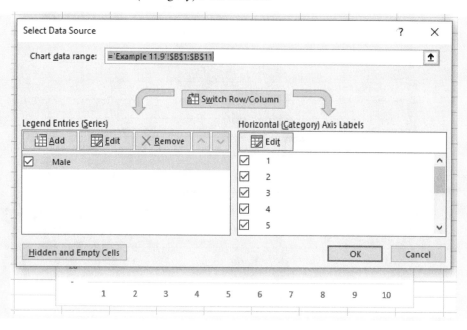

d. Select the values in the "Year" column. Select "OK."

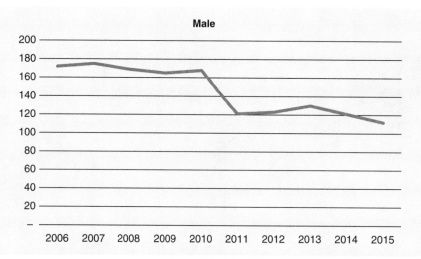

Step 4: Label the two axes and revise the title to be more descriptive of the data included in the chart.

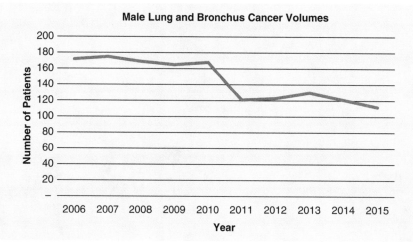

Scatter Diagram

A **scatter diagram** (also called a scatter plot) is used to graphically show the relationship between two numerical variables. A scatter diagram is used to determine whether there is a correlation, that is, a relationship, between two characteristics. Correlation implies that as one variable changes, the other also changes. This does not always mean that there is a cause-and-effect relationship between two variables because there may be other variables that could cause the change. If the two characteristics are somehow related, the pattern of points will show a tight clustering in a certain direction. The closer the points look like a line in appearance, the more the two characteristics are likely to be correlated. (See figure 11.8.) The different shapes in the scatter plot represent different subsets of the data.

The relationship between the values in figure 11.8 is positive. Notice that small values of the *x*-axis correspond to small values of the *y*-axis and large values of the *x*-axis correspond to large values of the *y*-axis; thus, a positive relationship is thought to exist.

In contrast, figure 11.9 shows a scatter diagram with a negative relationship. That is, the small values of the *x*-axis correspond to large values of the *y*-axis and large values of the *x*-axis correspond to small values of the *y*-axis. Additionally, the scatter diagram in figure 11.9 shows a strong correlation because the cluster of points is tight.

Figure 11.10 illustrates a scatter diagram with no relationship because the scatter points are plotted randomly on the graph.

Figure 11.8.   Sample scatter diagram showing a positive relationship

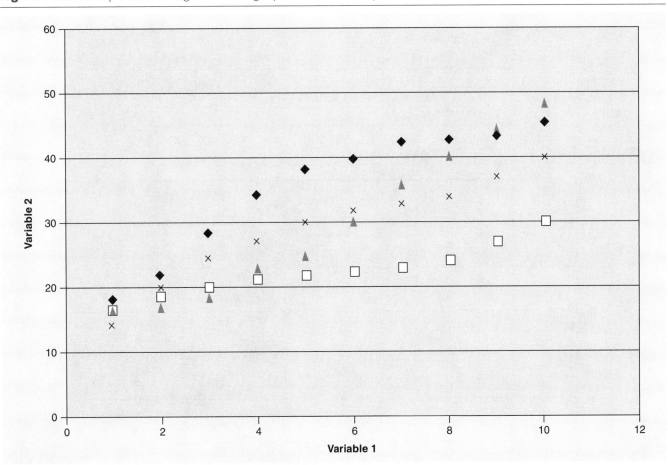

Figure 11.9.   Sample scatter diagram showing a negative relationship

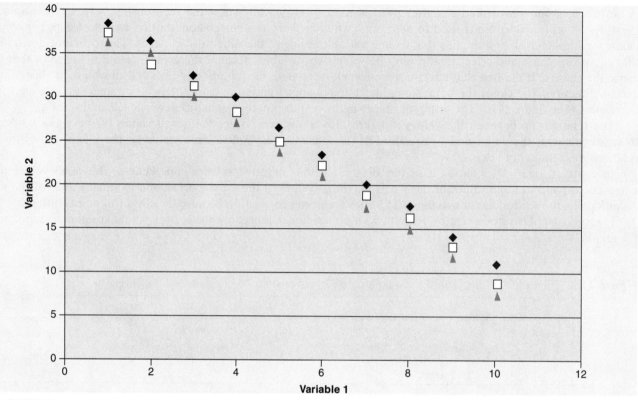

Source: ©AHIMA.

Figure 11.10.   Sample scatter diagram showing no relationship

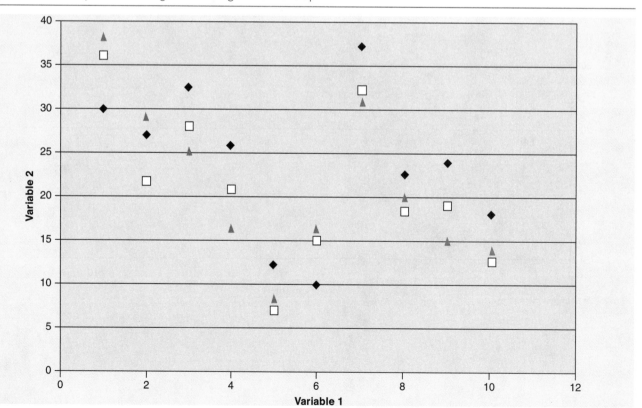

Source: ©AHIMA.

Example 11.10: The cardiology team at Community Hospital believes there is a relationship between the number of internal medicine transfers and cardiology transfers. Use Excel to create a scatter plot to investigate the relationship.

Month	Internal Medicine Transfers	Cardiology Transfers
January	15	20
February	14	18
March	13	15
April	13	20
May	14	14
June	13	19
July	8	14
August	9	15
September	4	20
October	9	22
November	8	21
December	12	19

Step 1: Select the data column of data for the internal medicine and cardiology transfers.
Step 2: Click on "'Insert" on the Excel menu and select the scatter chart.

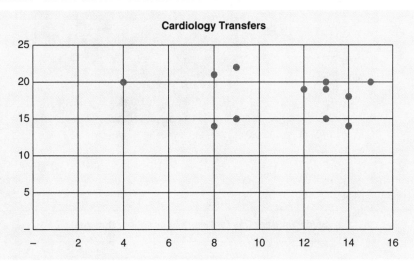

Step 3: Label the two axes and revise the titles. Since the internal medicine data are in the first column in the data table, they are on the *x*-axis (horizontal) and the cardiology transfers are on the *y*-axis.

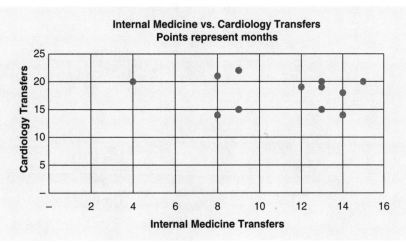

Is there a relationship between the two transfer rates? From the graph, it appears that there is not a strong positive or negative relationship between the two transfer counts.

Histograms

A **histogram** is a graph used to display frequency distributions for continuous numerical data (interval or ratio data). Histograms are created from frequency distribution tables. (See figures 11.11 and 11.12 for examples of histograms.) They look similar to bar graphs except that all the bars in a histogram are touching because they show the continuous nature of the distribution. In histograms the bars should be of equal width. Ordinarily in constructing a histogram, there should be no less than 4 and usually not more than 12 bars or classes, and the frequency groups should not overlap. Histograms are typically completed using a statistical program.

Figure 11.11. Sample histogram #1

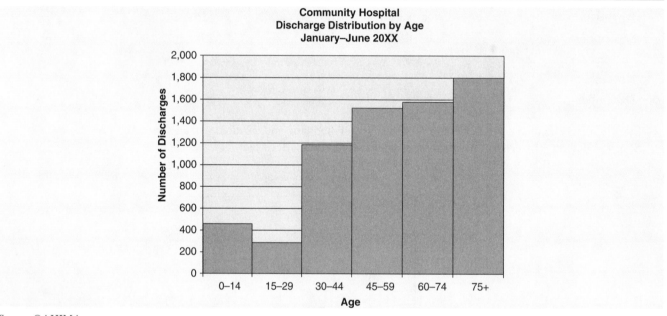

Source: ©AHIMA.

Figure 11.12. Sample histogram #2

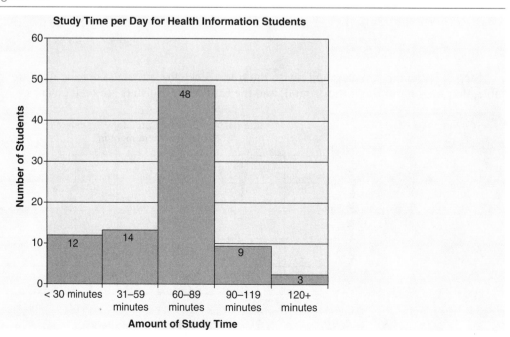

Source: ©AHIMA.

Frequency Polygon

A **frequency polygon** is similar to a histogram in that it is a graph depicting the frequency of continuous data; however, a frequency polygon is in line form instead of bar form. The advantage of a frequency polygon is that several of them can be placed on the same graph to make comparisons. A frequency polygon uses the same axes as the histogram; that is, the *x*-axis displays the scale of the variable and the *y*-axis displays the frequency. A dot is placed at the midpoint of the class interval or frequency. A line drawn from one point to the next then connects the dots. Because the *x*-axis represents the entire frequency distribution, the line starts at zero cases and is drawn from the last frequency to the *y*-axis to end with zero. (See figure 11.13.)

Pictogram

A **pictogram** is an attractive alternative type of bar graph in that it uses pictures to show the frequency of the data. For example, if you want to show the top five cancer site deaths, you might use stick people. If you need to show exact numbers, a pictogram will probably not be a good choice for your presentation; however, they are very good at catching the attention of your audience and will give them a good sense of your data. (See figure 11.14.)

Figure 11.13.   Sample Frequency polygon

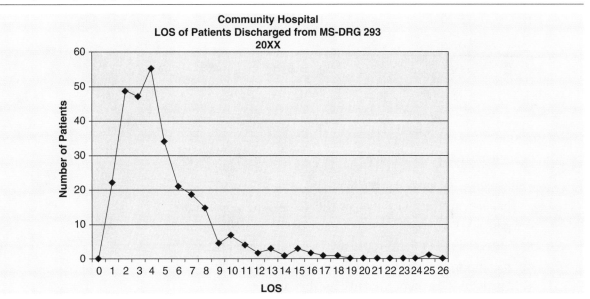

Source: ©AHIMA.

Figure 11.14.   Sample pictogram

University Medical Center
Cancer Registry
Number of Deaths, Top Five Cancer Sites, 20XX

Source: ©AHIMA.

Exercise 11.3

Complete the following exercises.

1. Indicate whether a table or a graph is the preferred method of presentation in the following situations:
    a. Distribution by site, sex, race, and time period of all cancers in your healthcare facility
    b. Survival trends over time by sex for lung cancer
    c. Display of prostate cancer stage of disease for a presentation at a professional conference
    d. Detailed treatment distribution of breast cancer for a physician on the staff of your hospital

2. Indicate which of the following categories (A, B, and C) are mutually exclusive and clearly defined.

A	B	C
0–15	≤ 10.0	0–10
15–30	10.1–20.0	11–20
30–45	20.1–30.0	21–30
45–60	30.1–40.0	31–40
60+	40.1–50.0	41–50
	50.1+	51+

3. In September 20XX, Community Hospital discharged 150 patients.

    - 105 patients were discharged home.
    - 6 patients were discharged home with follow-up home health.
    - 5 patients died.
    - 15 patients were transferred to a skilled nursing facility.
    - 7 patients were transferred to another acute-care facility.
    - 12 patients were transferred to a rehabilitation hospital.

    Use Excel to create a pie chart of this information.

4. Use the information in the table that follows to create a line graph of the data using Excel.

Community Hospital Number of Admissions to Cardiology Service January–June 20XX	
Month	**Number of Admissions**
January	120
February	125
March	130
April	119
May	121
June	130

Exercise 11.4

University Hospital Cancer Registry records show the following incidence of cancer in female patients for the past year. Construct an appropriate graph of the data using Excel.

University Hospital Cancer Registry 10 Most Prevalent Cancer Sites—Female Patients 20XX	
Site	**Number of Cases**
Breast	122
Lung and bronchus	52
Colorectal	34
Uterus	25
Thyroid	21
Melanoma	15
Lymphoma	14
Kidney	12
Ovary	11
Pancreas	4

Preparing Reports

Writing reports for your workplace is not the same as writing an article for a professional journal or preparing a report for an assignment in one of your classes, but the goal is the same. Communication is the goal, and it is achieved when you write your report in the style your audience prefers. Often your healthcare administration will let you know how reports are prepared and presented in your facility, or you could review previous reports that have been given to committees or your administration to use as a guide. Some reports are more formal than others. For example, for a committee meeting you may just provide some data in the form of graphs or tables to share with the members, whereas for a cancer conference, where information may be shared with the community, a more formal report will be in order.

Here are some general guidelines to follow:

- Include a title for the report.
- If your report is long, consider placing a paginated list of contents in the front of the report to make details easier to locate.
- If you are writing a formal report, include an introduction explaining the purpose of the report.
- The body of the report will include the narrative and any tables and graphs. These could be divided with titles.
  - Tables and graphs are great tools for presenting data. Tables show summarized and more detailed data, and graphs are useful for presenting relationships in visual form. The question of which to use depends on the audience.
  - Take a few minutes before you prepare a report to think about who will be reading or seeing your presentation. Will you be presenting information to your administrator about the need for new equipment in your department, will it be to a team who is deciding whether or not to investigate the need for a new service in your facility, or will it be to a committee evaluating the quality of care provided in your hospital? Determine what you are trying to say to this person or group. Determine what details must be included; then decide what types of tables or graphs you want to provide.

- Tables have several advantages over graphs:
  - More information can be presented in a table.
  - Exact values in tables can be helpful.
  - Ordinarily, less work is involved in creating a table.
- Graphs, on the other hand, also have advantages:
  - Graphs are more attention-grabbing than tables.
  - Graphs show trends more clearly.
  - Graphs bring out facts that will stimulate thinking.
- A narrative report will make the presentation more understandable and can explain what the values mean.
  - Narrative reports can include historical information; for instance, what the data have shown over a specific period of time.
  - The narrative can include factors that may influence the data, such as seasonal changes in the patient population or reasons for significant increases or decreases in the data.
- Ensure your data points are correct because inaccurate data may lead to inaccurate decisions.
- Include the sources of the data.
- Write to the style of your workplace.
  - Be objective. Report all the pertinent information, both positive and negative points.
  - Use bias-free language. Avoid words such as "awesome" or "incredible."
  - Write in an impersonal style. Do not start your sentences with "I compared …", but rather, "A comparison showed …"
  - Be concise and strive for clarity.
  - Explain any abbreviations or acronyms.
- Proofread your document; improve your grammatical skills.
  - Read your report carefully to ensure the graphs and tables make sense and are easy to understand.
    - You might even consider reading the report out loud to see how it sounds.
  - It is a good idea to ask another individual, another colleague or supervisor, to read your report to be certain it contains no mistakes and is logical.

Chapter 11   Matching Quiz

Match the definitions with the terms.

Definitions:

a. A graphic technique used to display frequency distributions of nominal or ordinal data that fall into categories; also called bar graph

b. Data that may be displayed by units of equal size and placed on a scale starting with zero and thus can be manipulated mathematically

c. An organized arrangement of data, usually in columns and rows

d. A graph that visually displays the linear relationships among factors

e. A type of data that represents observations that can be measured on an evenly distributed scale beginning at a point other than true zero

f. Four types of data (nominal, ordinal, interval, and ratio) that represent values or observations that can be sorted into a category; also called scales of measurement

g. A graphic technique used to illustrate the relationship between continuous measurements; consists of a line drawn to connect a series of points on an arithmetic scale and is often used to display time trends

h. A type of graph that shows data points collected over time and identifies emerging trends or patterns

i. A graphic technique in which the proportions of a category are displayed as portions of a circle

j. A graphic technique used to display the frequency distribution of continuous data (interval or ratio data) as either numbers or percentages in a series of bars

Terms:

1. _____ Histogram

2. _____ Interval data

3. _____ Run chart

4. _____ Ratio data

5. _____ Line graph

6. _____ Table

7. _____ Pie chart

8. _____ Bar chart

9. _____ Scatter diagram

10. _____ Categorical data

Chapter 11   Review

Complete the following exercises.

1. Which of the following graphs would be best to use to display the percentages of diagnoses seen at your mental health center?
   a. Frequency polygon
   b. Pie graph
   c. Bar graph
   d. Line graph

2. Physicians from the Community Physician's Clinic would like to demonstrate to the Community Hospital administration that additional exam rooms are needed to accommodate their patients. They ask the HIM manager to construct a graph showing the number of patients seen in the last year by the clinic physicians. The categories they wish to have displayed are primary care, 5,736; medical specialties, 2,473; surgical specialties, 2,022; and hospital outpatients, 984. Which type of graph would be appropriate?
   a. Line graph
   b. Bar graph
   c. Pie chart
   d. Scatter diagram

3. The administration at Community Physician's Hospital is interested in determining if they need to increase the number of physicians in order to see patients in a timely manner. The administrator asks the HIM manager to construct a graph that will show the following percentages about appointments in the following categories: patients who waited two to four weeks to see the physician, patients who waited one to two weeks to see a physician, patients who waited one week or less, and patients who were able to have an appointment on the day they called. Which would be the best graph to show this information?
   a. Line graph
   b. Bar graph
   c. Pie chart
   d. Scatter diagram

4. What type of numerical data contains only a finite number of results?

   a. Continuous

   b. Discrete

   c. Interval

   d. Ratio

5. When creating histograms, which is a true statement?

   a. Form classes of equal width.

   b. Always form frequency groups that do not overlap.

   c. Establish between 4 and 12 frequency groups.

   d. All the above

6. What do the wedges or divisions in a pie graph represent?

   a. Frequency groups

   b. Various data

   c. Percentages

   d. Classes

7. The following graph shows:

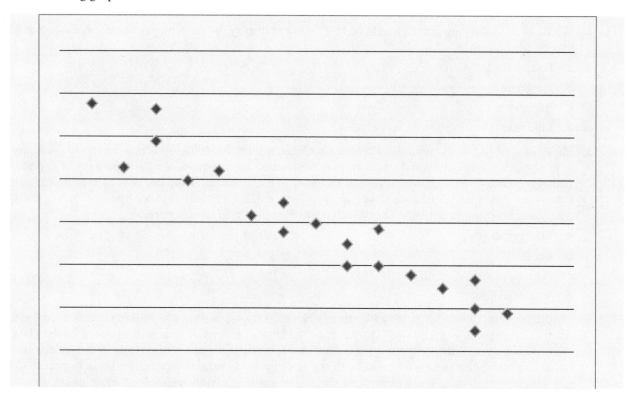

   a. Strong positive correlation

   b. Strong negative correlation

   c. Moderately positive correlation

   d. Moderately negative correlation

8. Which graph displays vertical bars to depict frequency distributions for continuous data?

   a. Histogram

   b. Line graph

   c. Pie graph

   d. Frequency distribution table

9. What is one of the simplest types of categorical data in which the values fall into unordered categories?

   a. Ordinal

   b. Nominal

   c. Ratio

   d. Interval

10. Which of the following graphs would be best for the cancer registrar to use to display the five-year survival rates of lung cancer patients in the years 20XX to 20XX at your hospital?

    a. Frequency polygon

    b. Bar graph

    c. Line graph

    d. Histogram

11. Which of the following graphs would be best to use to display the number of discharges by medical service for the past year?

    a. Line graph

    b. Bar graph

    c. Histogram

    d. Frequency polygon

12. A physician on your staff asked you to help her collect information on the effects of drinking alcohol during pregnancy and the birth weight of babies. You were asked to collect the following information.
    Did the mothers drink alcohol during pregnancy? (yes or no)
    Birth weight of the baby
    Apgar score at one minute
    Apgar score at five minutes
    The scales of these variables would be:

    a. Nominal, ordinal, interval, ratio

    b. Nominal, ratio, ordinal, ordinal

    c. Ordinal, nominal, ratio, interval

    d. Ratio, ordinal, interval, nominal

13. The family practice department at University Medical School offered the following information to its advisory board about placement of family practice graduates in your state for the past five years: Year 1 = 55 positions offered and 46 positions filled, Year 2 = 50 positions offered and 46 positions filled, Year 3 = 52 positions offered and 40 positions filled, Year 4 = 61 positions offered and 58 positions filled, and Year 5 = 64 positions offered and 62 positions filled. What type of graph would be most appropriate?

    a. Line graph

    b. Bar graph

    c. Pie chart

    d. Scatter diagram

14. When preparing a report for presentation, which of the following should be included?

    1. Title of the report
    2. Graphs will give more detail than tables
    3. Narrative will be helpful if included
    4. Content page must be included

    a. 1, 2, and 3
    b. 1 and 3
    c. 2, 3, and 4
    d. All the above

15. In creating a frequency distribution table, which of the following statements is not a basic rule to follow?

    a. Choose classes that cover the smallest and largest values.
    b. Make certain that each item can go into only one class.
    c. As a general rule, use between 10 and 15 classes.
    d. Do not produce gaps between classes.

CHAPTER 12 | Basic Research Principles

Learning Objectives

At the conclusion of this chapter, you should be able to do the following:

- Compare and contrast quantitative research and qualitative research
- Distinguish among the types of research, research methods, samples, data collection techniques, and data interpretation issues
- Determine the steps in the research process
- Explain the role of the Institutional Review Board (IRB) in research in healthcare facilities
- Comply with ethical guidelines in the use of statistics

Key Terms

Alternative hypothesis
Applied research
Basic research
Cluster sampling
Convenience sampling
Correlational research
Data collection
Descriptive research
Ethnography
Evaluation research
Experimental research
Exploratory research
Fabrication
Falsification
Historical research

Hypothesis
Individually identifiable health
   information
Informed consent
Institutional Review Board (IRB)
Instrument
Judgment sampling
Literature review
Naturalistic inquiry
Null hypothesis
Observation
Observational research
Plagiarism
Primary data source
Qualitative research

Quantitative research
Quota sampling
Reliability
Research
Sample
Sample size
Secondary data source
Simple random sampling (SRS)
Stratified random sampling
Structured interview
Survey
Systematic random sampling
Unrestricted question
Validity

Research is an inquiry process aimed at discovering new information about a subject or revising old information. It includes investigation or experimentation aimed at the discovery of new facts, revision of accepted theories or law in light of these new facts, or practical application using the new facts. Health information research examines all aspects of health and can include studies on human subjects as well as public policy. The goal of health information research is to make discoveries that will benefit health information professionals.

Basic Research Principles

Research is the search toward the solution of problems. It answers questions that you or others may have and calls attention to theories that may be helpful in predicting future experiences.

Research is done in many fields and may be done in a variety of ways. Health research covers the wide gamut of laboratory research, clinical trials, and public health issues. This chapter covers the basic types of research and the steps in the research process, including data-collection techniques and the different types of sampling methods.

Types of Research

There are generally two types of research: basic and applied. **Basic research** is a type of research that focuses on the development and refinement of theories. The investigator is not concerned with the immediate applicability of his or her results but, rather, tries to look for understanding of natural processes. **Applied research** is a type of research that focuses on the use of scientific theories to improve actual practice as in medical research applied to the treatment of patients. In this case, the investigator has some kind of application in mind and wants to discover information about it that can be used to solve a problem or in some way contribute to society; it is more practical in nature.

Research Methodology

Research methodology is a set of procedures or strategies used by researchers to collect, analyze, and present data. At a higher and more general level, researchers in research methodology have described two overarching approaches to research: the qualitative approach and the quantitative approach.

Qualitative research describes events, persons, activities, processes, and the like without the use of numerical data. It is generally aimed at understanding the experiences and attitudes of patients, the community, or healthcare workers (McCusker and Gunaydin 2015).

An example of qualitative research would be interviews with health information practitioners to determine whether their past healthcare experiences affected their decision to enter the health information field or interviews with mothers of handicapped infants to determine how their lives were affected by the birth of their children. Qualitative research consists of interviews, observations, and written documents that may be used individually or in combination.

Quantitative research uses quantitative methods, or numbers, to describe a study, including some comparisons of the population and statistical analysis to describe the results. Quantitative research consists of observations, experiments, structured interviews, and **surveys**.

Table 12.1 illustrates some characteristics of quantitative and qualitative research.

Table 12.1. Characteristics of quantitative and qualitative research

Quantitative Research	Qualitative Research
Uses quantitative methods, including observations, structured interviews, experiments, and surveys	Describes observations without the use of numerical data, including interviews, observations, and written documents
Is objective	Is subjective
Sample is generally randomly selected	Sample is typically purposefully selected, but may be randomly selected
Uses controlled measurements	Uses uncontrolled observations
Researcher is removed from the data; is an outside observer	Researcher is close to the data; has an inside perspective
Can be generalized and replicated	Is not generalized and may not be replicable
Is outcome oriented	Is process oriented

There is a trend toward combining the two methods, called mixed methods research. It is an approach in which researchers mix or combine quantitative and qualitative research techniques, methods, concepts, or language within one study and across related studies (Watzlaf and Forrrestal 2017, 15). Mixed methods research holds strong potential for contributing to better understanding of problems and holds untapped potential that warrants further investigation (Poth and Onwuegbuzie 2015).

One example of a technique that often uses both types of research methodologies is survey research. A single survey will often contain questions that result in both quantitative and qualitative data. For example, you might want to study the effects of a hospital's implementation of the electronic health record (EHR). Your survey could contain questions that require the interviewee to answer, "On a scale of 1 to 5 with 1 being very good and 5 being very poor, how would you describe the implementation process of the new software for your facility's EHR?" The same survey may very well contain additional questions such as, "In what ways would you change the process to better take into consideration the process used in your department?"

Exercise 12.1

Match the attributes of quantitative research or qualitative research.

- **a.** Qualitative research
- **b.** Quantitative research
- **c.** Mixed methods research

1. Researcher often has an inside perspective
2. Uses controlled measurements
3. Uses numbers to describe the results
4. The sample is purposefully selected
5. The study is process oriented
6. Structured interviews are used

The Research Process

Although there are as many descriptions of the types of research as there are textbooks and articles about the subject, most agree that the research process involves the following six major steps:

1. Define the problem.
2. Review the literature.
3. Design the research.
4. Collect the data.
5. Analyze the data.
6. Draw conclusions.

Defining the Problem

Problem definition refers to forming a question regarding a topic you would like to study. The most important thing is to be clear about what you want to study. Often an analysis of historical data, also called secondary information, has gone into the problem definition.

Historical data analysis simply means looking at the past to see what has been done before; it prevents reinventing the wheel. In previous research, an investigator may have made recommendations for future studies. In addition, problems may be broken down into subcomponents or smaller problems. Figure 12.1 demonstrates an example of a problem and its possible subcomponents.

Figure 12.1.   Example of a research problem and its subcomponents

Problem/Question: Should a physician clinic in your community put an organized health information department into operation?

- Subcomponent 1. What are the health information services that could be provided?
- Subcomponent 2. What types of employees should be employed in this department?
- Subcomponent 3. What amount of space is needed for the department?
- Subcomponent 4. Where should the health information department be located?
- Subcomponent 5. What equipment does the department need to be operation?
- Subcomponent 6. What would be the total estimated cost of the project

Source: ©AHIMA.

The definition also may define the scope of the study; that is, who or what will be included in the study. For example, a study that includes hospitals may be defined as including only those hospitals with fewer than 100 beds, a study that involves patients may include only those patients who are age 60 and over, or a study may include female patients only.

Reviewing the Literature

A **literature review** is an investigation of all the information about a topic. It is important to start any study with a review of literature on the research you want to conduct for three important reasons:

- To determine whether research has already been done on the question
- To determine whether any data sources can be used in the study
- To help make the hypothesis more specific

There are many sources of previous research. These may include journals, books, position papers, conference presentations, videos, interviews, and online databases, to name just a few. Google Scholar is an excellent resource to search when performing a literature review (scholar.google.com).

Designing the Research and Collecting the Data

There are several types of research design, including the following:

- **Exploratory research** is often initially undertaken when a topic is not clearly defined. The researcher has an idea that there may be a question that he would like answered and wants to find out more about that topic. This type of research allows the researcher to study a topic and gather information. It may generate a hypothesis. Exploratory research is generally informal and relies on literature review and informal discussions with others to find out more about a problem. Although exploratory research may not help answer the problem, it may provide insights into the problem. For example, a health information management (HIM) director may want to find out why claims are not being billed within the three-day requirement or why employees are coming to work late.
- **Historical research** involves an investigation and analysis of past events. This type of research also allows the researcher to apply previous researchers' experiences and conclusions in their professional practice. Researchers examine primary and secondary sources. Primary sources can include original documents, such as health records, meeting minutes, certificates, newspaper and journal articles, eyewitness accounts, pictures, recordings, and research reports. Secondary data sources include data that are derived from a primary source such as indices, reports of a person who relates the testimony of an eyewitness, textbooks, and reliable websites.
- **Descriptive research**, also called statistical research, provides data about the population you are studying, including the frequency that something occurs. These data might include studies on the status of the composition of the HIM workforce, employee morale in departments, coding accuracy, or the effects of EHR implementation. The most common collection techniques for descriptive research are case studies, observations, and surveys.
- **Correlational research** refers to studies that try to discover a relationship between variables. A variable is anything under study. In correlational research, the strength of the relationship is measured and there may

be a positive or a negative relationship between variables. Correlational research determines only if there is a relationship between two or more variables; it does not determine the cause of those relationships. If a strong relationship is found, experimental research can be carried out to determine causality. This type of research uses questionnaires, observations, and secondary data as data-collection methods. Examples of correlational research might include studying whether there is a relationship between watching violence on television and behavior, whether graduating with a 4.0 grade point average from college affects the type of job a student gets after graduation, or whether there is a relationship between eating eggs and cholesterol levels.

- **Evaluation research** is a process used to determine what has happened during a given activity or in an institution. The purpose of evaluation research is to lead to a better understanding of whether a program is effective, whether a policy is working, or whether something that was agreed upon is the most cost-effective way of doing something. For example, evaluation research may be done each year to determine whether your school's health information program is meeting its goals.

- **Experimental research** is used to establish cause and effect; also, a controlled investigation in which subjects are assigned randomly to groups that experience carefully controlled interventions that are manipulated by the experimenter according to a strict protocol; also called experimental study. In experimental research, certain variables are kept constant and an independent or experimental variable is manipulated. Researchers select both independent and dependent variables. Independent variables are the factors that researchers manipulate directly; dependent variables are the measured variables. Examples of experimental research include studies such as determining whether a certain medication is effective in treating Parkinsonism or studying whether the use of robotic technology in the operating suite is more beneficial to patients than the traditional surgical approach. Experimentation provides a context for hypothesis testing. Experimentation is the classic method of research where elements are manipulated, and effects are observed. Quasi-experimental research is similar to experimental research but does not include randomization of participants. This research provides control of when and to whom the measurement is applied, but because there is not random assignment to experimental and control groups, the equivalence of the groups is not assured.

- **Observational research** requires researchers to observe, document, and analyze events and behaviors. This is part of qualitative research design. Qualitative researchers also use a technique referred to as triangulation or multiple data collection techniques. In this process, data are verified through other data that were collected from other sources, other researchers, or different procedures. This type of research often uses administrative data or data extracted from an EHR.

Exercise 12.2

Match the research methods with the descriptions:

   a. Exploratory research

   b. Historical research

   c. Descriptive research

   d. Causal research

   e. Correlational research

   f. Evaluation research

   g. Experimental research

1. _____ A health information manager would like more information about a new supervisory technique, so he organizes a focus group of supervisors in the facility to generate ideas and clarify concepts.

2. _____ The wellness department director of your facility wants to test the effectiveness of an herbal supplement in the group of employees attending her weight management class. She divides the employees into two groups at random and each employee is given a pill to take every day, but the employees do not know what kind of pill they are taking; one is a sugar pill (the placebo) and one is the herbal supplement. The employees are evaluated after one month and no differences are found in the management of their weight, leading her to conclude that the herbal supplement was not effective.

3. _____ The behavioral health department at Community Hospital is interested in studying whether the smoking-cessation program they instituted for the employees is working.

4. _____ A researcher in your community is studying why there are differences in the number of lung cancer cases in your community versus the community 10 miles from your facility. The researcher surveyed residents in each community about their lifestyle choices. He found that citizens of your community smoke more than the other community.

5. _____ A researcher found that greater use of the internet can decrease social support and lead to depression and loneliness.

6. _____ A researcher wants to study if eating too much sugar causes childhood diabetes.

7. _____ A health information researcher reviews the past 30 years of the *Journal of AHIMA* to identify health information managers' concerns in the workplace.

Statement of the Hypothesis

In formal research, a **hypothesis** is formed. A hypothesis is a statement of the predicted relationship among variables in measurable terms. It is a proposed solution or explanation the researcher has reached through the literature review, observation, theory, or models. More simply stated, it is the tentative answer to the question being studied.

The statement of the hypothesis is important because it allows the researcher to think about the variables and type of research design to use in the study. The research tests the hypothesis, proving it to be positive or negative (correct or incorrect). The fact that a hypothesis is rejected (that is, proven incorrect) does not necessarily mean that the research is poor but, rather, only that the results are different from what was expected. The formulation of the hypothesis in advance of the data-gathering process is necessary for an unbiased investigation.

There are two types of hypotheses:

- The **null hypothesis** is a statement of the status quo or default situation. It may state that there is no difference between the population means or proportions being compared or that there is no association between the two variables being compared. For example, in a clinical trial of a new medication, the null hypothesis is as follows: The new medication is no better than the current medication. A detailed discussion of the null hypothesis is given in chapter 13, *Inferential Statistics in Healthcare*.

- The **alternative hypothesis** is a statement of what the study is set up to establish. It states what the predicted association or difference between the variables is. For example, in the clinical trial of a new medication, the alternative hypothesis is as follows: The new medication is better than the current medication.

 The null and alternative hypotheses are complements of each other. In other words, they should cover the entire set of situations that could be concluded for the variable of interest. In practice, it is much easier to define the alternative hypothesis first and then make the null hypothesis the complement or opposite situation.

Data-Collection Techniques

Data collection, the process by which data are gathered, includes **primary data sources**, the data obtained from observations and surveys and interviews. It also includes **secondary data sources**, which is data derived from the primary patient record, such as an index or database. Regardless of the data-collection method used, the research must be valid and reliable.

- **Validity** is the degree to which scientific observations actually measure or record what they purport to measure. For example, if the researcher is using a written questionnaire to collect data, he or she will pretest it by giving it to someone who may have been included in the subject population in order to determine whether it is well written, clear, and inclusive of everything the researcher is studying.

- **Reliability** is a measure of consistency of data items based on their reproducibility and an estimation of their error of measurement. With reliability, the major question is, can another researcher reproduce the study using a similar instrument and get similar results? A study may be reliable but not valid. That is, the study may be able to be replicated and yet not answer the research question.

The type of data-collection technique used depends on the type of research the investigator wishes to conduct. If the researcher wants to establish a causal relationship, he or she should conduct one of the experimental studies. However, if the researcher is breaking new ground in a poorly understood area of practice, he or she may want to consider an exploratory study in a qualitative design.

Some examples of data-collection methods include:

- Surveys: The survey method gathers data from a relatively large number of cases at a particular time. Surveys can include interviews and questionnaire surveys. In either case, the questions should be well thought out to ensure that they answer the questions of the research study. The questions can be restricted (structured) or closed ended when the investigator only wants certain answers. For example, "Yes" and "No" answers fall into this category. It is a good idea to provide for unanticipated responses. Providing an "Other" category permits respondent to indicate what might be their most important response, one the questionnaire builder had not anticipated.

- **Unrestricted questions**: This method may also be referred to as open-ended questions, allow the participant to express a freer response in his or her own words. Open-ended questionnaires are generally easier to write but require qualitative techniques to analyze. If the researcher wishes to use quantitative techniques, it may be better to take additional time to write a closed-ended type of questionnaire. When standardized questions are used in the interview process, this is referred to as a **structured interview**. This will ensure every participant in the study receives the same questions in the same order. In this type of interview, the data are collected by an interviewer rather than a questionnaire. The interviewer reads the question exactly as it appears on the survey along with the answer choices. Open-ended questions may be included, and the interviewer must be able to capture the responses given exactly as they are given. The order of the questions is also important. Each participant must receive the questions in the same order. In this way there would be little impact of contextual effects, where the answers given to a survey question may depend on the previous question.

- **Observation**: Instead of asking questions, the investigator observes the participant.
  - In nonparticipant observation, the researcher is a neutral observer who does not interact with the participants.
  - In participant observation, the researcher may participate in the actions being observed but tries to maintain his or her objectivity.
  - Another type of observation is called **ethnography**, also called **naturalistic inquiry**. An ethnography is method of observational research that investigates culture in naturalistic settings using both qualitative and quantitative approaches. Using this method of observation, the researcher observes, listens to, and sometimes converses with the subjects in as free and natural an atmosphere as possible. The assumption is that the most important behavior of individuals in groups is a dynamic process of complex interactions and consists of more than one set of facts, statistics, or even discrete incidents. A position of neutrality, that is, when the researcher observes, listens, and will occasionally talk with the participants but never guides them to give certain answers, is important in this type of research.

- *Experimental study*: This type of data collection technique includes the manipulation of the variable of interest while controlling other variables that may not be of interest to the researcher. Clinical trials for new drugs are an example of an experimental study. There are many types of experimental studies, and a complete discussion would be too lengthy and complex for this introductory section. Experimentation is a sophisticated technique for the collection of data and may not be appropriate for the beginning investigator.

Selection of an Instrument

The **instrument**, also called a tool, is a consistent way to collect data. Many different types of instruments are used in research studies, and whatever type is used should be one that fits the purpose of the research. The most common instrument encountered in applied research is a survey.

Researchers sometimes use instruments that have been published in databases and occasionally publish their own instrument with their research. However, researchers should not develop an instrument until they have established that one does not already exist. If you decide to develop your own instrument, develop the questions carefully and be sure to test them to ensure that you are gathering what you need to answer the question in your research problem. It is a good idea to have someone review the questions to be sure that the questionnaire is easily read and understood and will give you the information you wish to collect. It would be too costly and time consuming to have to repeat a survey because a question or two had been neglected or were not clearly worded.

Selection of Samples

Another consideration in data collection is the selection of subjects for the study. For example, a study on health information departments in the US could try to include every HIM department in the nation, but it would likely prove impractical and could be costly and time consuming. The next best thing is to use a **sample**. When chosen correctly, samples are considered to be representative of the population.

Generally, there are two types of sampling techniques: probability sampling and nonprobability sampling. Probability sampling uses some form of random selection. Probability sampling includes the following types:

- **Simple random sampling (SRS)**: This sampling technique involves choosing individuals from the population in such a way that every individual has an equal chance of being selected. SRS is the statistical equivalent of drawing sampling units from a hat. The sample can be chosen through a random drawing or by numbering the population and making choices using random number tables or a random number generator (White 2013).

- **Systematic random sampling**: In this type of sampling, the process of selecting a sample of subjects for a study by drawing every nth unit on a list. For example, if you were choosing from a list of patients discharged during the past month, you might choose the first patient randomly and every fifth patient thereafter. In this sample, choice of the first patient determines the others. Systematic random sampling is a useful tool if the sampling frame is not available electronically. For instance, if a random sample of patients is to be selected from a scanned roster of patients that signed in during one day at a clinic, then the listing of patients or sampling frame must be keyed into a spreadsheet for sorting. Instead of keying the patient identifiers or sequence numbers into a spreadsheet, systematic random sampling may be used to select the sample directly from the scanned roster (White 2013).

- **Stratified random sampling**: In stratified random sampling, the population is divided into similar groups or strata based on a set of criteria. Each unit in the population must be assigned to one and only one stratum. Therefore, the strata do not overlap. Once the population is divided into the strata, a simple random sample is selected from each of the strata. The number of units selected from each stratum is typically based on the size of the strata relative to the size of the population (White 2013). For example, you might want to select based on gender, by patients with private insurance, or by separating hospitals by the number of beds in the facility.

- **Cluster sampling**: In cluster random sampling, the population is divided into groups before the sample is selected. As in stratified random sampling, the groups or clusters must be mutually exclusive and exhaustive. That is, every unit in the population is assigned to one and only one cluster. Cluster sampling may be performed as single-stage or two-stage versions. In single-stage cluster sampling, clusters are selected at random and all units in that cluster are included in the sample. An example of single-stage cluster sampling is to randomly select a day in the month and select all cases coded on that day as the sample. In two-stage cluster sampling, the clusters are selected at random and then the units within the randomly selected clusters are selected at random. An example of two-stage cluster sampling is to randomly select three shifts occurring during the month and then randomly select records from the three selected shifts to make up the sample.

  Cluster sampling is useful when a sampling frame containing the entire population is not available, but natural groups of the population are available for selection. Care should be taken to ensure that clusters are homogenous. For instance, in the single-stage cluster example where days are selected at random from the month, the analyst may want to exclude weekends from the population of clusters. Specialized data analysis techniques are required to analyze the data resulting from a cluster sample (White 2013).

Almost all qualitative research methods rely on nonprobability sampling. Nonprobability sampling does not involve a random sampling of the population. Nonprobability sampling includes the following:

- **Judgment sampling**: In judgment sampling, the researcher relies on his or her own judgment to select subjects for a study. For example, in a study on health information departments in acute-care hospitals that are using an EHR, the researcher might use his or her judgment to select a specific hospital size for the study from among large, small, and medium-sized hospitals that use EHRs. Interviewers who stop individuals on the street in order to ask their opinion on a topic is a population example of this type of sampling. The interviewer makes the judgment on whom to interview.

- **Quota sampling**: In this type of sampling technique, the researcher first divides the population, as in stratified sampling, and then selects the number of subjects based on a specified proportion. In quota sampling, the selection of the sample is made by the researcher who has been given or decides on quotas to fill from the subgroup of the population. Continuing with the example of health information departments above, if 50 of the 100 hospitals in the state are using an EHR and 50 are not, the researcher may choose to base their study on 20 of the hospitals because that would be 20 percent of the total population of hospitals in the state. In simple terms, a quota sample involves getting participants when you can find them, keeping in mind that the participants will have certain common characteristics.

- **Convenience sampling**: In this sampling technique, selection is based on the availability of subjects who are "conveniently" available to participate in the study. Continuing with the example above, the researcher may decide to use only hospitals within a specific city or within a certain driving distance.

Once the sample has been selected, the researcher will choose a delivery method for the instrument. This could include an electronic or web-based survey, a paper-based survey that is mailed to participants, individual face-to-face interviews, telephone interviews, or focus groups, where participants meet together at one location to discuss a topic using the interview method with an interviewer or moderator.

Exercise 12.3

Match the type of sampling with the description:

- **a.** Simple random
- **b.** Systematic random
- **c.** Stratified random
- **d.** Cluster
- **e.** Judgment
- **f.** Quota
- **g.** Convenience

1. _____ A health information professional is gathering information for a study from the coding professionals in her department.

2. _____ The marketing department of your facility will choose 50 patient satisfaction surveys from patients age 35 to 45.

3. _____ A researcher will study the incidence of cancer in your state. First, he selects the city, then the hospitals, and finally the patients to study.

4. _____ Your college is conducting a study on study habits of students. The first thing they do is divide the student body into undergraduate and graduate students; then they select a random sample of each group to interview.

5. _____ You were asked by the health information committee to evaluate the discharge summaries on every tenth patient discharged last quarter.

6. _____ A health information researcher wants to report on the salary of professionals over the last year. She uses a database from the American Health Information Management Association in which every person has the same chance of being selected for the study.

7. _____ A health information researcher wants to study the effects of the Health Insurance Portability and Accountability Act (HIPAA) regulations on employees, so she selects privacy officers with at least five years of experience to interview.

Sample Size

Usually there is a trade-off between the desirability of a large sample and the feasibility of a small one. The sample size is the number of subjects needed in a study to represent a population. The ideal **sample size** is one that is large enough to serve as an adequate representation of the population about which the researcher wishes to generalize and small enough to be selected economically in terms of subject availability, expense in both time and money, and complexity of data analysis. Here are tips about sample size:

- The larger the sample, the smaller the magnitude of sampling error.
- Survey studies ordinarily have a larger sample size than experimental studies.
- Questionnaires that are mailed can have a response rate as low as 20 percent depending on the content of the questionnaire (Kelly et al. 2003) so a large initial sample is recommended.
- When planning to have subgroups from the study population, begin with a large group to ensure you have enough participants for the subgroups.

Analyzing the Data

In this step of the research process, the investigator tries to determine what the data report. Data analysis takes a fair amount of time and should be undertaken carefully. Most researchers use a variety of techniques to describe the data. Two types of statistical applications are relevant to most quantitative research studies:

- Descriptive statistics describe the data. Measures of central tendency and measures of variation are included in descriptive statistics. These are discussed in detail in chapter 10, *Descriptive Statistics in Healthcare*.
- Inferential statistics allow the researcher to make inferences about the population characteristics (parameters) from the sample's characteristics. Chi-square and *t* tests are examples of inferential statistics that are discussed in chapter 13, *Inferential Statistics in Healthcare*.

Qualitative research relies on non-numerical observations, which include words, gestures, activities, time, space, images, artifacts, and perceptions (Watzlaf and Forrrestal 2017, 255). Two methods of analysis for qualitative research include the following:

- Grounded theory is an approach for developing theory that is taken from data that have been systematically gathered and analyzed. This usually includes data that have been obtained from observation, interviews, and review of artifacts and texts (Cohen and Crabtree 2006). The researcher is continually moving in and out of the data. Using our example of HIM directors from above, the researcher may interview HIM directors and ask what their role in the development of the facility's EHR has been. After reviewing the data, the researcher may then decide to sample HIM directors with varying educational degrees to see if there are any differences. This constant moving in and out of the data is referred to as constant comparative method. This is only completed when there are no more ideas emerging from the data.
- Content analysis is the systematic and objective analysis of communication. Content analysis is used to examine a variety of communication in addition to written documentation including speech, body language, music, television shows, commercials, and movies. The purpose of content analysis is to study and predict behaviors (Watzlaf and Forrrestal 2017, 257). In a study of role-modeling in the operating room (OR), the researchers used content analysis and the identification of themes to systematically document the types of exemplary behaviors medical students saw when observing the OR team during their anesthesia rotation in the OR. The researchers found that there were several themes such as teamwork, calmness, cooperativeness, teaching, and communication with patients. The researchers concluded that this type of exemplary behavior would contribute to their understanding of how professional behavior is viewed and potentially emulated by medical students (Curry et al. 2011).

Statistics Software Packages

There are many software packages on the market to help researchers analyze both their qualitative and quantitative data. A search on the internet will return results showing many free software packages. These packages can help the researcher produce descriptive statistics along with charts or graphs. One such package is Epi-Info, which is free software from the Centers for Disease Control and Prevention (CDC). It includes a program to create questionnaires along with allowing entry of data and analysis and creation of graphs and charts.

Another package available from the CDC is EZ-Text, which helps researchers enter data, create a codebook for the participant responses, manage and analyze qualitative databases, and export data into a variety of formats for analysis.

SPSS Statistical Package for Social Sciences (SPSS) is a statistical package that supports many industries. It offers a variety of analytical and graphic software. It also is used by many industries for its predictive analytics to help users make decisions. Other software packages include Tableau, which transforms spreadsheets and documents into professional graphic presentations, and R software, a free downloadable language and software package for statistical computing and graphics.

Drawing Conclusions

In the discussion of the conclusions, the researcher will try to answer whether or not the results supported the hypothesis or, if using the qualitative approach, identified the problem. The results from each hypothesis should be described. In the conclusion researchers also explain the significance, implications, and consequences of the findings of their study (Watzlaf and Forrrestal 2017, 263). New knowledge about a particular issue is created. Researchers use this discussion to support their hypothesis or identified problem or explain how the findings do not support them and why. Any limitations discovered during data analysis are reported. For example, the study of health information departments mentioned earlier studied one city. That may be a limiting factor; that is, the conclusions may not apply to other geographical areas. In the presentation of the research findings, new hypotheses may be proposed if the data do not support the original hypothesis or if additional problems were identified, these are explained as well. Researchers usually include tables and graphs in this section of the research report to clarify and display the data. Researchers may also make recommendations for new research into areas where questions occurred or where data did not support the original hypothesis.

Data Interpretation Issues

It has been said that statistics can tell us anything we want them to or that it is easy to lie or mislead with statistics. Unfortunately, data can be misinterpreted in many ways. Sometimes misinterpretation is the result of mistakes made in calculation or presentation of the data. Other times techniques are used so that data are purposely misconstrued. HIM professionals have an ethical obligation to report data honestly and accurately. The Department of Health and Human Services (HHS) Office of Research Integrity (ORI) is responsible for developing policies, procedures, and regulations for detecting misconduct of research and overseeing projects from groups who receive federal money. Their Division of Investigative Oversight will monitor and investigate any reports of misconduct. Reports of misconduct and their resolutions are posted on their website. The ORI also offers a definition of research misconduct as including fabrication, falsification, and plagiarism. **Fabrication** means that the data or the reported results are made up. **Falsification** means that the research material, equipment, or processes were manipulated, the data were not accurately represented, or they were changed or omitted from the report, or the results were not accurately reported. **Plagiarism** refers to taking another person's ideas or words without giving them credit. Misconduct does not include making an honest mistake or having differing opinions.

The American Statistics Association's Guidelines for Statistics Practice is a good resource to read before undertaking any research. It outlines the researcher's responsibility to the research, the subject, the research team, employers, the publications, and other researchers.

Misleading Presentation of Numbers

Statistics can be very powerful. Health information practitioners are generally the first individuals called upon to retrieve data for a facility; therefore, it is important for any "statistical communication" to be correct (Gelman and Nolan 2002).

The easiest way to fabricate data is to simply make up the numbers. As reported by the US Public Health Service, this is what happened in the case of Jon Sudbo. It was determined that he fabricated results in the reporting of information in a grant application and in the grant's first-year progress report (ORI 2011). In another case investigated by the ORI, Dong Xiao, a cancer researcher, intentionally fabricated data in his findings, including graphs he created to describe a steroid that was being tested on prostate cancer growth (ORI 2015). It is misleading and dangerous for the public to trust the study results when data are untrue; it is also a waste of research funds.

Ignoring the Baseline

Another common error is comparing raw numbers without adjusting the baseline. For example, if Hospital A and Hospital B each had 40 deaths last month, do these data provide the best indication of the level of care given at Hospital A and Hospital B? A better comparison would be to look at the number of total discharges and deaths during the last month. If Hospital A had 200 total discharges and 40 deaths and Hospital B had 500 total discharges and 40 deaths, these additional data would change some inferences about each hospital. Knowing the case mix of each hospital (such as severity of cases and diagnoses) would provide additional data for a more accurate comparison.

Selection Bias

Statistical errors can also occur when a sample used in research does not represent the population. For example, if a report was generated on the length of stay of weekend admissions for the past year using as a sample patients admitted on Friday, Saturday, or Sunday, and compared with a similar report from the previous year that used as a sample patients admitted on Saturday or Sunday, then the comparison would be biased. Comparison of the results in this example could be biased because the samples used did not represent the same days of the week. Some types of samples are inherently biased, such as convenience sampling in which subjects who are chosen are conveniently available, or snowball sampling where the researcher must rely on a participant to refer another participant. The researcher should report the results but not imply that they reflect the whole population. In the case of Dong Xiao, the number of subjects (mice) was misrepresented. (He reported he studied the effects on 10 mice when there were only 4 in the experiment.)

Graphical Misrepresentations

Graphs can be manipulated to emphasize different points. For example, a bar graph can be designed so that the difference between bar heights is lessened. The smaller the increments on the *y*-axis, the more definition there is between the different bars. A pie chart can be manipulated to pull one wedge away from the rest of the chart. This would bring greater emphasis to that portion of the pie chart even though there may not be significant differences from the rest of the chart. It is also important to be careful with three-dimensional graphs as these may misrepresent data, causing the data to appear smaller or larger. In the case of Dong Xiao, a number of figures were also falsified to show that his results did have an effect on inhibiting cancer cells.

Sabotage

There are also cases of sabotage of a colleague's work. Vipul Bhrigu, a postdoctoral researcher, meticulously and systematically sabotaged the work of a graduate student in his lab by tampering with her experiments and poisoning her cell-culture media. The ORI judged this case as research misconduct, but this ruling has been challenged by at least one other researcher because it does not technically meet the definition of misconduct by the ORI (Rasmussen 2014, 412). Other cases of misbehavior in research have occurred. For example, in one survey that asked about the behavior of colleagues, "fabrication, falsification and modification had been observed, on average, by over 14 percent of respondents and other questionable practices by up to 72 percent" (Fanelli 2009). Moreover, he found that the researchers "admitted more frequently to have "modified" or "altered" research to "improve the outcome" than to have reported results they "knew to be untrue" (Fanelli 2009).

Importance of Data Validation

Computer-generated statistical reports are common in healthcare facilities. As discussed in chapter 9, *Statistics Computed within the Health Information Management Department,* when an HIM professional receives a statistical report, he or she should examine it carefully. The total number of admissions and discharges listed in a report should match coded records. The report should also be compared against the total number of discharges listed in the census data. If the totals do not match, it is important to determine the reasons for the discrepancies. Many reports give only whole numbers. The HIM professional may need to edit the report and its statistics to ensure consistency with usual reporting procedures, such as reporting numbers to the second decimal place. Doing so makes the information valuable to administration or medical staff.

Introduction to Institutional Review Boards

Healthcare organizations that conduct research on human subjects are required to have an **Institutional Review Board (IRB)**. The IRB is a committee primarily responsible for protecting the rights and welfare of research subjects. Professionals who serve on IRBs have extensive education and experience in clinical research. Most of these individuals have medical, doctoral, or other advanced degrees. IRB is a common term used in organizations; however, an institution may use whatever name it chooses. Some organizations refer to this group as an independent ethics committee, research ethics board, or human subjects committee.

The IRB functions as a kind of ethics committee that focuses on what is right or wrong and what is undesirable in order to protect the rights and welfare of anyone participating in the research study. Because human subjects may be involved, researchers are required to follow certain ethical principles that guide researcher behavior and morality. Research ethics provide the following:

- A structure for analysis and decision-making
- Support and reminders for researchers to protect human subjects
- Workable definitions of benefits and risks

Risk versus benefit is critical in weighing the advantages of biomedical research. A benefit may be specific to the individual subject or to others as a result of the research. Risks are considered minimal when the probability and magnitude of harm or discomfort anticipated in the proposed research are not greater than those encountered in daily life.

IRBs are responsible for reviewing the research procedures before the study is started and may require periodic reviews during the study. They may approve, modify, or deny requests for research in their facility. If a research project is denied by the IRB, they must notify the researcher and give him or her an opportunity to respond to the denial. Any research on humans must be done carefully to ensure that subjects are not abused in any way. Referring to the earlier example of a study consisting of interviews with mothers of handicapped infants, even though there would not be any physical pain to the mothers, questions asked in the study theoretically could cause the mothers emotional pain. The researcher must obtain permission from the IRB before any research study is started and prepare a plan for the research. This means that the researcher must have thought through the research carefully, prepared any questionnaires, and decided how to select a sample and how to collect data in order to prepare the documentation necessary for the IRB, including informed consent forms for the subjects to read and sign. The IRB should continually review research until it is completed.

In most cases, biomedical research requires that subjects give an informed consent. **Informed consent** is a person's voluntary agreement to participate in research or to undergo a diagnostic, therapeutic, or preventive procedure. It is based on adequate knowledge and an understanding of relevant information provided by the investigators. In giving informed consent, subjects do not waive any of their legal rights nor do they release the investigator, sponsor, or institution from liability for negligence. Federal regulations require that certain information be provided to each human subject, including the following:

- A statement that the study involves research, the purpose of the research, the expected time frame of their participation, a description of the procedures to be followed, and the identification of procedures that are experimental
- A description of reasonably foreseeable risks or discomforts
- A description of the benefits to the subject or others who may reasonably benefit from the research
- A disclosure of any appropriate alternative procedures or courses of treatment that might be advantageous to the subject

- A statement describing the extent to which confidentiality of records identifying the subject will be maintained
- For research involving more than minimal risk, an explanation of whether any compensation or medical treatments are available if injury occurs, and if so, what they consist of or where further information may be obtained
- An explanation of whom to contact for answers to pertinent questions about the research and whom to contact in the event of a research-related injury
- A statement that participation is voluntary, that refusal to participate will involve no penalty or loss of benefits to which the subject may be entitled, and that the subject may discontinue participation at any time without penalty or loss of benefits to which the subject may be entitled (HHS 2004)

Federal regulations also require that informed consent be in a language that is understandable to the subject. The consent form must be translated into that language. Subjects who are not literate in their language must have an interpreter present to explain the study and to translate questions and answers between subject and investigator. A model consent form appears in figure 12.2.

Figure 12.2. Template for informed consent for research involving human subjects

Consent to Investigational Treatment or Procedure

I, _____ , hereby authorize or direct _____ or associates of his/her choosing to perform the following treatment or procedure (describe in general terms), upon _____ (myself).

The experimental (research) portion of the treatment or procedure is:

1. Purpose of the procedure or treatment
2. Possible appropriate alternative procedure or treatment (not to participate in the study is always an option)
3. Discomforts and risks reasonably to be expected
4. Possible benefits for subjects/society
5. Anticipated duration of subject's participation (including number of visits)

I hereby acknowledge that _____ has provided information about the procedure described above, about my rights as a subject, and he/she answered all questions to my satisfaction. I understand that I may contact him/her at phone number _____ should I have additional questions. He/she has explained the risks described above, and I understand them; he/she has also offered to explain all possible risks or complications.

I understand that, where appropriate, the US Food and Drug Administration may inspect records pertaining to this study. I understand further that records obtained during my participation in this study that may contain my name or other personal identifiers may be made available to the sponsor of this study. Beyond this, I understand that my participation will remain confidential.

I understand that I am free to withdraw my consent and participation in this project at any time after notifying the project director without prejudicing future care. No guarantee has been given to me concerning this treatment or procedure.

I understand that in signing this form, beyond giving consent, I am not waiving any legal rights that I might have and I am not releasing the investigator, the sponsor, or institution or its agents from any legal liability for damages that they might otherwise have.

In the event of injury resulting from participation in this study, I also understand that immediate medical treatment is available at _____ and that the costs of such treatment will be at my expense; financial compensation beyond that required by law is not available. Questions about this should be directed to the Office of Research Risks _____.

I have read and fully understand the consent form. I sign it freely and voluntarily. A copy has been given to me.

Source: HHS 2004.

Privacy Considerations in Clinical and Biomedical Research

In response to a congressional mandate in HIPAA, the HHS issued regulations titled Standards for Privacy of Individually Identifiable Health Information. Known as the Privacy Rule, it protects health records and other **individually identifiable health information**, from being used or disclosed in any form. According to HIPAA privacy provisions, individually identifiable health information is that information which specifically identifies the patient to whom the information relates, such as age, gender, date of birth, and address. In other words, individually identifiable refers to whether someone could tell or in some way could determine to whom the information refers based on the data elements. The rule became effective on April 14, 2001, and organizations covered by the rule (covered entities) were expected to comply by April 14, 2003.

The Privacy Rule establishes a category of protected health information (PHI), which may be used or disclosed only in certain circumstances or under certain conditions. PHI is a subset of what is called individually identifiable health information. It includes what healthcare professionals typically regard as a patient's PHI, such as information in the patient's health records as well as billing information for services rendered. PHI also includes identifiable health information about subjects of clinical research. Patient information considered "protected" is listed on the HHS website (HHS 2016).

Health information is any information, oral or recorded in any form, that "(1) Is created or received by a health care provider, health plan, public health authority, employer, life insurer, school or university, or health care clearinghouse; and (2) Relates to the past, present, or future physical or mental health or condition of an individual; the provision of health care to an individual; or the past, present, or future payment for the provision of health care to an individual" (45 CFR 160.103).

The Privacy Rule defines the means by which human research subjects are informed of how their personal medical information will be used or disclosed. It also outlines their right to access the information. Further, it protects the privacy of individually identifiable information but ensures researchers continue to have access to the medical information they need to conduct their research. Investigators are permitted to use and disclose PHI for research with individual authorization or without individual authorization under limited circumstances.

A valid Privacy Rule authorization is an individual's signed permission allowing a covered entity to use or disclose the patient's PHI for the purpose(s) and to the recipient(s) stated in the authorization. When an authorization is obtained for biomedical research purposes, the Privacy Rule requires that it pertain only to a specific research study, not to future unspecified projects. The core elements of the Privacy Rule authorization are as follows:

- A description of the PHI to be used or disclosed, identifying the information in a specific and meaningful manner
- The names or other specific identification of the person or persons authorized to make the requested use or disclosure
- The names or other specific identification of the person or persons to whom the covered entity may make the requested use or disclosure
- A description of each purpose of the requested use or disclosure
- An authorization expiration date or expiration event that relates to the individual or to the purpose of the use or disclosure
- The signature of the individual and the date. If the individual's legally authorized representative signs the authorization, a description of his or her authority to act for the individual also must be provided

In addition, the authorization must include statements indicating the following:

- That the individual has the right to revoke the authorization at any time and must be provided with the procedure for doing so
- Whether treatment, payment, enrollment, or eligibility of benefits can be contingent upon authorization, including research-related treatment and consequences of refusing to sign the authorization, if applicable
- Any potential risk that the PHI will be redisclosed by the recipient and no longer protected by the Privacy Rule

Finally, the authorization must be written in plain language, and a copy must be provided to the individual. A model HIPAA consent form appears in figure 12.3; optional elements that may be included in the HIPAA consent form are listed in figure 12.4.

Figure 12.3. Model HIPAA consent: Required elements

**Authorization to Use or Disclose (Release) Health Information
That Identifies You for a Research Study**

If you sign this document, you give permission to ___(name of healthcare providers)___ at
___(name of covered entity)___ to use or disclose (release) your health information that identifies
you for the research study described here:

(provide a description of the research study, such as title and purpose)

The health information that we may use or disclose (release) for this research includes:

The health information listed above may be used by and/or disclosed (released) to:

___(name of covered entity)___ is required by law to protect your health information. By signing this

document, you authorize ___(name of covered entity)___ to use and/or disclose (release) your
information for this research. Those persons who receive your health information may not be
required by federal privacy laws (such as the Privacy Rule) to protect it and may share your
information with others without your permission, if permitted by laws governing them.

Please note that (include the appropriate statement):

- You do not have to sign this authorization, but if you do not, you may not receive research-related treatment.

  (when the research involves treatment and is conducted by the covered entity or when the covered entity provides healthcare solely for the purpose of creating protected health information to disclose to a researcher)

- (Name of covered entity) may not condition (withhold or refuse) treating you based upon whether you sign this authorization.

  (when the research does not involve research-related treatment by the covered entity or when the covered entity is not providing healthcare solely for the purpose of creating protected health information to disclose to a researcher)

Please note that (include the appropriate statement):

- You may change your mind and revoke (take back) this authorization at any time, except to the extent that (name of covered entity) has already acted based on this authorization. To revoke this authorization, you must write to (name of covered entity and contact information).

  (where the research study is conducted by an entity other than the covered entity)

- You may change your mind and revoke (take back) this authorization at any time. Even if you revoke this authorization, (name of persons at the covered entity involved in the research) may still use or disclose health information they already have obtained about you as necessary to maintain the integrity or reliability of the current research. To revoke this authorization, you must write to (name of covered entity and contact information).

This authorization does not have an expiration date.

Source: HHS 2004.

Some facilities may also have a research protocol monitoring committee that reviews any research before and during the study to ensure that there are no adverse effects on the participants. It may even recommend closure of research that is not meeting safety standards, does not have scientific merit, or is not meeting the goals of the research.

Ethical Guidelines in Statistics

The HIM professional has an obligation to follow ethical guidelines in statistical practice. Statistics play an important part in clinical and healthcare administrative decision-making. Therefore, statistical data collection, calculation, display, and interpretation must be appropriate and accurate. To help ensure data quality, HIM professionals should follow the edicts of the IRB at their facilities and follow accepted ethical practice. When using statistics, HIM professionals must assure that they understand the capabilities and limitations of statistics. They must also use appropriate statistical methods and techniques for the question under study.

The American Statistical Association (ASA) has developed Ethical Guidelines for Statistical Practice. They advocate for integrity in the professional work of researchers, particularly when private interests may inappropriately influence the reporting of statistics. Their guidelines in part read that statisticians should do the following:

Figure 12.4.   Model HIPAA consent: Optional elements

Authorization to Use or Disclose (Release) Health Information
That Identifies You for a Research Study

- Your health information will be used or disclosed when required by law.

- Your health information may be shared with a public health authority that is authorized by law to collect or receive such information for the purpose of preventing or controlling disease, injury, or disability, and conducting public health surveillance, investigations, or interventions.

- No publication or public presentation about the research described above will reveal your identity without another authorization from you.

- All information that does or can identify you is removed from your health information; the remaining information will no longer be subject to this authorization and may be used or disclosed for other purposes.

- **When the research for which the use or disclosure is made involves treatment and is conducted by a covered entity:** To maintain the integrity of this research study, you generally will not have access to your personal health information related to this research until the study is complete. At the conclusion of the research and at your request, you generally will have access to your health information that (name of covered entity) maintains in a designated record set that includes medical information or billing records used in whole or in part by your doctors or other healthcare providers at (name of covered entity) to make decisions about individuals. Access to your health information in a designated record set is described in the Notice of Privacy Practices provided to you by (name of covered entity). If it is necessary for your care, your health information will be provided to you or your physician.

- If you revoke this authorization, you may no longer be allowed to participate in the research described in this authorization.

Source: HHS 2004.

- Present their findings and interpretations honestly and objectively
- Avoid untrue, deceptive, or undocumented statements
- Disclose any financial or other interests that may affect, or appear to affect, their professional statements (ASA 2018)

Hopefully, one's research will raise new questions about what should be studied and suggest needs for future research. The researcher should always include conclusions about whether or not the problem is better understood or perhaps even resolved by the study.

Health information researchers provide other HIM professionals with knowledge and methods to answer questions and to decipher problems in the work setting. Researchers should be commended for their hard work because they must be very patient and unhurried. Research requires expertise and practice and is rarely spectacular work. However, it has contributed not only to a better place to practice HIM but also to a better place to live and a greater understanding of the world around us.

Those students who would like to be involved in research and who need to develop skills in research should follow these steps:

1. Take at least one course in statistics and research methodologies.
2. Begin to read research studies in professional journals to see how others have performed their research.
3. Agree to work with a skilled health information researcher on a study to gain experience. You can find this information by contacting the author of a research study that you enjoyed reading. It is highly likely he or she will be performing another research study.
4. Learn how to present data effectively both in written form and verbally.

Exercise 12.4

Put the steps of the research process in order.

Order	Description
	Analyze the data
	Design the research
	Define the problem
	Draw conclusions
	Review the literature
	Collect the data

Chapter 12   Matching Quiz

Match the definitions with the terms.

Definitions:

a. The process of selecting subjects for a sample from each cluster within a population

b. A type of research instrument with which the members of the population being studied are asked questions and respond orally

c. A systematic investigation of all the knowledge available about a topic from sources such as books, journal articles, theses, and dissertations

d. The appropriation of another person's ideas, processes, results, or words without giving appropriate credit

e. An administrative body that provides oversight for the research studies conducted within a healthcare institution

f. A statement that describes a research question in measurable terms

g. Making up data or results and recording or reporting them

h. A sample in which every element in the population has an equal chance of being selected

i. The use of subjects who are nearby or at hand

j. A technique where the population is first segmented into mutually exclusive subgroups, and then judgment is used to select the subjects or units from each segment based on a specified proportion

Terms:

1. _____ Cluster sampling   6. _____ Literature review

2. _____ Fabrication   7. _____ Plagiarism

3. _____ Hypothesis   8. _____ Random sample

4. _____ Institutional Review Board   9. _____ Quota sampling

5. _____ Convenience sampling   10. _____ Survey

Chapter 12   Review

Complete the following exercises.

1. The degree to which scientific observations actually measure or record what they purport to measure is referred to as _____.
   a. Integrity
   b. Validity
   c. Reliability
   d. Theory

2. The type of research that uses methods or numbers, including comparisons of the population and statistical analysis, to describe results is called _____.
   a. Qualitative research
   b. Quantitative research
   c. Hypothetical research
   d. Theoretical research

3. This type of sample consists of individuals from the population chosen in such a way that every individual has an equal chance of being selected.
   a. Cluster sample
   b. Quota sample
   c. Simple random sample
   d. Judgment sample

4. A statement of the predicted relationship of what the researcher is studying is called a(n) _____.
   a. Educated guess
   b. Essay
   c. Theory
   d. Hypothesis

5. Data can be misinterpreted in which of the following ways except?
   a. Fabrication of data
   b. Graphical misrepresentations
   c. Selection bias
   d. Selection of an instrument

6. The portion of the research in which the researcher explains the significance and findings of the study is called _____.
   a. Analyzing the data
   b. Drawing conclusions
   c. Sample selection
   d. Selecting the instrument

7. Which type of research entails manipulation of a situation in some way in order to test a hypothesis?
   a. Correlational research
   b. Experimental research
   c. Evaluation research
   d. Hypothetical research

8. Which of the following is the repeatability of scientific observations?
   a. Reliability
   b. Validity
   c. Theory
   d. Integrity

9. Which data-collection method gathers data from a relatively large number of cases at a particular time?
   a. Survey
   b. Observation
   c. Essay
   d. Experimental study

10. In which type of sample does the researcher rely on his or her opinion to select the subjects?
    a. Simple random sample
    b. Judgment sample
    c. Cluster sample
    d. Quota sample

11. A tool used by the researcher to collect data is referred to as the _____.
    a. Survey
    b. Instrument
    c. Research mechanism
    d. Apparatus

12. The type of research describing events, persons, and so on without the use of numerical data is called _____.
    a. Qualitative research
    b. Quantitative research
    c. Theoretical research
    d. Hypothetical research

13. A committee within an organization whose primary responsibility is to protect the rights and welfare of research subjects is referred to as _____.
    a. Research committee
    b. Health information committee
    c. Institutional review board
    d. Therapeutics committee

14. What are generally the two types of research?

    a. Quantitative and qualitative

    b. Basic and applied

    c. Scientific and hypothetical

    d. Theory and hypothesis

15. A method of observation in which the researcher observes and often speaks with the subjects in as free and natural an atmosphere as possible is called _____.

    a. Freedom of inquiry

    b. Conclusive inquiry

    c. Ethnography

    d. Controlled research

13 Inferential Statistics in Healthcare

Learning Objectives

At the conclusion of this chapter, you should be able to do the following:

- Explain inferential statistics
- Compare and contrast descriptive and inferential statistics
- Interpret the standard error of the mean and confidence intervals
- Identify and describe the null hypothesis
- Understand the importance of *t* tests and the chi-square

Key Terms

Chi-square	*p*-value	Type I error
Confidence interval	Standard error of the mean	Type II error
Inferential statistics	*t* test	

In health information management (HIM) practice, descriptive statistics, covered in chapter 10, *Descriptive Statistics in Healthcare,* are most often used in an HIM department. Terms such as mortality and morbidity are examples of descriptive statistics. Healthcare researchers, in contrast, are interested in understanding the characteristics of and reaching conclusions about a population from a sample, which is called **inferential statistics**. We will see the use of this type of statistic in health information research as well.

Inferential Statistics

In chapter 10 we learned that descriptive statistics describe a population and are used to describe data in ways that are manageable and easily understood. Inferential statistics allow us to generalize data from a sample to a population with a certain amount of confidence regarding our findings. Without inferential statistics, it would be very difficult, short of conducting a census, to describe the characteristics of a population. The ability to interpret inferential statistics requires a understanding of descriptive statistical measures and computations.

Errors in sampling procedures are inevitable. The use of random sampling limits the types of errors, but there is no guarantee that the sample drawn will be exactly the same as the population. For this reason, inferential statistics are limited to certain amounts of confidence.

This chapter discusses the interpretation of common inferential statistical measures, including standard error of the mean, confidence intervals, hypothesis testing, *t* tests, and chi-square.

It is not the intention of this chapter to replace a general statistics course. This chapter merely provides a review of concepts you have learned in that course with exercises from a healthcare perspective. An exhaustive explanation of these concepts, including mathematical computation, is beyond the scope of this book.

Confidence Intervals

When trying to determine the characteristics of a population, the mean or average from one sample may not be sufficient because of the potential for a random sampling error. A more accurate representation could be found by taking many large samples, calculating the mean for each sample, and then finding the standard deviation of all the sample means. This value is called the **standard error of the mean**, abbreviated SE_m, and comes from the standard deviation of many sample means. Because of a statistical theory called the central limit theorem, the distribution of all the sample means is a normal distribution when the sample size is reasonably large. An in-depth discussion of this concept is beyond the scope of this text, but this underlying theorem is the basis for much of inferential statistics.

Finding the SE_m in the manner described above can be tedious, and it may not be realistic to find the SE_m of the sample means. For this reason, statisticians have found a formula for approximating the SE_m from only one random sample:

$$SE_m = \frac{Standard\ deviation\ of\ the\ sample}{Square\ root\ of\ the\ sample\ size} \ or\ \frac{sd}{\sqrt{n}}$$

Example 13.1: Use the data that follows to calculate the SE_m mean = 150, sd = 10 for a sample of size 75. Round to two decimal places.

$$\bar{x} = 150, sd = 10, n = 75$$

$$SE_m = \frac{sd}{\sqrt{n}} = \frac{10}{\sqrt{75}} = \frac{10}{8.66} = 1.154$$

Rounded to two decimal places: 1.15.

In inferential statistics, the SE_m may be used to calculate a range of potential values for the population mean. This is called a **confidence interval** (abbreviated CI). Confidence intervals have probabilities associated with them that assess the certainty that the actual population mean (which we cannot observe) is included in the interval.

In a normal distribution, confidence intervals are calculated by adding one standard error of the mean to and subtracting one from the mean, then adding two standard errors of the mean to and subtracting two from the mean, and so on. The percentages below come from a normal distribution (see chapter 10 for more information about normal distribution):

- 68 percent of all scores in a normal distribution fall within + or – 1 standard deviation away from the mean.
- 95 percent of all scores in a normal distribution fall within + or – 2 standard deviations away from the mean.
- 99.7 percent of all scores in a normal distribution fall within + or – 3 standard deviations away from the mean.

Example 13.2: Use the statistics from example 13.1 to calculate 68 percent and 95 percent confidence intervals for the population mean.

68% CI:
$$150 - 1.15 = 148.85$$
$$150 + 1.15 = 151.15$$

95% CI:
$$150 - (2 \times 1.15) = 147.70$$
$$150 + (2 \times 1.15) = 152.30$$

It is important to note that the larger the sample size, the more confidence there is in the mean and the smaller the chance for sampling errors, meaning a smaller SE_m. Further, the more homogenous a population (less variation), the smaller the SE_m. In fact, if a population were all the same (no variation) the SE_m would be zero.

Exercise 13.1

Given the information below, find the 68 percent, 95 percent, and 99.7 percent confidence intervals. Round to one decimal place.

$$\bar{x} = 14, sd = 2, n = 30$$

68% CI = _____

95% CI = _____

99.7% CI = _____

Hypothesis Testing

As presented in chapter 12, *Basic Research Principles,* the null hypothesis is the default situation or status quo. When comparing two populations, it may state that the difference between two population means is zero. Hypothesis testing is a technique that allows the researcher to assess the likelihood that the null hypothesis is true given the sample data collected during the study.

Suppose we obtain a sample of the length of stay (LOS) at University Hospital and Community Hospital. The mean LOSs are as follows:

University Hospital (Group U): $\bar{X}_u = 3.9\ days$

Community Hospital (Group C): $\bar{X}_c = 3.5\ days$

From these results, it would appear that the LOS at University Hospital is longer than the LOS at Community Hospital. However, this may not be true; in fact, the difference may be due to errors in sampling, and the population mean of the LOS of patients at University Hospital may equal the population mean of the LOS of patients at Community Hospital. Hypothesis testing can help answer this question because it takes into consideration the sample mean, the sample standard deviation, and the size of the sample.

The null hypothesis is that the two hospitals' mean LOSs are equal and can be expressed as follows:

$$H_0 : \mu_u = \mu_c \ or \ \mu_u - \mu_c = 0$$

When conducting research, most researchers are searching for differences in population means and are therefore not looking to confirm the null hypothesis. In fact, hypothesis testing will only allow the researcher to either reject or not reject the null hypothesis. Therefore, researchers must also develop an alternative hypothesis to test against the null. The alternative hypothesis can be expressed either as a one-sided alternative

$$H_0 : \mu_u < \mu_c$$

or

$$H_0 : \mu_u > \mu_c$$

or a two-sided alternative

$$H_0 : \mu_u \neq \mu_c$$

The first alternative hypothesis states that group U is larger than group C; this would be the same as the samples would imply, that the LOS at University Hospital is longer than the LOS at Community Hospital. The second alternative hypothesis states that group U is smaller than group C; this would indicate the samples do not represent the population, and that the LOS at University Hospital is no longer than the LOS at Community Hospital. The third alternative hypothesis states that group U and group C are different, but there is not enough information to determine which population of patients has the longer mean LOS.

Because there is always a chance that the null hypothesis is true, testing it will lead to a probability (p) that it is true. The smaller the *p*-**value** (probability that the null hypothesis is true given the sample data), the more evidence that we should reject the null hypothesis. As a rule of thumb accepted by most statisticians in hypothesis testing, if the probability that the null hypothesis is true is 5 percent or less, the null hypothesis is rejected. The threshold for rejecting the null hypothesis (5 percent) is called the alpha level. Therefore, if the *p*-value is less than that alpha level (5 percent or 0.05) then the null hypothesis should be rejected.

In hypothesis testing, rejecting the null hypothesis with this level of confidence is, in effect, describing the relationship between the means as statistically significant. This is generally the manner in which the null hypothesis is discussed in academic journals.

Dealing with levels of uncertainty in hypothesis testing creates two types of errors: Type I errors and Type II errors. A **Type I error** occurs when the null hypothesis is rejected, yet it is actually true. A **Type II error** occurs when the null hypothesis is not rejected, yet it is false. Following are examples of both types of errors.

Type I Error

According to the National Cancer Institute, a woman's chance of being diagnosed with breast cancer from age 50 through age 59 is 2.38 percent (NCI 2012). With this knowledge, going to see a doctor because of a lump on her breast presents a risk that the doctor will diagnose the patient with breast cancer even if she does not have breast cancer. Consider the following null hypothesis: there is no difference between women diagnosed with breast cancer and women not diagnosed with breast cancer. Rejecting the null hypothesis in this instance would be assuming that the doctor will not diagnose her with breast cancer, as there is a difference between the two populations (women diagnosed with breast cancer and women not diagnosed with breast cancer). However, if she is diagnosed with breast cancer, this would be an example of a Type I error. Simply said, the patient could receive a positive test result when, in fact, she does not have breast cancer.

Type II Error

A Type I error is controlled by the researcher setting the acceptable error rate. A Type II error is driven by the sample size and the particular test used. Suppose a drug company has developed a new drug for a serious disease and the new drug is effective. If, however, the null hypothesis is not rejected because the drug company selected a level of significance that is too high, the results of the study will have to be described as insignificant and the drug may not receive government approval (Pyrczak 2010, 83). This is an example of a Type II error.

When describing the null hypothesis, it is never "accepted." Rather, we say "reject the null hypothesis" or "fail to reject the null hypothesis."

Exercise 13.2

Use the following information to provide an example of a Type I and Type II error.

A pharmaceutical company tests a promising new medicine designed to lower cholesterol when taken daily. The pharmaceutical company conducts a study to determine the effectiveness of the medication against a placebo. Consider the null hypothesis: there is no difference between the effectiveness of the new medication and the placebo in lowering cholesterol.

    Type I error: _____
    Type II error: _____

 The calculation of the actual test statistic is not presented in this text. Instead, the practical interpretation of the results is presented.

t Test

A *t test* is an example of a test of the null hypothesis regarding two population means to determine if a set of results is statistically significant. As mentioned previously, for the results to be considered statistically significant, the probability that the null hypothesis is true should be 5 percent or less. The results of a *t* test can be written several ways. Consider the following example.

Example 13.3:

Group	$\bar{x}$	Standard Deviation (*sd*)	n
A	5.3	1.6	10
B	6.6	1.0	10

With this group of data, the results of the t test (calculate using Excel or a calculator) can be written as follows:

The null hypothesis: There is no difference between the groups.

$$H_0: \mu_1 - \mu_2 = 0 \text{ (the difference between the means is zero)}$$

1. Statistically significant ($t = 2.18$, $df = 18$, $p < 0.05$)

2. Statistically significant at the 0.05 level ($t = 2.18$, $df = 18$)

3. Reject H_0 at the 0.05 level ($t = 2.18$, $df = 18$)

Where: t = the value produced by the t test

        df = The degrees of freedom are found by taking $n - 1$ for the number of groups. In the sample above, there are two groups, therefore:

$$df = (n_1 - 1) + (n_2 - 1)$$
$$df = (10 - 1) + (10 - 1) = 18$$
$$df = 18$$

Statements 1 through 3 above all reject the null hypothesis and say that there is a statistically significant difference between the population means of Group A and Group B ($5.3 - 6.6 = -1.3$ days).

However, the sample data may not support the conclusion that there is a statistically significant difference between the means. Consider the following example.

Example 13.4:

Group	$\bar{x}$	Standard Deviation (*sd*)	*n*
A	25	3	8
B	24	3	8

$$H_0: \mu_1 - \mu_2 = 0 \text{ (the difference between the means is zero)}$$

1. Not statistically significant ($t = 0.67$, $df = 14$, $p > 0.05$)

2. H_0 is not rejected at the 0.05 level ($t = 0.67$, $df = 14$)

These statements do not reject the null hypothesis and say that the difference between the sample means is not statistically significant ($25 - 24 = 1$). The null hypothesis is not rejected because the probability of incorrectly rejecting the null hypothesis and stating the means are different is greater than 5 percent; for this reason, the difference between the means is not statistically significant.

Example 13.5:

Group	$\bar{x}$	Standard Deviation (*sd*)	*n*
A	18	2.5	7
B	17	8	7

The null hypothesis: There is no difference between the groups.

$H_0: \mu_1 - \mu_2 = 0$ (the difference between the means is zero)

($t = 0.32$, $df = 12$, $p > 0.05$) Do not reject the null hypothesis.

Exercise 13.3

Given the information in the example above, would you reject the null hypothesis or not? How would you state your findings?

It is important to note that understanding the computation involved in testing the null hypothesis is reserved for an advanced statistics course and is not part of the daily activities of a healthcare practitioner. How to interpret the results of these tests, however, is important. For this reason, a section on chi-square is briefly introduced.

Chi-Square

Chi-square (represented by the symbol χ^2) is a test of significance that deals with nominal data and frequencies, specifically data where the standard deviation and mean are not meaningful descriptions. Note that calculation is possible, just not meaningful. Using computer software to conduct a chi-square test is simple and quickly yields results. Consider the following example.

Example 13.6: Employees at a large healthcare facility were randomly asked whether they smoked and whether they had parents who smoked. The results of the 150 employees sampled were as follows:

	Parents Who Smoke	**Parents Who Do Not Smoke**
Employee smokes	45	25
Employee does not smoke	30	50

The data in this table suggest that those employees with parents who did not smoke were likelier not to smoke (50 versus 25) than were those employees with parents who smoked (30 versus 45). From this sample alone, there appears to be a relationship between smoking and having parents who smoke. However, there is a possibility that the null hypothesis, that the relationship does not exist in this population, is true. A chi-square test can determine whether the relationship is statistically significant. A chi-square test using the values above yielded these results:

$$\chi^2 = 10.71, df = 1, p < 0.01$$

Based on the results, there is a less than 1 percent chance of making a mistake by rejecting the null hypothesis. Said another way, the results are statistically significant; there is a relationship between employees who do not smoke having parents who do not smoke.

Notice below that the degrees of freedom are determined differently for chi-square. The degrees of freedom are found by taking $(r-1) \times (c-1)$ for the number of categories, where r = the number of rows and c = the number of columns.

$$df = (r-1)(c-1)$$
$$df = (2-1)(2-1) = (1)(1) = 1$$
$$df = 1$$

Chapter 13 Matching Quiz

Match the definitions with the term.

Definitions:

a. A test of significance, represented by χ^2, that deals with nominal data and frequencies, specifically data where the standard deviation and mean are not meaningful descriptions

b. A healthcare statistic that is calculated from the standard error of the mean, it is an estimate of the true limits within which the true population mean lies; the range of values that may reasonably contain the true population mean

c. Statistics that are used to make inferences from a smaller group of data to a large one

d. A hypothesis that states there is no association between the independent and dependent variables in a research study

e. A value that is found by taking many large samples, calculating the mean for each sample, and then finding the standard deviation of all the sample means

f. A test of the null hypothesis to determine if a set of results is statistically significant

g. Occurs when the null hypothesis is rejected, yet it is actually true

h. Occurs when the null hypothesis is not rejected, yet it is false

Terms:

1. _____ Type II error
2. _____ Null hypothesis
3. _____ Confidence interval
4. _____ Type I error

5. _____ Standard error of the mean
6. _____ t test
7. _____ Chi-square
8. _____ Inferential statistics

Chapter 13   Review

1. Define the term inferential statistics.

2. Explain the difference between descriptive and inferential statistics.

3. Identify which choices would be considered descriptive statistics and which would be considered inferential statistics.

   Of 500 randomly selected people in New York City, 210 people had O+ blood.

   a. "42 percent of the people in New York City have O+ blood." Is the statement descriptive statistics or inferential statistics?

   b. "58 percent of the people of New York City do not have type O+ blood." Is the statement descriptive statistics or inferential statistics?

   c. "42 percent of all people living in New York State have type O+ blood." Is the statement descriptive statistics or inferential statistics?

4. Identify which choices would be considered descriptive statistics and which would be considered inferential statistics.

   On the last three Friday evenings, City Hospital diagnosed a number of heroin overdoses. There were four on January 14, 20XX, two on January 21, 20XX, and six on January 28, 20XX.

   a. "City Hospital averaged four heroin overdoses in their ED for the last three Friday evenings."

   b. "City Hospital never has more than six heroin overdoses on Friday evenings."

   c. "Friday nights are the busiest time for heroin overdoses at City Hospital."

5. The standard error of the mean comes from the standard deviation of many population means.

   a. True

   b. False

6. Create a null hypothesis for the following research question: What are the differences between ED shifts on medication errors?

7. Create a null hypothesis for the following research question: On a clinical trial of a new drug, what will be the effects compared to a currently used drug?

8. Reword the following research hypothesis to a null hypothesis: Smoking during pregnancy increases the risk of a child being born prematurely.

9. Reword the following research hypothesis to a null hypothesis: Regular exercise in older adults decreases blood pressure levels.

10. Based on the results below, how would you describe the relationship between heart attack patients being treated with aspirin and whether or not they lived?

	Male Heart Attack Patients Treated with Aspirin	Male Heart Attack Patients Not Treated with Aspirin
Male patients who lived	15	4
Male patients who did not live	2	8

$$\chi^2 = 9.39, df = 1, p \le 0.01$$

11. Use the information in the table that follows to determine if the differences between the means are significant.

Medical Terminology Class

Group A = Number of word elements remembered by students using flash cards

Group B = Number of word elements remembered by students not using flash cards

Group	$\bar{x}$	Standard Deviation (sd)	n
A	75	2.0	10
B	50	3.5	10

The null hypothesis: There is no difference between the groups.

$$H_0: \mu_1 - \mu_2 = 0 \text{ (the difference between the means is zero)}$$

$$(t = 19.61, df = 18, p < 0.01)$$

12. Given the following p values, which would be considered more significant?

   a. $p \le 0.3$

   b. $p \le 0.02$

   c. $p \le 0.25$

13. Given the following null hypothesis, give an example of a Type I error.

   H_0: There is no difference between the number of males or females who go to their primary care physician for an annual exam.

14. Given the following null hypothesis, give an example of a Type II error.

   H_0: There is no difference in the level of understanding of this chapter between students who have previously taken a statistics course and students who have not previously taken a statistics course.

15. Given the following information, determine the 68 percent, 95 percent, and 99.7 percent confidence intervals. Round to two decimal places.

$$\bar{x} = 4.33, SE_m = 3$$

APPENDIX A | An Introduction to Data Analytics

With the advent of electronic health records (EHRs), a new field of information science has emerged that is concerned with the management of health data—data analytics. This field combines information technology with healthcare and develops ways to control stored health information. Because of the proliferation of data and the need to make it meaningful, the next challenge for healthcare is the move toward data analytics. This area will make it possible for data analysts to use the data from the EHRs along with data from other systems, such as research results, to provide better care for patients and monitor the cost of that care more closely.

What Is Data Analytics?

Healthcare is a business that relies on tremendous amounts of decision-making, both in the clinical and administrative aspects of healthcare. EHRs have expanded the amount of data available to physicians and administrators. Big data is a term used for the massive amounts of information that can be interpreted by analytics to provide an overview of trends or patterns. The primary purpose of any healthcare data should be to help healthcare practitioners provide the best care available to patients. A trend in healthcare is to move toward evidence-based medicine, which involves systematically reviewing clinical data and making treatment decisions based on the best available information (Kayyoll et al. 2013). This would be tedious and most impossible for a physician to complete manually.

Healthcare administrators also use data to make sound business decisions regarding financial aspects of the facility. Data analysis is defined as the task of transforming, summarizing, or modeling data to allow the user to make meaningful conclusions. For example, data analytics can help healthcare administrators identify fraud in their billing claims. Data analytics can link various components, including provider and equipment supplier names, aliases, and demographic data, to detect unusual or hidden relationships.

Health data analysts are responsible for taking health data and transforming it into information that is easily understood. The American Health Information Management Association (AHIMA) offers a credential called certified health data analyst (CHDA). Practitioners who earn this credential have the knowledge to acquire, manage, analyze, interpret, and transform data into accurate, consistent, and timely information, while balancing the "big picture" strategic vision with day-to-day details (AHIMA 2015). Individuals with this credential are prepared for the role of data analyst or content analyst. A data analyst works with policies and procedures on how data will be acquired and studies the data to translate it into information that administrators can use to make business decisions, while a content analyst is responsible for supporting the development and design of clinical information systems by working with clinicians to determine what they need to make good clinical decisions. Another role could be an informaticist who is responsible for tracking outcomes for analysis and billing.

Data analytics is the science of examining raw data with the purpose of drawing conclusions about that information. Analytics can be descriptive, predictive, or prescriptive.

- Descriptive analytics is just the summarization of data.
- Predictive analytics is a branch of data mining concerned with the prediction of future probabilities and trends, also called forecasting.

- Prescriptive analytics is related to descriptive and predictive analytics, but it tries to automatically process new data to improve the accuracy of predictions and provide better decision options (SearchCIO 2012).

Types of Healthcare Data

Healthcare data are divided into two broad categories of quantitative and qualitative data. Quantitative data are numeric while qualitative data describe observations. Quantitative data can be numerically counted. They deal with measurements. Quantitative data are categorized into the categories of interval and ratio. As covered in chapter 11 of this text, *Presentation of Data,* interval data are numeric, in which we know the order and the differences between the values. Ratio data have a defined unit of measure, and the intervals between successive values are equal.

Qualitative data are divided into the nominal scale and ordinal scale. Observations are organized into categories in which there is no recognition of order, and ordinal data are types of data where the values are in ordered categories and the order of the numbers is meaningful, but not the numbers themselves.

Data are also categorized in terms of internal and external data. Internal data sources are those which are obtained from inside an organization. In healthcare this includes health records, registries, surveys taken of patient satisfaction or other performance improvement studies, annual or other reports, and committee minutes.

External data sources refer to data collected outside an organization. For example, a census, reports from the Centers for Medicare and Medicaid Services (CMS) or the Centers for Disease Control (CDC), economic databases, journals, and even social media have links to outside data. Healthcare organizations use both internal and external data to help them in decision-making.

Data analytics relies on both descriptive and inferential statistics. Remember from chapter 10 of this text, *Descriptive Statistics in Healthcare,* that descriptive statistics describe a population. The typical value may be described by using the mean, median, or mode. The spread of the data may be described using range, variance, and standard deviation. Inferential statistics, which is discussed in chapter 13 of this text, allow us to generalize from a sample to a population with a certain amount of confidence regarding our findings. Inferential statistics are used to test hypotheses or make decisions about the population. These statistics have a probability of making an error. This was referred to as a Type I or Type II error. Inferential statistics offers a confidence level; that is, the probability that the value of a parameter falls within a specified range of values. For example, a confidence level of 95 percent means that there is a probability of at least 95 percent that the result is reliable.

Most studies conducted by a health data analyst require a type of sample. These were covered in detail in chapter 12 of this text, *Basic Research Principles.* The most common type of probability sample used is the random sample. These include simple, stratified, systematic, and cluster sampling. The sample size is determined by the amount of precision desired for the study. There are a number of software tools available to help analysts calculate the size; Statistical Package for the Social Sciences (SPSS) and Statistical Analysis System (SAS) are common. Another program that is often used is called RAT-STATS. It is free to download from the Office of Inspector General's Office of Audit Services. This statistical software program helps facilities perform billing reviews by generating random numbers to random samples, evaluate sample results, and estimate a sample size.

Types of Data Analytics

Healthcare facilities use data analytics to help them make business and clinical decisions. However, new technologies will allow data to be used immediately. This immediate use of data will permit facilities to stay competitive and flexible.

Descriptive Analytics

Descriptive analytics describe raw data. This type of analytics is useful because it helps us see what was done in the past. We can learn from our past behaviors and begin to look at how we can effect some change in the future. Most of the statistics used in healthcare fall into this category. This type of analytics is used to understand at an aggregate level what is happening with patients in healthcare facilities.

Predictive Analytics

Predictive analytics are about understanding the future, keeping in mind that nothing can predict the future with 100 percent certainty. This type of analytics takes the information the healthcare facility has in its EHRs and data warehouses and tries to make the best guess based on patterns. Facilities use this type of analytics when they want to look into the future. Called forecasting, this type of analytics helps determine the probability that something will happen.

Data Mining

Data mining is the process of extracting and analyzing large volumes of data from a database for the purpose of identifying hidden and sometimes subtle relationships or patterns and using those relationships to predict behaviors. Data mining uses both graphical techniques and descriptive statistics to identify trends and patterns in data (White 2013, 7).

For example, data mining can be used to determine which type of patients are using the most resources or abusing resources or to help healthcare facilities make management decisions and help physicians make good clinical decisions for patients.

Data mining has successfully helped healthcare organizations fight healthcare fraud. The National Healthcare Anti-Fraud Association (NHCAA) estimated that fraudulent payments for healthcare services accounts for about 3 percent of the total health expenditures in 2007. They place the range of fraud to be from $70 billion to over $200 billion (Lamont 2009, 1). Fraud in healthcare includes a variety of activities, such as charging for services that were never performed, assigning codes that would receive a higher reimbursement, or creating nonexistent patients. Data mining can detect patterns that do not match what would typically be seen in certain claims—higher than average charges, tests and services that are not usually performed, treatments that do not match the diagnosis, and demographics to identify patients that lead the facility to suspect identity theft.

Clinical Data Warehouse

A clinical data warehouse is a collection of data that reflects all aspects of hospital operations and that is used for reporting and analysis. Rather than backing up data, a warehouse lets users find subject-oriented information on demand (Byer 2011). Warehouses are found in many departments in the healthcare facility including the pharmacy, registration, accounting services, and the laboratory. Combining these data into a warehouse allows for many users of the data. The clinical data warehouse can make patient care more efficient and quality outcomes easier to assess. They can also use the warehouse for gathering data for grant-funded research studies. Because of the volume of data available in the health record along with articles in medical journals, researchers will be able to identify associations, trends, and patterns in the data more easily.

Predictive Modeling

Predictive modeling is a statistical method that uses historical data to identify patterns that can be used to determine the odds of a particular outcome based on the observed data. That is, statistics from the past are reviewed to determine what is likely to happen in the future. Predictive modeling is used by many companies that want to predict future trends. For example, insurance companies use predictive modeling, or analysis, to determine how insurance policies will be priced. They "investigate thousands of predictors—including such things as what other policies an insured [individual] has, whether they pay their bills on time, and various characteristics of the area in which the risk is located" (Insurance Journal 2012). The auto insurance industry is also able to use telematics—the computer and electronic technology involved in our cars—to record driving behavior data from its customers (Insurance Journal 2012). In the case of healthcare, predictive modeling statistical techniques are used to determine the likelihood of certain events occurring together (White 2011).

Predictive modeling can help healthcare organizations reduce costs and improve patient care. For example, many health insurance companies use predictive modeling techniques to identify claims that are suspicious in order to have them reviewed for accuracy. CMS has moved toward predictive modeling to detect improper Medicare claims. Predictive modeling flags suspicious claims and requires them to be reviewed individually. In 2015, in an effort to improve patient care and prevent one million heart attacks and strokes by 2017, the Department of Health and Human Services (HHS) launched its Million Hearts: Cardiovascular Disease Risk Reduction Model (Letourneau 2015).

Predictive modeling goes beyond just collecting data. At Advocate Health Care, a large health system based in Illinois, a predictive analytics project identifies which patients might be readmitted within 30 days after discharge. Another project they have undertaken includes an initiative to identify patients who are likely candidates for interventions to prevent disease, better manage their health conditions outside the hospital, and prevent future hospitalizations, all of which could save insurers and the system money (Evans 2014).

Real-Time Analytics

Unlike retrospective analytical tools, such as predictive modeling, real-time analytics refers to data that can be accessed as they come into a computer system. Real-time analytics, also referred to as streaming analytics, implies instantaneous results; however, the data may not be immediately available, but rather within a few minutes. The most valuable data in this category are those that are collected and analyzed during the customer interaction, not the review afterward. The analysis that counts is not the results of the last three months, or even the last three days, but the last 30 seconds—probably less (Babcock 2015). The University of Texas Southwestern Medical Center in Dallas is analyzing data from their EHRs to study readmissions of congestive heart failure patients. The EHR analytics model used in the study draws on 29 clinical, social, and behavioral factors within 24 hours of a patient's admission for heart failure, making it possible to match the intensity of the readmission intervention to the patient's risk of readmission on any given day. This real-time program allows physicians to focus on the patients with the highest risk of readmission and has been successful in reducing the number of hospital returns (Bresnick 2013).

Prescriptive Analytics

Prescriptive analytics is a relatively new field of analytics that allows users to prescribe a number of different possible actions. This type of analytics predicts what will happen, but also provides recommendations that will take advantage of the predictions. By providing information about the possible future, this allows facilities to look at the predicted outcomes and come to a decision. Because this is relatively new, most companies are not yet using this technique in their daily course of business (Halo 2014).

Using Data Analytics for Decision-Making

Healthcare organizations are beginning to rely on data analytics to learn about their patient populations. The more information they have, the more they can make informed decisions.

Data analytics can help healthcare providers in clinical decision support. For example, data analytics can be used to help physicians search through past cases to make an informed decision on one particular patient. Having all patient information, such as lab and x-ray results, medications, and physician orders, on one electronic dashboard (or e-dashboard) can improve how physicians view the data and make decisions about their patients. A dashboard is a visual display of the most important information that a physician would need to see about the physician's patients. These can usually be customized by facility or an individual. Data analytics can also help facilities with coordinating a patient's care; that is, monitoring when patients are transferred to other physicians or services. Healthcare providers can use data analytics to help illness from recurring by looking for patterns in the data that are linked to an illness.

Data analytics can also help healthcare executives in a variety of ways. For example, employees can monitor hospital inventory so they will know when to order materials rather than keep a large inventory on hand. Organizations can also compare their facilities with others and then establish benchmarks to improve care. Something as simple as determining wait times in clinics can have a financial impact on the organization. When a facility falls short of its benchmarks, it can apply educational programs to teach employees how to improve processes.

Data analytics is one of the most useful tools available to a health information professional. A health information management (HIM) professional's educational background and experience makes them particularly adept at dealing with data analytics. AHIMA's *Healthcare Data Analysis Toolkit* lists a number of skills needed to be successful as a data analyst, including the following:

- Understands coding systems (CPT/HCPCS, DRG, ICD-10-CM, ICD-10-PCS, National Drug Code [NDC])
- Demonstrates strong verbal and written communication skills
- Demonstrates excellent organizational and time-management skills
- Exhibits keen attention to detail and problem-solving skills
- Knows Microsoft Office, especially Excel and Access (Bronnert et al. 2011)

Health information professionals are in a unique position because they understand coding systems in which all diseases are categorized and can communicate with the many departments of the healthcare facility, including the administrative and clinical sides of healthcare. Their educational programs require computer skills. HIMS programs are one of the few allied health fields that requires a statistics course in their educational requirements.

Big data is growing exponentially. For example, some companies have developed ways to track patients with their smartphones or other medical devices to determine how patients are behaving. One example is from Propeller Health, a company that developed a GPS-enabled software that keeps track of patients with chronic respiratory diseases. It keeps track of medications and inhaler use and can be used with rescue and controller medications for tracking symptoms. The sensor on the inhaler wirelessly connects to the patient's smartphone to record data, which can be shared with the patient's physician.

Reminders that can be sent to patients with chronic diseases to remind them to take their medications or make an appointment to have lab tests completed are all part of big data in healthcare. There will be many more opportunities to help patients in the future. The potential for cutting healthcare costs also is possible. It is estimated that $300 billion to $450 billion in reduced healthcare spending could be conservative, as many insights and innovations are still ahead (Kayyoll et al. 2013). Facilities and individuals willing to put in the time and energy to learn more about data analytics will reap the rewards.

In Medicine 2064, Dr. Daniel Kraft explains his vision of healthcare, in which patients work together with their physicians in participatory medicine to create specialized medications specifically for them. He states we are on the technological cusp now with the big data we are collecting. It will not be necessary to wait for a patient to get sick to provide treatment; physicians will be able to know how to prevent disease before it happens (Kraft 2014).

Information Governance

As EHRs continue to evolve, and as data analytics continue to develop more information, healthcare facilities will need to organize and manage this information. An initiative that is gaining momentum in this area is information governance (IG). IG is defined as an organization-wide framework for managing information throughout its lifecycle and supporting the organization's strategy, operations, and regulatory, legal, and environmental requirements. IG applies to all information kept in a facility. IG includes policies, procedures, and processes developed in a healthcare facility that support the facility's efforts to gain value from and understand its information in order to meet the organization's goals as well as protect itself against legal action. It includes more than traditional HIM practices but also information security, compliance, quality management, and risk management. IG ensures the trustworthiness of information.

APPENDIX B | References

45 CFR 160.103: General Administrative Requirements Definitions Subpart A. 2013. http://www.ecfr.gov/cgi-bin/text-idx?node=se45.1.160_1103&rgn=div8.

Agency for Healthcare Research and Quality. 2017 (February). Preventing Avoidable Readmissions. Accessed from Agency for Healthcare Research and Quality: Advancing Excellence in Health Care: https://www.ahrq.gov/professionals/quality-patient-safety/patient-safety-resources/resources/impptdis/index.html.

American College of Surgeons. 2019 (March 02). Apply for Accreditation. Accessed from Commission on Cancer: https://www.facs.org/quality-programs/cancer/coc/apply.

American Health Information Management Association (AHIMA). 2017. *Pocket Glossary of Health Information Management and Technology,* 5th ed. Chicago: AHIMA.

American Health Information Management Association (AHIMA). 2015. Certified health data analyst (CHDA). www.ahima.org/certification/cdha.

American Statistical Association. 2018. Ethical guidelines for statistical practice. https://www.amstat.org/ASA/Your-Career/Ethical-Guidelines-for-Statistical-Practice.aspx.

Babcock, C. 2015 (June 23). Big data moves toward real-time analysis. http://www.informationweek.com/big-data/software-platforms/big-data-moves-toward-real-time-analysis/a/d-id/1320952.

Barfield, W. 2016 (April 18). Standard Terminology for Fetal, Infant and Perinatal Deaths. *Pediatrics* 2016; 137(5): e20160551. doi:10.1542/peds.2016-0551.

Bowden, J. 2008. *Writing a Report: How to Prepare, Write and Present Really Effective Reports*. Oxford, UK: How to Books Ltd.

Bresnick, J. 2013 (August 2). Real-time EHR data analytics helps reduce readmissions by 5%. *EHR Intelligence.* https://ehrintelligence.com/news/real-time-ehr-data-analytics-helps-reduce-readmissions-by-5/.

Bronnert, J., J. Clark, L. Hyde, J. Solberg, S. White, and M. Wolin. 2011. *Health Data Analysis Toolkit*. Chicago: AHIMA.

Byer, C. 2011 (October 25). Using health care data analytics to improve information management. *Tech Target.* http://searchhealthit.techtarget.com/tutorial/Using-health-care-data-analytics-to-improve-information-management.

Casto, A. 2018. *Principles of Healthcare Reimbursement,* 6th ed. Chicago: AHIMA.

Centers for Disease Control and Prevention (CDC). 2019 (January 23). About CDC 24-7. https://www.cdc.gov/about/organization/cio.htm.

Centers for Disease Control and Prevention (CDC). 2019 (February 21). National Vital Statistics System. https://www.cdc.gov/nchs/nvss/index.htm.

Centers for Disease Control and Prevention (CDC). 2019a. National Healthcare Safety Network (NHSN) overview. https://www.cdc.gov/nhsn/pdfs/pscmanual/1psc_overviewcurrent.pdf.

Centers for Disease Control and Prevention (CDC). 2019b. National Healthcare Safety Network: Surgical site infection (SSI) event. http://www.cdc.gov/nhsn/PDFs/pscManual/9pscSSIcurrent.pdf.

Centers for Disease Control and Prevention (CDC). 2019. Most Recent National Asthma Data. https://www.cdc.gov/asthma/most_recent_national_asthma_data.htm.

Centers for Disease Control and Prevention (CDC). 2018 (March 23). Cancer Prevention and Control. https://www.cdc.gov/cancer/dcpc/about/.

Centers for Disease Control and Prevention (CDC). 2018 (August 8). National Vital Statistics System. https://www.cdc.gov/nchs/nvss/fetal_death.htm

Centers for Disease Control and Prevention (CDC). 2017 (March 31). National Center for Health Statistics Infant Health. https://www.cdc.gov/nchs/fastats/infant-health.htm.

Centers for Disease Control and Prevention (CDC). 2016a. CDC Wonder. Underlying causes of death, 2010. http://wonder.cdc.gov/controller/datarequest/D76.

Centers for Disease Control and Prevention (CDC). 2016. Deaths and mortality: FastStats. http://www.cdc.gov/nchs/fastats/deaths.htm.

Centers for Disease Control and Prevention (CDC). 2015. National Healthcare Safety Network. http://www.cdc.gov/nhsn/index.html.

Centers for Disease Control and Prevention. 2013. Deaths and mortality: Final data for 2013. http://www.cdc.gov/nchs/data/nvsr/nvsr64/nvsr64_02.pdf.

Centers for Disease Control and Prevention (CDC). National Center for Health Statistic. (n.d.). Underlying Cause of Death 1999-2017 on CDC WONDER Online Database, released December 2018. Data are from the Multiple Cause of Death Files, 1999-2017, as compiled from data provided by the 57 vital statistics jurisdictions.

Cohen D., and B. Crabtree. 2006 (July). Qualitative research guidelines project. Robert Wood Foundation. http://www.qualres.org/HomeGrou-3589.html.

Curry, S., C. Cortland, and M. Graham. 2011. Role-modelling in the operating room: Medical student observations of exemplary behavior. *Medical Education* 45(9):946–957.

Department of Health and Human Services (HHS). 2016. Guidance regarding methods for de-identification of protected health information in accordance with the Health Insurance Portability and Accountability Act (HIPAA) Privacy Rule. http://www.hhs.gov/hipaa/for-professionals/privacy/special-topics/de-identification/index.html.

Department of Health and Human Services (HHS). 2014. The health consequences of smoking—50 years of progress: A report of the Surgeon General, 2014: 677. http://www.surgeongeneral.gov/library/reports/50-years-of-progress/full-report.pdf.

Department of Health and Human Services (HHS). 2004. HIPAA authorization for research: NIH Publication Number 04-5529. https://privacyruleandresearch.nih.gov/pdf/authorization.pdf.

Dudovskiy, J. 2011. Research Methods. http://research-methodology.net/.

Evans, M. 2014 (July 12). Data collection could stump next phase of predictive analytics. *Modern Healthcare.* http://www.modernhealthcare.com/article/20140712/MAGAZINE/307129969.

Fanelli, D. 2009. How many scientists fabricate and falsify research? A systematic review and meta-analysis of survey data. *PLoS ONE* 4(5):e5738. doi: 10.1371/journal.pone.0005738. http://journals.plos.org/plosone/article?id=10.1371/journal.pone.0005738.

Folkerts, B. Coordinator, HIM Program, Hutchinson Community College. 2016 (January 19). E-mail exchange to author.

Gelman, A. and D. Nolan. 2002. *Teaching Statistics: A Bag of Tricks.* New York: Oxford University Press. http://stat.columbia.edu/~gelman/bag-of-tricks/chap10.pdf.

Halo Business Intelligence. 2014. Descriptive, predictive, and prescriptive analytics explained: the two-minute guide to understanding and selecting the right analytics. https://halobi.com/2014/10/descriptive-predictive-and-prescriptive-analytics-explained/.

Hoyert, D. 2011. The changing profile of autopsied deaths in the United States, 1972-2007. *NCHS Data Brief, 2011*(67), 1–8.

Huffman, E. K. 1994. *Health Information Management.* Berwyn, IL: Physician's Record Company.

Insurance Journal. 2012. How predictive modeling has revolutionized insurance. http://www.insurancejournal.com/news/national/2012/06/18/251957.htm.

Kalra, A., R. Fisher, and P. Axelrod. 2010. Decreased length of stay and cumulative hospitalized days despite increased patient admissions and readmissions in an area of urban poverty. *Journal of General Internal Medicine* 25(9):930–935. http://www.ncbi.nlm.nih.gov/pmc/articles/PMC2917661/.

Kayyoll, B., D. Knott, and S. VanKulken. 2013. The big-data revolution in US healthcare: Accelerating value and innovation. http://www.mckinsey.com/insights/health_systems_and_services/the_big-data_revolution_in_us_health_care.

Kelly, K., B. Clark, V. Brown, and J. Sitzia. 2003. Good practice in the conduct and reporting of survey research. *International Journal for Quality in Health Care* 15(3):261–266. http://intqhc.oxfordjournals.org/content/15/3/261.

Kotabagi RB, Charati, SC, Jayachandar D. (2011). Clinical Autopsy vs Medicolegal Autopsy. *Med J Armed Forces India,* 2011(3), 258–63. doi:10.1016/S0377-1237(05)80169-8

Kraft, D. 2014. (September 16). Alger YouTube video: Medicine 2064. https://www.youtube.com/watch?v=iOgt85cPU8Q &feature=youtu.be.

Lamont, J. 2009 (June). KM challenges fraud. *KM World* 18:6. http://www.kmworld.com/Articles/Editorial/Features/KM-challenges -fraud-53982.aspx.

Watzlaf, V. and E. Forrestal. 2017. *Health Informatics Research Methods: Principles and Practice*. Chicago: AHIMA.

Letourneau, R. 2015 (October 2). "How CMS aims to prevent 1M heart attacks, strokes." *Health Leaders Media*. http://healthleadersmedia .com/content/QUA-321274/How-CMS-Aims-to-Prevent-1M-Heart-Attacks-Strokes.html.

Martin, J.A., B.E. Hamilton, S.J. Ventura, M.J.K. Osterman, E. Wilson, and T.J. Mathews. 2012. Births: Final data for 2010. National vital statistics reports; vol 61, no 1. Hyattsville, MD: National Center for Health Statistics.

McCusker, K. and S. Gunaydin. 2015. Research using qualitative, quantitative or mixed methods and choice based on the research. *Perfusion* 30(7):537–542.

Miller, P.J. and F.L. Waterstraat. 2004. Apples to apples: Using auto benchmarking to measure productivity. *Journal of AHIMA* 75(1):44–49.

National Center for Health Statistics. 2015 (November 6). e-Vital Standards Initiatives. National Vital Statistics System: https://www .cdc.gov/nchs/nvss/evital_standards_intiatives.htm.

National Conference of State Legislatures. 2019 (February 28). CON-Certificate of Need State Laws. http://www.ncsl.org/research/ health/con-certificate-of-need-state-laws.aspx.

National Center for Health Statistics. 2011 (August). The changing profile of autopsied deaths in the United States, 1972–2007. NCHS Data Brief 67. http://www.cdc.gov/nchs/data/databriefs/db67.pdf.

National Cancer Institute. 2012 (September 24). Breast cancer risk in American women. http://www.cancer.gov/types/breast/risk-fact -sheet.

National Conference of State Legislatures (NCSL). 2015 (September). Certificate of need: State health laws and programs. http://www .ncsl.org/research/health/con-certificate-of-need-state-laws.aspx.

The Office of Research Integrity. 2015 (January 22). Case summary: Xiao, Dong. http://ori.hhs.gov/content/case-summary-xiao-dong.

The Office of Research Integrity. 2011 (April 19). Case summary: Sudbo, Jon. http://ori.hhs.gov/content/case-summary-sudbo-jon.

Onwuegbuzie, A. and C. Poth. 2015. Afterword. *International Journal of Qualitative Methods* 14(2):122–125.

Optum. 2012 (February 3). An inpatient prospective payment system refresher: MS-DRGs. *Advance Healthcare Network for Health Information Management Professionals*. http://health-information.advanceweb.com/Web-Extras/CCS-Prep/An-Inpatient-Prospective -Payment-System-Refresher-MS-DRGs-2.aspx.

Pendergrass, J. 2015. Interviewed by L. Horton. Personal interview. October 8. Hutchinson Regional Medical Center, Hutchinson, Kansas.

Poth, C. and A. Onwuegbuzie. 2015. Editors' introduction. *International Journal of Qualitative Methods* 14(2):1–4.

Pronovost, P., D. Angus, T. Dorman, K. Robinson, T. Dremsizov, and T. Young. 2002. Physician staffing patterns and clinical outcomes in critically ill patients. *JAMA* 288(17): 2151–2162.

Pyrczak, F. 2010. *Making Sense of Statistics: A Conceptual Overview*. Los Angeles: Pyrczak Publishing.

Rasmussen, L. 2014. The case of Vipul Bhrigu and the federal definition of research misconduct. *Science and Engineering Ethics* 20(2):411–421.

SearchCIO. 2012. Predictive analytics. http://searchcio.techtarget.com/definition/Prescriptive-analytics.

Shambaugh, E., J.L. Young, C. Zippin, D. Lum, C. Akers, and M.A. Weiss. 1994. SEER Program Self-Instructional Manual for Cancer Registrars—Book 7: Statistics and Epidemiology for Cancer Registries. Publication No. 94-3766. Washington, DC: US Department of Health and Human Services.

US Census Bureau. 2013. American Fact Finder. American estimate of the resident population: April 1, 2010 to July 1, 2013. 2013 population estimates." http://factfinder.census.gov/faces/tableservices/jsf/pages/productview.xhtml?src=bkmk.

Voth, K. 2015 (October 6). Interviewed by L. Horton. Personal interview. Hutchinson Clinic, Hutchinson, Kansas.

WebMD. 2014 (September 9). Types of anesthesia. http://www.webmd.com/pain-management/tc/anesthesia-topic-overview.

White, S. 2016. *A Practical Approach to Analyzing Healthcare Data*. 3rd ed. Chicago: AHIMA.

White, S. 2011 (September). Predictive modeling 101. *Journal of AHIMA* 82(9):46–47.

World Health Organization. 2019 (March 1). Poliomyelitis. https://www.who.int/news-room/fact-sheets/detail/poliomyelitis.

World Health Organization. 2019 (March 2). What we do. Accessedhttps://www.who.int/about/what-we-do.

World Health Organization. (n.d.). Health statistics and information systems. Accessed March 16, 2019.https://www.who.int/healthinfo/statistics/indmaternalmortality/en/.

World Health Organization. (n.d.). Maternal, newborn, child and adolescent health. Accessed March 17, 2019. https://www.who.int/maternal_child_adolescent/topics/maternal/maternal_perinatal/en/.

APPENDIX C

Formulae

Formulae listed alphabetically by name

Statistic	Numerator	Denominator	Chapter
Adjusted hospital autopsy rate	Total number of hospital autopsies including ED, OP and home healthcare patients for a given period	Total number of deaths of hospital patients whose bodies are available for autopsy	7
Anesthesia mortality rate	Number of deaths caused by anesthesia agents for a period	Number of anesthetics administered for the same period	6
Average daily inpatient census	Total number of inpatient service days for a given period	Total number of days for the same period	3
Average daily inpatient census for NBs	Total number of NB inpatient service days for a given period	Total number of days for the same period	3
Average daily inpatient census for a PCU	Total number of inpatient service days for a PCU for a given period	Total number of days for the same period	3
ALOS	Total LOS (discharge days) for a given period	Total number of discharges, including deaths, for the same period	5
ALOS for NBs or ANLOS	Total LOS (discharge days) for all NB discharges and deaths for a given period	Total number of NB discharges, including deaths, for the same period	5
Bed turnover rate (direct Formula)	Number of discharges (including deaths) for a period	Average bed count during the period	4
Bed turnover rate (indirect Formula)	Occupancy rate × number of days in period	Average length of stay for period	4
Cancer case fatality rate	Number of deaths from cancer during a period	Number of discharges for cancer during a period	6
Cancer mortality rate	Number of deaths from cancer during a period	Number in population at risk during a period	6
C-section rate	Total number of C-sections for a period	Total number of deliveries (including C-sections) in the same period	8

(continued on next page)

Statistic	*Numerator*	*Denominator*	*Chapter*
Complication rate	Total number of complications for a period	Total number of discharges (including deaths) for the same period	8
Consultation rate	Total number of patients receiving consultations for a period	Total number of discharges (including deaths) for the same period	8
Fetal autopsy rate	Total number of autopsies on intermediate and late fetal deaths for a given period	Total number of intermediate and late fetal deaths for the same period	7
Fetal mortality rate	Number of intermediate and late fetal deaths for a period	Number of live births plus number of intermediate and late fetal deaths for the same period	6
Gross autopsy rate	Total number of autopsies on inpatient deaths for a given period	Total number of inpatient deaths for the same period	7
Gross mortality rate (hospital mortality rate)	Number of inpatient deaths, including NBs, for a period	Number of discharges, including deaths and NB, for the same period	6
Infant mortality rate	Number of infant deaths during a period	Number of live births during same period	6
Infection rate	Total number of infections for a period	Total number of discharges (including deaths) for the same period	8
Inpatient bed occupancy rate	Total number of inpatient service days for a given period	Total number of inpatient bed count days for the same period	4
Maternal mortality rate	Number of maternal deaths for a period	Number of live births, for the same period	6
Net autopsy rate	Total number of autopsies on inpatient deaths for a given period	Total number of inpatient deaths minus not autopsied coroner or medical examiner cases for the same period	7
Net mortality rate (institutional mortality rate)	Number of inpatient deaths, including NBs, minus deaths < 48 hours for a period	Number of discharges, including deaths and NB, minus deaths < 48 hours for the same period	6
NB autopsy rate	Total number of autopsies on newborn deaths for a given period	Total number of newborn deaths for the same period	7
Newborn bassinet occupancy rate	Total number of newborn inpatient service days for a given period	Total number of bassinet bed count days for the same period	4
Newborn mortality rate	Total number NB deaths for a period	Number of NB discharges, including deaths, for the same period	6
OB case fatality rate	Number of direct maternal deaths for a period	Number of OB discharges for the same period	6
Postoperative infection rate	Total number of infections in clean surgical cases for a period	Number of surgical operations for the same period	8
Postoperative mortality rate	Number of deaths within 10 days after surgery for a period	Number of patients operated on for the same period	6
Readmission rate	Number of patients readmitted within 30 days of the previous discharge	Total patients discharged (excluding deaths)	8

Formulae listed by chapter

Chapter 3

Indicator	Numerator	Denominator
Average daily inpatient census	Total number of inpatient service days for a given period	Total number of days for the same period
Average daily inpatient census for NBs	Total number of NB inpatient service days for a given period	Total number of days for the same period
Average daily inpatient census for a PCU	Total number of inpatient service days for a PCU for a given period	Total number of days for the same period

Chapter 4

Statistic	Numerator	Denominator
Inpatient bed occupancy rate	Total number of inpatient service days for a given period	Total number of inpatient bed count days for the same period
Newborn bassinet occupancy rate	Total number of newborn inpatient service days for a given period	Total number of bassinet bed count days for the same period
Bed turnover rate (direct Formula)	Number of discharges (including deaths) for a period	Average bed count during the period
Bed turnover rate (indirect Formula)	Occupancy rate x number of days in period	Average length of stay for period

Chapter 5

	Numerator	Denominator
ALOS	Total LOS (discharge days) for a given period	Total number of discharges, including deaths, for the same period
ALOS for NBs or ANLOS	Total LOS (discharge days) for all NB discharges and deaths for a given period	Total number of NB discharges, including deaths, for the same period

Chapter 6

Statistic	Numerator	Denominator
Gross mortality rate (hospital mortality rate)	Number of inpatient deaths, including NBs, for a period	Number of discharges, including deaths and NB, for the same period
Net mortality rate (institutional mortality rate)	Number of inpatient deaths, including NBs, minus deaths < 48 hours for a period	Number of discharges, including deaths and NB, minus deaths < 48 hours for the same period
Postoperative mortality rate	Number of deaths within 10 days after surgery for a period	Number of patients operated on for the same period
Anesthesia mortality rate	Number of deaths caused by anesthesia agents for a period	Number of anesthetics administered for the same period

(continued on next page)

Statistic	Numerator	Denominator
Maternal mortality rate	Number of maternal deaths for a period	Number of live births, for the same period
OB case fatality rate	Number of direct maternal deaths for a period	Number of OB discharges for the same period
Newborn mortality rate	Total number NB deaths for a period	Number of NB discharges, including deaths, for the same period
Infant mortality rate	Number of infant deaths during a period	Number of live births during same period
Fetal mortality rate	Number of intermediate and late fetal deaths for a period	Number of live births plus number of intermediate and late fetal deaths for the same period
Cancer mortality rate	Number of deaths from cancer during a period	Number in population at risk during a period
Cancer case fatality rate	Number of deaths from cancer during a period	Number of discharges for cancer during a period

Chapter 7

Rate	Numerator	Denominator
Gross autopsy rate	Total number of autopsies on inpatient deaths for a given period	Total number of inpatient deaths for the same period
Net autopsy rate	Total number of autopsies on inpatient deaths for a given period	Total number of inpatient deaths minus not autopsied coroner or medical examiner cases for the same period
Adjusted hospital autopsy rate	Total number of hospital autopsies including ED, OP and home healthcare patients for a given period	Total number of deaths of hospital patients whose bodies are available for autopsy
NB autopsy rate	Total number of autopsies on newborn deaths for a given period	Total number of newborn deaths for the same period
Fetal autopsy rate	Total number of autopsies on intermediate and late fetal deaths for a given period	Total number of intermediate and late fetal deaths for the same period

Chapter 8

Rate	Numerator	Denominator
Infection rate	Total number of infections for a period	Total number of discharges (including deaths) for the same period
Postoperative infection rate	Total number of infections in clean surgical cases for a period	Number of surgical operations for the same period

(continued on next page)

Rate	Numerator	Denominator
Complication rate	Total number of complications for a period	Total number of discharges (including deaths) for the same period
C-section rate	Total number of C-sections for a period	Total number of deliveries (including C-sections) in the same period
Consultation rate	Total number of patients receiving consultations for a period	Total number of discharges (including deaths) for the same period
Readmission rate	Number of patients readmitted within 30 days of the previous discharge	Total patients discharged (excluding deaths)

APPENDIX D

Glossary of Healthcare Services and Statistical Terms

Accuracy: A characteristic of data that are free from significant error, up to date, and representative of relevant facts.

Adjusted hospital autopsy rate: The proportion of hospital autopsies performed following the deaths of patients whose bodies are available for autopsy.

Admission date: The year, month, and day a patient first enters the hospital as an inpatient.

Agency for Healthcare Research and Quality (AHRQ): An agency within the Department of Health and Human Services whose mission is to produce evidence to make healthcare safer, higher quality, more accessible, equitable, and affordable, and to work within the US Department of Health and Human Services and with other partners to make sure that the evidence is understood and used.

Aggregate data: Data extracted from individual health records and combined to form de-identified information about groups of patients that can be compared and analyzed.

Alternative hypothesis: A statement of what the study is set up to establish. It states what the predicted association or difference between the variables is.

Ambulatory care facility: A healthcare facility that provides preventive or corrective healthcare services on a nonresident basis in a provider's office, clinic setting, or outpatient setting.

Analysis of variance (ANOVA): Test used to assess the differences among more than two means.

Ancillary service visit: The appearance of an outpatient in a unit of a hospital or outpatient facility to receive services, tests, or procedures that ordinarily are not counted as encounters for healthcare services.

Ancillary services: Tests and procedures ordered by a physician to provide information for use in patient diagnosis or treatment.

Anesthesia: Loss of feeling or awareness, as when an anesthetic is administered before surgery.

Anesthesia mortality rate: The ratio of deaths caused by anesthetic agents to the number of anesthetics administered during a specified period of time.

Applied research: A type of research that focuses on the use of scientific theories to improve actual practice as in medical research applied to the treatment of patients.

Arithmetic mean length of stay (AMLOS): The average length of stay for all patients.

Autopsy: The postmortem examination of the organs and tissues of a body to determine the cause of death or pathological conditions.

Autopsy rate: The proportion or percentage of deaths in a healthcare organization that are followed by the performance of an autopsy.

Average: The value obtained by dividing the sum of a set of numbers by a count of the number of values in the set.

Average daily inpatient census: The average or mean number of inpatients present in the hospital each day for a given period of time.

Average duration of hospitalization: *See* **average length of stay**

Average length of stay (ALOS):   The average number of days that inpatients discharged during the period under consideration stayed in the hospital.

Bar chart: A graphic technique used to display frequency distributions of nominal or ordinal data that fall into categories; also called *bar graph.*

Bar graph: *See* **bar chart**

Basic research: A type of research that focuses on the development and refinement of theories.

Bed capacity: The number of beds that a facility has been designed and constructed to house, rather than the actual number of beds set up and staffed for use.

Bed count: The number of inpatient beds set up and staffed for use on a given day; also called an inpatient bed or bed complement.

Bed count day: A unit of measure that denotes the presence of one inpatient bed (either occupied or vacant) set up and staffed for use in one 24-hour period.

Bed occupancy percentage: The bed occupancy ratio expressed as a percentage.

Bed occupancy ratio: The proportion of beds occupied, defined as the ratio of inpatient service days to bed count days during a specified period of time.

Bed size: The total number of inpatient beds for which a facility is equipped and staffed to provide patient care services.

Bed turnover rate: The average number of times a bed changes occupants during a given period of time.

Big data: Massive amounts of information that can be interpreted by analytics to provide an overview of trends or patterns.

Boarder: An individual such as a parent, caregiver, or other family member who receives lodging at a healthcare facility but is not a patient.

Boarder baby: A newborn who remains in the nursery following discharge because the mother is still hospitalized, or a premature infant who no longer needs intensive care but remains for observation.

Budget: A plan that converts the organization's goals and objectives into targets for revenue and spending.

Calculation of inpatient service days: The measurement of the services received by all inpatients in one 24-hour period.

Cancer mortality rate: The proportion of patients who die from cancer.

Cancer registrar: An individual who is responsible for capturing a complete summary of the history, diagnosis, treatment and disease status for every cancer patient.

Cancer registry: A collection of information about the occurrence of cancer, the types of cancers that occur and their locations within the body, the extent of cancer at the time of diagnosis (disease stage), and the kinds of treatment that patients receive.

Capital budget: The allocation of resources for long-term investments and projects.

Case fatality rate: The total number of deaths due to a specific illness during a given time period divided by the total number of cases during the same period.

Case-mix: A method of grouping patients according to a predefined set of characteristics

Case management: *See* **Utilization management**

Categorical data: Data collected and then sorted or divided into groups.

Cause-specific mortality rate: The total number of deaths due to a specific illness during a given time period divided by the estimated population for the same time period.

Census: A survey of a population.

Census day: *See* **inpatient service day**

Census statistics: Statistics that examine the number of patients being treated at specific times, the lengths of their stay, and the number of times a bed changes occupant.

Census survey: A survey that collects data from all the members of a population.

Centers for Disease Control and Prevention (CDC):   A division of the Department of Health and Human Services (HHS) that is recognized as the lead agency responsible for protecting the health of the US population by providing credible information to help individuals make the right healthcare decisions and promoting quality of life through the prevention and control of disease, injury, and disability.

Centers for Medicare and Medicaid Services (CMS):   The division of the Department of Health and Human Services that is responsible for developing healthcare policy in the United States and for administering the Medicare program and the federal portion of the Medicaid program.

Certificate of need: A state-directed program that requires healthcare facilities to submit detailed plans and justifications for the purchase of new equipment, new buildings, or new service offerings that cost in excess of a certain amount.

Cesarean section: A surgical operation for delivering a child by cutting through the wall of the mother's abdomen.

Cesarean section rate: The ratio of all C-sections to the total number of deliveries, including C-sections, during a specified period of time.

Chi-square test: A test of significance, represented by χ^2, that deals with nominal data and frequencies, specifically data where the standard deviation and mean are not meaningful descriptions.

Chronic: Chronic is something considered lasting for a long duration.

Clean surgical case: A surgical case in which no infection existed prior to surgery.

Clinical autopsy: An autopsy in which permission is granted by the next of kin and is primarily performed to confirm the cause of death or identify any other diseases that may have contributed to the death.

Clinical data warehouse: A collection of data that reflects all aspects of hospital operations that is used for reporting and analysis.

Clinic outpatient: A patient who is admitted to a clinical service of a clinic or hospital for diagnosis or treatment on an ambulatory basis.

Clinical research: A specialized area of research that primarily investigates the efficacy of preventive, diagnostic, and therapeutic procedures; also called medical research.

Cluster sampling: The process of selecting subjects for a sample from each cluster within a population (for example, a family, school, or community).

Community-acquired infection: An infectious disease contracted as the result of exposure before or after a patient's period of hospitalization.

Complete master census: A total census for a facility showing the names and locations of patients present in the hospital at a particular point in time and their location.

Complication: A medical condition that arises during an inpatient hospitalization (for example, a postoperative wound infection).

Complication rate: The total number of hospital inpatients with a complication for a given period divided by the total number of discharges and deaths for the same period.

Concomitant: Concomitant refers to taking place at the same time.

Confidence interval: An interval that has probability associated with it that assess the certainty that the actual population mean (which we cannot observe) is included in the interval.

Consultation: The response by one healthcare professional to another healthcare professional's request to provide recommendations and/or opinions regarding the care of a particular patient or resident.

Consultation rate: The total number of hospital inpatients receiving consultations for a given period divided by the total number of discharges, including deaths, for the same period.

Continuous data: Data that represent measurable quantities but are not restricted to certain specified values.

Control group: A comparison study group whose members do not undergo the treatment under study.

Convenience sampling: A sampling technique where the selection of units from the population is based on easy availability and/or accessibility.

Coroner: The official (elected or appointed, physician or nonphysician) who is responsible for determining the cause, time, and manner of death in unattended, violent, or unexplained deaths, or in cases in which a law may have been broken.

Correlational research: Research design to discover a relationship between variables. A variable is anything under study.

Cost–benefit analysis: A process that uses quantitative techniques to evaluate and measure the benefit of providing products or services compared to the cost of providing them.

Crude birth rate: The number of live births divided by the number of deliveries.

Daily census: The number of inpatients present at the census-taking time each day, plus any inpatients who were both admitted after the previous census-taking time and discharged before the next census-taking time.

Daily inpatient census: A statistic that measures the number of inpatients admitted to the hospital or unit at any time during a given day. It includes the number of inpatients present at census-taking time each day, plus any inpatients who were both admitted and discharged after the census-taking time the previous day.

Dashboard: A visual display of the most important information needed to achieve one or more objectives; consolidated and arranged on a single screen so the information can be monitored at a glance.

Data: The dates, numbers, images, symbols, letters, and words that represent basic facts and observations about people, processes, measurements, and conditions.

Data accuracy: The extent to which data are free of identifiable errors.

Data analysis: The task of transforming, summarizing, or modeling data to allow the user to make meaningful conclusions.

Data analytics: The science of examining raw data with the purpose of drawing conclusions about that information.

Data collection: The process by which data are gathered.

Data mining: The process of extracting and analyzing large volumes of data from a database for the purpose of identifying hidden and sometimes subtle relationships or patterns and using those relationships to predict behaviors.

Data warehouse: A repository of historical data organized for reporting and analysis. It facilitates data access by having data from many sources in one place, linked together, and easily searchable.

Date of encounter (outpatient and physician services):   The year, month, and day of a visit or other healthcare encounter.

Date of procedure: The year, month, and day of each significant procedure.

Date of service (DOS):   The date a test, procedure, or service was rendered.

Days of stay: *See* length of stay

Dead on arrival (DOA):   The condition of a patient who arrives at a healthcare facility with no signs of life and who was pronounced dead by a physician.

Death rate: *See* mortality rate.

Decile: Data divided into 10 equal parts.

Decimal: A quotient derived from a fraction where the denominator is a multiple of 10.

Delivery: The process of delivering a liveborn infant or dead fetus (and placenta) by manual, instrumental, or surgical means.

Denominator: The part of a fraction that is below the line. The denominator tells us how many equal parts a whole is broken into.

Dependent variable: A measurable variable in a research study that depends on an independent variable.

Descriptive analytics: The summarization of data.

Descriptive research: A type of research that provides data about the population you are studying, including the frequency that something occurs.

Descriptive statistics: Describes what the data show about the characteristics of a group or population; in other words, they may be used to describe a particular population.

Discharge date: The year, month, and day that an inpatient is formally released from the hospital.

Discharge days: *See* **length of stay** and **total length of stay**

Discharge diagnosis list: A complete set of discharge diagnoses applicable to a single patient episode, such as an inpatient hospitalization.

Discharge transfer: The transfer of an inpatient to another healthcare institution at the time of discharge.

Discrete data: Data that are typically whole numbers; that is, they can have only a finite number of specified values.

Disposition: For outpatients, the healthcare practitioner's description of the patient's status at discharge (no follow-up planned, follow-up planned or scheduled, referred elsewhere, expired), for inpatients, a core health data element that identifies the circumstances under which the patient left the hospital (discharged alive, discharged to home or self-care, discharged and transferred to another short-term general hospital for inpatient care, discharged and transferred to a skilled nursing facility, discharged and transferred to an intermediate care facility, discharged and transferred to another type of institution for inpatient care or referred for outpatient services to another institution, discharged and transferred to home under care of an organized home health services organization, discharged and transferred to home under care of a home intravenous therapy provider, left against medical advice or discontinued care, expired, status not stated).

Duration of inpatient stay: *See* **length of stay**

Early fetal death: The death of a product of human conception that is fewer than 20 weeks of gestation and 500 grams or less in weight before its complete expulsion or extraction from the mother.

Electronic health record (EHR):   A computerized record of health information and associated processes; also called computer-based patient record.

Electronic medical record (EMR):   A form of computer-based health record in which information is stored in whole files instead of by individual data elements.

Electronic signature: Any representation of a signature in digital form, including an image of a handwritten signature.

Emergency department: The department of a hospital responsible for the provision of medical and surgical care to patients arriving at the hospital in need of immediate care. The emergency department is also called the *emergency room* or *ER*.

Emergency department patient: A patient who is admitted to the emergency department of a hospital for the diagnosis and treatment of a condition that requires immediate medical, dental, or allied health services in order to sustain life or to prevent critical consequences.

Encounter: The direct personal contact between a patient and a physician or other person authorized by state licensure law and, if applicable, by medical staff bylaws to order or furnish healthcare services for the diagnosis or treatment of the patient.

Episode of care: A period of relatively continuous medical care performed by healthcare professionals in relation to a particular clinical problem or situation.

Ethnography: A method of observational research that investigates culture in naturalistic settings using both qualitative and quantitative approaches.

Evaluation research: A process used to determine what has happened during a given activity or in an institution.

Evidence-based medicine: The judicious use of the best current available scientific research in making decisions about the care of patients.

Exacerbation: To make more violent, bitter, or severe.

Experimental research: A research design used to establish cause and effect; also, a controlled investigation in which subjects are assigned randomly to groups that experience carefully controlled interventions that are manipulated by the experimenter according to a strict protocol; also called *experimental study.*

Exploratory research: A research design used because a problem has not been clearly defined or its scope is unclear.

Fabrication: The data or the reported results are made up.

Falsification: The research material, equipment, or processes were manipulated, the data were not accurately represented, or they were changed or omitted from the report, or the results were not accurately reported.

Fetal autopsy rate: The rate of autopsies performed on intermediate and late fetal deaths for a given time period divided by the total number of intermediate and late fetal deaths for the same time period.

Fetal death: The CDC defines fetal death as the spontaneous intrauterine death of a fetus at any time during pregnancy. Fetal deaths later in pregnancy (at 20 weeks of gestation or more, or 28 weeks or more, for example) are also sometimes referred to as "stillbirths."

Fetal mortality rate: A proportion that compares the number of intermediate and/or late fetal deaths to the total number of live births and intermediate or late fetal deaths during the same period of time.

Fiscal year: Any consecutive 12-month period an organization uses as its accounting period.

Forensic autopsy: An autopsy in which a legal representative has ordered an autopsy to be performed.

Fraction: One or more parts of a whole.

Frequency distribution: Shows the values that a variable can take, and the number of observations associated with each value.

Frequency distribution table: A table consisting of a set of classes or categories along with the numerical counts that correspond to nominal and ordinal data.

Frequency polygon: A graph depicting the frequency of continuous data; however, a frequency polygon is in line form instead of bar form.

Full-time equivalent employees (FTEs):   The total number of workers, including part-time, in an area as the equivalent of full-time positions.

Gender: The biological sex of the patient as recorded at the start of care.

General anesthesia: One of three major types of anesthesia that when administered patient is unconscious and has no sensations.

Graph: A graphic tool used to show numerical data in a pictorial representation.

Gross autopsy rate: The ratio of all inpatient autopsies to all inpatient deaths during any given period. Outpatients are not included in this autopsy statistic.

Gross mortality rate: The number of inpatient deaths that occurred during a given time period divided by the total number of live discharges and deaths for the same time period.

Health data analysts: Individuals responsible for taking health data and transforming it into information that is easily understood.

Histogram: A graph used to display the frequency distributions for continuous numerical data (interval or ratio data). Histograms are created from frequency distribution tables.

Historical research: A research design to investigate and analyze of past events.

Home health (HH):   An umbrella term that refers to the medical and nonmedical services provided to patients and their families in their places of residence; also called home care.

Home health agency (HHA):   A program or organization that provides a blend of home-based medical and social services to homebound patients and their families for the purpose of promoting, maintaining, or restoring health or of minimizing the effects of illness, injury, or disability.

Home healthcare: Home healthcare is healthcare that is provided by a home health agency and occurs within one's home.

Home healthcare patient: A patient who receives care within their own home provided by a home health agency.

Hospice care: The medical care provided to persons with life expectancies of six months or less who elect to forgo standard treatment of their illness and to receive only palliative care.

Hospice patients: Patients receiving an interdisciplinary program of palliative care and supportive services that addresses the physical, spiritual, social, and economic needs of terminally ill patients and their families.

Hospital: A healthcare entity that has an organized medical staff and permanent facilities that include inpatient beds and continuous medical and nursing services and that provides diagnostic and therapeutic services for patients, as well as overnight accommodations and nutritional services.

Hospital-acquired infection (HAI):   *See* **nosocomial infection**

Hospital-acquired infection rate: *See* **nosocomial infection rate**

Hospital ambulatory care: All hospital-directed preventive, therapeutic, and rehabilitative services provided by physicians and their surrogates to patients who are not hospital inpatients.

Hospital autopsy: A postmortem (after-death) examination performed on the body of a person who has at some time been a hospital patient by a hospital pathologist or a physician of the medical staff who has been delegated the responsibility.

Hospital autopsy rate: The total number of autopsies performed by a hospital pathologist for a given time period divided by the number of deaths of hospital patients (inpatients and outpatients) whose bodies were available for autopsy for the same time period.

Hospital inpatient: A patient who is provided with room, board, and continuous general nursing services in an area of an acute care facility where patients generally stay at least overnight.

Hospital inpatient autopsy: A postmortem (after-death) examination performed on the body of a patient who died during an inpatient hospitalization by a hospital pathologist or a physician of the medical staff who has been delegated the responsibility.

Hospital inpatient bed: Accommodations with supporting services (such as food, laundry, and housekeeping) for hospital inpatients, excluding those for the newborn nursery, but including incubators and bassinets in nurseries for premature or sick newborn infants.

Hospital live birth: In an inpatient facility, the complete expulsion or extraction of a product of human conception from the mother, regardless of the duration of pregnancy, which, after such expulsion or extraction, breathes or shows any other evidence of life, such as beating of the heart, pulsation of the umbilical cord, or definite movement of voluntary muscles.

Hospital mortality rate: *See* **gross mortality rate**

Hospital newborn bassinet: Accommodations including incubators and isolettes in the newborn nursery with supporting services (such as food, laundry, and housekeeping) for hospital newborn inpatients.

Hospital newborn inpatient: A patient born in the hospital at the beginning of the current inpatient hospitalization.

Hospital outpatient: A hospital patient who receives services in one or more of a hospital's facilities when he or she is not currently an inpatient or a home care patient.

Hospital outpatient care unit: An organized unit of a hospital that provides facilities and medical services exclusively or primarily to patients who are generally ambulatory and who do not currently require or are not currently receiving services as an inpatient of the hospital.

Hospitalization: The period during an individual's life when he or she is a patient in a single hospital without interruption.

Hybrid health record: A combination of paper and electronic records.

Hypothesis: A statement that describes a research question in measurable terms.

Iatrogenic: Induced inadvertently by a physician or surgeon or by medical treatment or diagnostic procedures.

Incidence rate: A computation that compares the number of new cases of a specific disease for a given time period to the population at risk for the disease during the same time period.

Individually identifiable health information: According to HIPAA privacy provisions, that information which specifically identifies the patient to whom the information relates, such as age, gender, date of birth, and address.

Induced termination of pregnancy: The purposeful interruption of an intrauterine pregnancy that was not intended to produce a liveborn infant and that did not result in a live birth.

Infant death: The death of a liveborn infant at any time from the moment of birth to the end of the first year of life (364 days, 23 hours, 59 minutes from the moment of birth).

Infant mortality rate: The number of deaths of individuals under one year of age during a given time period divided by the number of live births reported for the same time period.

Infection rate: The number of infections for the period divided by the number of discharges, including deaths for the period.

Inferential statistics: Statistics that are used to make inferences or decisions about a larger group of data by drawing conclusions from a small group of the population. The smaller group selected from the population is called a *sample*.

Information: Data that have been deliberately selected, processed, and organized to be useful.

Information governance: An organization-wide framework for managing information throughout its lifecycle and supporting the organization's strategy, operations, and regulatory, legal, and environmental requirements.

Informed consent: A person's voluntary agreement to participate in research or to undergo a diagnostic, therapeutic, or preventive procedure.

Inpatient: *See* **hospital inpatient**

Inpatient admission: When an acute care facility formally accepts a patient who is to be provided with room, board, and continuous nursing service in an area of the facility where patients generally stay at least overnight.

Inpatient bed occupancy rate: The total number of inpatient service days for a given time period divided by the total number of inpatient bed count days for the same time period; also called *percentage of occupancy*.

Inpatient census: The number of inpatients present in a healthcare facility at any given time.

Inpatient days of stay: *See* **length of stay**

Inpatient discharge: The termination of hospitalization through the formal release of an inpatient from a hospital.

Inpatient service day: A unit of measure denoting the services received by one inpatient in one 24-hour period or any portion of that 24-hour period. Also referred to as **patient day** or **census day.**

Institutional mortality rate: *See* **net mortality rate**

Institutional Review Board (IRB):   The IRB is a committee primarily responsible for protecting the rights and welfare of research subjects. Professionals who serve on IRBs have extensive education and experience in clinical research.

Instrument: A standardized and uniform way to collect data.

Interhospital transfer: When a patient leaves one hospital and is immediately admitted to another hospital or healthcare facility.

Intermediate fetal death: The death of a product of human conception before its complete expulsion or extraction from the mother that has completed 20 weeks of gestation (but less than 28 weeks) and weighs 501 to 1,000 grams.

Internal validity: An attribute of a study's design that contributes to the accuracy of its findings.

Interval data: A type of data that represents observations that can be measured on an evenly distributed scale beginning at a point other than true zero.

Interview guide: A list of written questions to be asked during an interview.

Intrahospital transfer: Transfers within the hospital from one patient care unit to another during an inpatient admission.

Intranet: A private network that works like the Internet but can only be accessed by certain individuals, such as employees of a company.

Intrarater reliability: A measure of a research instrument's reliability in which the same person repeating the test will get reasonably similar findings.

Judgment sampling: A sampling technique where the researcher relies on his or her own judgment to select the subjects for a study.

Knowledge: The information, understanding, and experience that give individuals the power to make informed decisions.

Late fetal death: The death of a product of human conception that is 28 weeks or more of gestation and weighs 1,001 grams or more before its complete expulsion or extraction from the mother.

Leave of absence: A physician-authorized absence of an inpatient from a hospital or other facility for a specified period of time occurring after admission and prior to discharge.

Length of stay (LOS):   The total number of patient days for an inpatient episode, calculated by subtracting the date of admission from the date of discharge.

Line graph: A graphic technique used to illustrate the relationship between continuous measurements; consists of a line drawn to connect a series of points on an arithmetic scale and is often used to display time trends.

Literature review: A systematic investigation of all the knowledge available about a topic from sources such as books, journal articles, theses, and dissertations.

Live birth: According to the World Health Organization (WHO), a live birth refers to the complete expulsion or extraction from its mother of a product of conception, irrespective of the duration of the pregnancy, which, after such separation, breathes or shows any other evidence of life—for example, beating of the heart, pulsation of the umbilical cord, or definite movement of voluntary muscles—whether or not the umbilical cord has been cut or the placenta is attached. Each product of such a birth is considered live born.

Local anesthesia: One of three major types of anesthesia that when administered numbs a small area of the body.

Low-birth-weight neonate: Any newborn baby, regardless of gestational age, whose weight at birth is less than 2,500 grams.

Managed care: A generic term for reimbursement and delivery systems that integrate the financing and provision of healthcare services by means of entering contractual agreements with selected providers to furnish comprehensive healthcare services and developing explicit criteria for the selection of healthcare providers, formal programs of ongoing quality improvement and utilization review, and significant financial incentives for members to use providers associated with the plan.

Managed care organization (MCO):   A type of healthcare organization that delivers medical care and manages all aspects of the care or the payment for care by limiting providers of care, discounting payment to providers of care, or limiting access to care.

Maternal death: The death of any woman while pregnant or within 42 days of termination of pregnancy, from any cause, related to or aggravated by pregnancy or its management (regardless of duration or site of pregnancy), but not from accidental or incidental causes.

Maternal mortality rate: For a hospital, the total number of maternal deaths directly related to pregnancy for a given time period divided by the total number of obstetrical discharges for the same time period (aka. OB case fatality rate);

for a community, the total number of deaths attributed to maternal conditions during a given time period in a specific geographic area divided by the total number of live births for the same time period in the same area.

Mean: A measure of central tendency that is determined by calculating the arithmetic average of the observations in a frequency distribution.

Measure: A term referring to the quantifiable data about a function or process.

Measures of central tendency: The typical or average numbers that are descriptive of the entire collection of data for a specific population.

Median: The midpoint (center) of the distribution of values, or the point above and below which 50 percent of the values fall.

Medical examiner: *See* **coroner**

Medical services: The activities relating to medical care performed by physicians, nurses, and other healthcare professional and technical personnel under the direction of a physician.

Medicare-severity diagnosis related groups (MS-DRG): Payment groups designed for the Medicare population that recognize severity of illness, resource use, and patient complexity. Patients who have similar clinical characteristics and similar costs are assigned to an MS-DRG, which is linked to a fixed payment amount based on the average cost of patients in the group. Patients can be assigned to an MS-DRG based on diagnosis, surgical procedures, age, and other administrative information.

Medio-Legal (ML) autopsy: *See* **forensic autopsy**

Method: A way of performing an action or task; also, a strategy used by a researcher to collect, analyze, and present data.

Military time: Time measured in hours numbered to 24 (as 0100 or 2300) from one midnight to the next.

Mode: A measure of central tendency that is value that occurs most frequently in the data.

Morbidity: The state of being diseased or the number of sick persons including illness, injury, or deviation from normal health.

Morgue: The place where the bodies of persons who have died are kept until identified and claimed by relatives or released for burial.

Mortality: A term referring to the incidence of death in a specific population; also, the loss of subjects during the course of a clinical research study, or attrition.

Mortality rate: A rate that measures the risk of death for the cause under study in a defined population during a given time period. *Also called* **death rate.**

MS-DRGs: Payment groups, designed for the Medicare population, that recognize severity of illness, resource use, and patient complexity.

Multivariate: In reference to research studies, a term meaning that many variables were involved.

Naturalistic observation: A type of nonparticipant observation in which researchers observe certain behaviors and events as they occur naturally.

Necropsy: *See* **autopsy**

Neonatal death: The death of a liveborn infant within the first 27 days, 23 hours, and 59 minutes following the moment of birth.

Neonatal mortality rate: The number of deaths of infants under 28 days of age during a given time period divided by the total number of births for the same time period.

Neonatal period: The period of an infant's life from the hour of birth through the first 27 days, 23 hours, and 59 minutes of life.

Net autopsy rate: The ratio of inpatient autopsies compared to inpatient deaths calculated by dividing the total number of inpatient autopsies performed by the hospital pathologist for a given time period by the total number of inpatient deaths minus not autopsied coroners' or medical examiners' cases for the same time period.

Net mortality rate: The total number of inpatient deaths, including newborns, minus the number of deaths that occurred more than 48 hours after admission divided by the total number of inpatient discharges including deaths.

Newborn (NB):   An inpatient who was born in a hospital at the beginning of the current inpatient hospitalization.

Newborn autopsy rate: The number of autopsies performed on newborns who died during a given time period divided by the total number of newborns who died during the same time period.

Newborn bassinet count: The number of available hospital newborn bassinets, both occupied and vacant, on any given day.

Newborn bassinet count day: A unit of measure that denotes the presence of one newborn bassinet, either occupied or vacant, set up and staffed for use in one 24-hour period.

Newborn death: The death of a liveborn infant born during the same admission as their birth.

Newborn mortality rate: The number of newborns who died divided by the total number of newborns, both alive and dead.

Nominal data: The lowest level of measurement. The word *nominal* means "pertaining to a name." In the nominal scale, observations are organized into categories in which there is no recognition of sequential order.

Normal distribution of data: Most of the values in a set of data are close to the "average" and relatively few values tend to one extreme or the other, creating a bell-shaped distribution curve.

Nosocomial infection: An infection acquired by a patient while receiving care or services in a healthcare organization; also called hospital-acquired infection.

Nosocomial infection rate: The number of hospital-acquired infections for a given time period divided by the total number of inpatient discharges for the same time period.

Null hypothesis: A hypothesis that states there is no association between the independent and dependent variables in a research study.

Numerator: The part of a fraction that is above the line and signifies the number of parts of the denominator taken.

Numerical data: Data that include discrete data and continuous data.

Nursing facility: A comprehensive term for long-term care facilities that provide nursing care and related services on a 24-hour basis for residents requiring medical, nursing, or rehabilitative care.

OB Case Fatality Rate: The total number of maternal deaths directly related to pregnancy for a given time period divided by the total number of obstetrical discharges for the same time period (aka. hospital maternal mortality rate).

Obstetrical discharges: The discharges of women while pregnant or within 42 days of termination of the pregnancy.

Observation: Research technique where the investigator observes the participant.

Observation patient: A patient with a medical condition that imposes a significant degree of instability and disability and who needs to be monitored, evaluated, and assessed to determine whether he or she should be admitted for inpatient care or discharged for care in another setting.

Observational research: A research method that requires researchers to observe, document, and analyze events and behaviors.

Occasion of service: A specified, identifiable service that involves the care of a patient but is not an encounter (for example, a lab test ordered during an encounter).

Occupancy percent/ratio: *See* **bed occupancy ratio**

Operation: *See* **surgical operation**

Operational budget: A type of budget that allocates and controls resources to meet an organization's goals and objectives for the fiscal year.

Ordinal data: A type of data that represents values or observations that are in ordered categories.

Outlier: An extreme statistical value that falls outside the normal range and may distort its representation of the central tendency of a set of numbers.

Outpatient: A patient treated in a hospital setting such as the emergency department or clinic.

_p_-value: Probability that a null hypothesis is true given the statistics derived from the sample data.

Patient: A living or deceased individual who is receiving or has received healthcare services.

Patient care unit (PCU): An organizational entity of a healthcare facility organized both physically and functionally to provide care.

Patient day: _See_ **inpatient service day**

Payback period: A financial method used to evaluate the value of a capital expenditure by calculating the time frame that must pass before inflow of cash from a project equals or exceeds outflow of cash.

Percentage: A value computed on the basis of the whole divided into 100 parts.

Percent/percentage of occupancy: _See_ **inpatient bed occupancy rate**

Perinatal death: An all-inclusive term that refers to both stillborn infants and neonatal deaths.

Pictogram: A type of bar graph that uses pictures to show the frequency of the data.

Pie chart: A method of displaying data as component parts of a whole. It is an easily understood chart in which the sizes of the slices of the pie show the proportional contribution of each part.

Pie graph: _See_ **pie chart**

Plagiarism: The appropriation of another person's ideas, processes, results, or words without giving appropriate credit.

Population: The universe of data under investigation from which a sample is taken.

Postmortem examination: _See_ **autopsy**

Post-neonatal death: The death of a liveborn infant from 28 days to the end of the first year of life (364 days, 23 hours, and 59 minutes from the moment of birth).

Post-neonatal mortality rate: The number of deaths of persons aged 28 days up to, but not including, one year during a given time period divided by the number of live births for the same time period.

Postoperative infection rate: The number of infections that occur in clean surgical cases for a given time period divided by the total number of operations within the same time period.

Postoperative mortality rate: The ratio of deaths within 10 days after surgery to the total number of operations performed during a specified period of time.

Postpartum: The time after childbirth.

Postterm neonate: Any neonate whose birth occurs from the beginning of the first day of the 43rd week (295th day) following onset of the last menstrual period.

Predictive analytics: A branch of data mining concerned with the prediction of future probabilities and trends; also called forecasting.

Predictive modeling: A process used to identify patterns that can be used to predict the odds of a particular outcome based on the observed data.

Pre-existing condition: Any injury, disease, or physical condition occurring prior to an arbitrary date.

Prepartum: The time occurring before childbirth; also called _antepartum_.

Prescriptive analytics: Data analytics technique that tries to determine the best solution or outcome among various choices.

Preterm infant: An infant with a birth weight between 1,000 and 2,499 grams and/or a gestation between 28 and 37 completed weeks.

Preterm neonate: Any neonate whose birth occurs through the end of the last day of the 38th week (266th day) following onset of the last menstrual period.

Primary data source: The data obtained from observations, and surveys and interviews.

Procedure: *See* **surgical procedure**

Productivity: A unit of performance defined by management in quantitative standards.

Profiling: A measurement of the quality, utilization, and cost of medical resources provided by physicians, or groups of physicians, that is made by employers, third-party payers, government entities, and other purchasers of healthcare.

Proportion: A type of ratio in which x is a portion of the whole $(x + y)$.

Puerperal: The period immediately following childbirth.

Qualitative research: Research that describes events, persons, activities, processes, etc. and the like without the use of numerical data.

Quantitative research: Research that uses quantitative methods, or numbers, to describe a study, including some comparisons of the population and statistical analysis to describe the results.

Quartile: Data organized in order of magnitude can be divided into four equal parts, or quartiles.

Questionnaire: A type of survey in which the members of the population are questioned through the use of electronic or paper forms.

Quota sampling: A sampling technique where the researcher first divides the population, as in stratified sampling, and then selects the number of subjects based on a specified proportion. The selection of the sample is made by the researcher who has been given or decides on quotas to fill from the subgroup of the population.

Quotient: The number obtained by dividing the numerator of a fraction by the denominator.

Random sampling: An unbiased selection of subjects that includes methods such as simple random sampling, stratified random sampling, systematic sampling, and cluster sampling.

Randomization: The assignment of subjects to experimental or control groups based on chance.

Range: The simplest measure of spread. It represents the difference between the largest and smallest values in a frequency distribution.

Ranked data: A type of ordinal data where the observations are first arranged from highest to lowest according to magnitude and then assigned numbers that correspond to each observation's place in the sequence.

Rate: A measure used to compare an event over time; a comparison of the number of times an event did happen (numerator) with the number of times an event could have happened (denominator).

Ratio: A number found by dividing one quantity by another; also, a general term that can include a number of specific measures such as proportion, percentage, and rate.

Ratio data: The highest level of measurement. On the ratio scale, there is a defined unit of measure, a real zero point, and the intervals between successive values are equal.

Real-time analytics: Data that can be accessed is it comes into a computer system.

Recap: Abbreviation of *recapitulation*.

Recapitulation: A concise summary of data.

Recurrence: To occur again after an interval.

Regional anesthesia: One of three major types of anesthesia that when administered patient is awake or may be sedated.

Release of information: The process of disclosing patient information from the medical record to another party. Federal, state and local regulations exist to govern the release of a patient's medical record information.

Relevance: How applicable information is to some matter.

Reliability: A measure of consistency of data items based on their reproducibility and an estimation of their error of measurement.

Research: An inquiry process aimed at discovering new information about a subject or revising old information. It includes investigation or experimentation aimed at the discovery of new facts, revision of accepted theories or law in light of these new facts.

Research data: Data used for the purpose of answering a proposed question or testing a hypothesis.

Rounding: The process of approximating a number to a level of precision that is meaningful for the application.

Run chart: A type of graph that shows data points collected over time and identifies emerging trends or patterns.

Sample: A set of units selected for study that represents a population.

Sample size: The number of subjects needed in a study to represent a population.

Sample size calculation: The qualitative and quantitative procedures to determine an appropriate sample size.

Sample survey: A type of survey that collects data from representative members of a population.

Scales of measurement: *See* **categorical data**

Scatter diagram: A graph used to visually display the linear relationships between two numerical variables. A scatter diagram is used to determine whether there is a correlation, that is, a relationship, between two characteristics. Also called a *scatter plot*.

Secondary data source: Data derived from primary sources and may be collected by someone other than the primary user.

Secondary record: A record derived from the primary record and containing selected data elements.

Simple random sampling (SRS):   A sampling technique that involves choosing individuals from the population in such a way that every individual has an equal chance of being selected. SRS is the statistical equivalent of drawing sampling units from a hat.

Skewness: The horizontal stretching of a frequency distribution to one side or the other so that one tail is longer than the other.

Spreadsheet: Worksheet into which text, numbers, and formulas are entered to assist with calculations.

Standard deviation (SD):   A measure of variability that describes the deviation from the mean of a frequency distribution in the original units of measurement; the square root of the variance.

Standard error of the mean: This value comes from the standard deviation of many sample means. Because of a statistical theory called the central limit theorem, the distribution of all the sample means is a normal distribution when the sample size is reasonably large.

Statistics: A branch of mathematics concerned with collecting, organizing, summarizing, and analyzing data.

Stillbirth: The birth of a fetus, regardless of gestational age, that shows no evidence of life (such as heartbeats or respirations) after complete expulsion or extraction from the mother during childbirth.

Stratified random sampling: The process of selecting the same percentages of subjects for a study sample as they exist in the subgroups (strata) of the population.

Structured interview: An interview format that uses a set of standardized questions that are asked of all applicants.

Surgical mortality rate: *See* **postoperative mortality rate**

Surgical operation: One or more surgical procedures performed at one time for one patient via a common approach or for a common purpose.

Surgical procedure: Any single, separate, systematic process upon or within the body that can be complete in itself; is normally performed by a physician, dentist, or other licensed practitioner; can be performed with or without instruments; and is performed to restore disunited or deficient parts, remove diseased or injured tissues, extract foreign matter, assist in obstetrical delivery, or aid in diagnosis.

Surgical site infection (SSI):   *See* **postoperative infection**

Surgical site infection (SSI) rate: *See* **postoperative infection rate**

Survey: A type of research instrument with which the members of the population being studied are asked questions and respond orally.

Swing bed hospital: A hospital participating in Medicare that has approval to provide post-hospital skilled care; the hospital can use its beds, as needed, for either acute care or skilled nursing care.

Systematic random sampling: The process of selecting a sample of subjects for a study by drawing every *n*th unit on a list.

***t* test:**   An example of a test of the null hypothesis regarding two population means to determine if a set of results is statistically significant.

Table: An organized arrangement of data, usually in columns and rows.

Term neonate: Any neonate whose birth occurs from the beginning of the first day of the 39th week (267th day) through the end of the last day of the 42nd week (294th day) following onset of the last menstrual period.

Total bed count days: The sum of inpatient bed count days for each of the days during a specified period of time.

Total discharge days: *See* **total length of stay**

Total inpatient service days: The sum of all inpatient service days for each of the days during a specified period of time.

Total length of stay: The sum of the days of stay of any group of inpatients discharged during a specific period of time; also called *discharge days.*

Transfer: The movement of a patient from one treatment service or location to another; *See* **intrahospital transfer**

Tumor registry: *See* **Cancer registry**

Type I error: A Type I error occurs when the null hypothesis is rejected, yet it is actually true.

Type II error: A Type II error occurs when the null hypothesis is not rejected, yet it is false.

Unit labor cost: Cost determined by dividing the total annual compensation by total annual productivity.

Unrestricted question: A type of question that allows the participant to express a freer response in his or her own words; also called *open-ended question.*

Utilization management: A program that evaluates the healthcare facility's efficiency in providing necessary services in the most resource-effective manner, while also evaluating the level of care required.

Validity: The degree to which scientific observations actually measure or record what they purport to measure.

Variability: The difference between each score and every other score in a frequency distribution.

Variable: A characteristic or property that may take on different values.

Variance: The square of the standard deviation or the average of the squared deviation from the mean.

Variance analysis: An assessment of a department's financial transactions to identify differences between the budget amount and the actual amount of a line item.

Visit: A single encounter with a healthcare professional that includes all the services supplied during the encounter.

Vital statistics: Data related to births, deaths, marriages, divorces, and fetal deaths.

Well newborn: A newborn born at term, under sterile conditions, with no diseases, conditions, disorders, syndromes, injuries, malformations, or defects diagnosed, and no operations other than routine circumcision performed.

Whole number: The portion of the decimal to the left of the decimal point (.).

World Health Organization (WHO):   The international organization founded by the United Nations (UN), is the directing and coordinating authority on international health within the UN's system. This organization is also responsible for a number of international classifications, including *The International Statistical Classification of Diseases & Related Health Problems* (ICD-10) and *The International Classification of Functioning, Disability & Health* (ICF).

APPENDIX E

Answers to Odd-Numbered Chapter Exercises

Chapter 1

Exercise 1.1

Type of Healthcare Information	Type of Data Source
1. Productivity reports pulled from patient visit report	Secondary
2. Tumor registry	Secondary
3. State vital statistics	Primary
4. Hospital census	Primary
5. Hospital disease index	Secondary
6. Patient health record	Primary
7. Health insurance data pulled from national census	Primary

Chapter 2

Exercise 2.1

1. $\dfrac{1}{2}$

   Divide numerator and denominator by common factor (20)

2. $\dfrac{2}{3}$

   Divide the numerator and denominator by common factor (2)

3. $\dfrac{2}{9}$

   Divide the numerator and denominator by common factor (6)

4. $\dfrac{2}{3}$

    Divide the numerator and denominator by common factor (4)

5. $\dfrac{4}{7}$

    Divide the numerator and denominator by common factor (4)

Exercise 2.3

1. 40
    42 is closer to 40 than 50, so round to 40.

2. 340
    338 is closer to 340 than 330, so round to 440.

3. 220
    217 is closer to 220 than 210, so round to 220.

4. 6,990
    6,989 is closer to 6,990 than 6,980, so round to 6,990.

5. 8,530
    8,532 is closer to 8,530 than 8,540, so round to 8,530.

6. 200
    156 is closer to 200 than 100, so round to 200.

7. 300
    321 is closer to 300 than 400, so round to 300.

8. 3,800
    3,807 is closer to 3,800 than 3,900, so round to 3,800.

9. 4,400
    4,357 is closer to 4,400 than 4,300, so round to 4,400.

10. 8,200
    8,175 is closer to 8,200 than 8,100, so round to 8,200.

11. 38
    The 1 in the tenths position is less than 5, so round to 38.

12. 56
    The 6 in the tenths position is more than 5, so round to 56. Note that the 9 in the hundredths digit does not impact the rounding.

13. 15
    The 7 in the tenths position is more than 5, so round to 15.

14. 625
    The 2 in the tenths position is less than 5, round to 625.

15. 101
    The 5 in the tenths position is greater to or equal to 5, round to 101.

16. 19.8
    The 6 in the hundredths position is greater than or equal 5, so round to 19.

17. 34.6
    The 2 in the hundredths position is less than 5, round to 6.

18. 172.9
    The 7 in the hundredths position is more than 5 so round to 9.

19. 100.0

The 8 in the hundredths position is more than 5, so round to 100.0. Notice here that the 9 in the tenths position will be rounded to a 10—the 0 will go in the tenths position, then the 1 is added to 99 to get 100.

20. 126.0

The 6 in the hundredths position is more than 5, so round to 126.0.

21. 8.37

The 8 in the thousandths position is more than 5, so round to 8.37.

22. 14.53

The 6 in the thousandths position is more than 5, so round to 14.53.

23. 0.88

The 6 in the thousandths position is more than 5 so round up. Also, remember when requested to round to decimal places and your answer is less than a whole number, add the "0" to the left of the decimal point.

24. 28.00

The 9 in the thousandths position is more than 5 so round up. Notice here that the 9 in the tenths position will be rounded to a 10—the 0 will go in the tenths position, then the 1 is added to 27 to get 28.

25. 15.90

The 1 in the thousandths position is less than 5, so round down.

Exercise 2.5

1. a. 2:24 = 1:12

Divide both numbers by common factor (4) then by the common factor (2). Or divide by the common factor (8).

b. 1:5

Divide both numbers by common factor (3).

c. 1:2

Divide both numbers by common factor (8).

d. 1:6

Divide both numbers by common factor (12).

e. 5:7

There is no common factor by which to divide, so the ratio is already in its simplest form.

2. # of Men: # of Women or 15:20 = 3:4

Divide both numbers by common factor (5).

3. 320:1,000 = 32:100 = 8:25

Divide both numbers by common factor (10) then by the common factor (4). Or, divide by the common factor (40).

4. 12 total instructors – 5 male = 7 female. Ratio is 5:7

There is no common factor by which to divide, so the ratio is already in its simplest form.

5. 12 total instructors – 3 with MS and 9 with BS. Ratio is 9:3 = 3:1

Divide both numbers by common factor (3).

6. 16 total births – 4 male and 12 female. Ratio is 4:12 = 1:3

Divide both numbers by common factor (4).

Exercise 2.7

1. $(6.9 + 3.7 + 7.7 + 6.6 + 7.3 + 5.5 + 9.9 + 7.0 + 5.5 + 7.7) = \dfrac{67.8}{10} = 6.78$ lbs .

Using Excel:

	A
1	6.9
2	3.7
3	7.7
4	6.6
5	7.3
6	5.5
7	9.9
8	7
9	5.5
10	7.7
11	=AVERAGE (A1:A10)

2. $(101.7 + 100.4 + 98.9 + 100.2 + 98.6) = \dfrac{499.8}{5} = 99.96$ degrees

Using Excel:

	A
1	101.7
2	100.4
3	98.9
4	100.2
5	98.6
6	=AVERAGE (A1:A5)

3. $\dfrac{(164 + 155 + 172 + 145 + 138 + 136 + 142)}{7} = \dfrac{1{,}052}{7} = 150.28$ round to 150

Using Excel:

	A
1	164
2	155
3	172
4	145
5	138
6	136
7	142
8	=AVERAGE (A1:A7)

4. 127

Excel formula version:

	A
1	130
2	135
3	132
4	126
5	120
6	122
7	124
8	=AVERAGE (A1:A7)
9	

Excel calculated version:

	A	B
1	130	
2	135	
3	132	
4	126	
5	120	
6	122	
7	124	
8	127	Average

5. $\dfrac{(\$13.87 + \$14.02 + \$15.56 + \$15.75 + \$16.32)}{5} = \dfrac{75.52}{5} = \$15.10$

	A	B
1	13.87	
2	14.02	
3	15.56	
4	15.75	
5	16.32	
6	=AVERAGE(A1:A5)	Average
7		

Excel formula version:

	A	B
1	13.87	
2	14.02	
3	15.56	
4	15.75	
5	16.32	
6	15.104	Average
7		

Excel calculated version:

Round using Excel formatting

	A	B
1	13.87	
2	14.02	
3	15.56	
4	15.75	
5	16.32	
6	15.10	Average
7		

Chapter 3

Exercise 3.1

1. Yes. *The counts could have differed. Any number of admissions, discharges, or transfers could have occurred between 12 midnight and 1 a.m. on either day.*

2. No. *The total hospital census would be inconsistent. Every PCU in the hospital should follow the same administrative procedure.*

3. No. *The patient cannot be in two places at the same time. If both units are counting heads only once a day at midnight, the patient is counted as being present in unit A only. The patient should be indicated in unit B's census as a transfer.*

4. Intrahospital transfer

5. 124 patients. *Hospitals include only inpatients in the inpatient census calculations.*

Exercise 3.3

Census = The number of inpatients present in a healthcare facility at any given time

Inpatient census = Same as census

Daily inpatient census = Number of inpatients present at census time plus any inpatient who subsequently is both admitted and discharged prior to the next inpatient census.

Inpatient service day = A unit of measure equivalent to the services received by one inpatient during one 24-hour period

The figure representing an inpatient service day will be the same as the figure for the daily inpatient census. (It may be the same as the inpatient census, provided there were no patient admitted/discharged on the same day.)

Exercise 3.5

1. Excel formula version:

B	C	D	E	F	G	H	I	J	K	L	M	N	O	P
12:01 a.m. Census		Adm		Trf	Total		Dis	Dis	Trf	11:59 p.m. Census			Serv Days	
A/C	NB	A/C	Bir	in	A/C	NB	A/C	NB	out	A/C	NB	A/D	A/C	NB
48	2	2	1	1	51	3	1	2	1	49	1			
=L4	=M4	3	1	2	=B5+D5+F5	=C5+E5	4	1	2	=G5-I5-K5	=H5-I5			

Excel calculated version:

	A	B	C	D	E	F	G	H	I	J	K	L	M	N	O	P
1		12:01 a.m.		Adm		Trf	Total		Dis	Dis	Trf	11:59 p.m.			Serv	
2		Census										Census			Days	
3	Day	A/C	NB	A/C	Bir	in	A/C	NB	A/C	NB	out	A/C	NB	A/D	A/C	NB
4	1-Jun	48	2	2	1	1	51	3	1	2	1	49	1			
5	2-Jun	49	1	3	1	2	54	2	4	1	2	48	1			
6																

2. June 3 will begin with 48 and 1.

The 11:59 p.m. census at the close of one day is the inpatient census at the beginning of the next day.

3.

	A	B	C	D	E	F	G	H	I	J	K	L	M	N	O	P
1		12:01 a.m.		Adm		Trf	Total		Dis	Dis	Trf	11:59 p.m.			Serv	
2		Census										Census			Days	
3	Day	A/C	NB	A/C	Bir	in	A/C	NB	A/C	NB	out	A/C	NB	A/D	A/C	NB
4	1-Jun	48	2	2	1	1	51	3	1	2	1	49	1			
5	2-Jun	49	1	3	1	2	54	2	4	1	2	48	1			
6	3-Jun	48	1	3	1	2	53	2	4	1	2	47	1			

The following data elements for June 3 must be updated with the values presented in exercise 3.6.

1. Cell D6 = 1

2. Cell E6 = 1

3. Cell F6 = 1

4. Cell I6 = 3

5. Cell J6 = 0

6. Cell K6 = 1

7. Cell N4 = 1

8. Cell N5 = 1

9. Cell N6 = 0

	A	B	C	D	E	F	G	H	I	J	K	L	M	N	O	P
1		12:01 a.m.		Adm		Trf	Total		Dis	Dis	Trf	11:59 p.m.			Serv	
2		Census										Census			Days	
3	Day	A/C	NB	A/C	Bir	in	A/C	NB	A/C	NB	out	A/C	NB	A/D	A/C	NB
4	1-Jun	48	2	2	1	1	51	3	1	2	1	49	1	1	50	1
5	2-Jun	49	1	3	1	2	54	2	4	1	2	48	1	1	49	1
6	3-Jun	48	1	3	1	2	53	2	4	1	2	47	1	0	46	2

The patients admitted and discharged on the same day should be added to the 11:59 p.m. census data for each day to compute the inpatient service days. If you arrived at a different answer, you should review the following steps:

   a. *Begin June 2 with the number of patients remaining (11:59 p.m. census), not the number of inpatient service days.*

   b. *Add the number of admissions and transfers in and subtract the number of discharges and transfers out.*

   c. *Add the number of remaining patients admitted and discharged on the same day to the 11:59 p.m. census at the end of each day for the inpatient service days without newborns.*

   d. *Carry the newborns from the 11:59 p.m. census to the inpatient service days column. Each newborn is counted as a service day, too.*

   e. *Begin June 3 with the patients remaining (11:59 p.m. census) from the previous day. June 3 should read across: 48 A/C, 1 NB; 1 A/C; 1 bir; 1 trf in; 50 A/C; 2 NB; 3 dis A/C; 0 NB dis; 1 trf out; 46 A/C; 2 NB; 0 A/D.*

   f. *Because no patients were admitted and discharged on June 3, the 11:59 p.m. census equals inpatient service days for June 3.*

  4. *Yes, if he or she were born and died between census-taking times on two successive days. A newborn transferred out of or discharged from the hospital on the same day he or she was born also could be considered an A/D.*

  5. Calculate the inpatient service days for each of the remaining 27 days of June, and then total the data from the column of inpatient service days for all 30 days of the month.

Exercise 3.7

  1. *(250 + 1,353) – 1,348 = (1,603 – 1,348) = 255*

  2. (23 + 73) – 65 = (96 – 65) = 31

  3. Inpatient service days cannot be computed from the information given because the total number of patients admitted and discharged on the same day is needed to calculate inpatient service days.

  4.

Day	12:01 a.m. Census	Adm	Trf in	Total	Dis	Trf out	11:59 p.m. Census	A/D	Inpt. Serv Days
$\frac{8}{1}$	20	4	2	26	2	8	16	1	16

The data are not correct.

The inpatient service days should be 17. The patient who was admitted and discharged on the same day should be added to the service days.

  5. (15 + 240) – 232 = (255 – 232) = 23

Exercise 3.9

1. **a.** 171

   If you arrived at any other answer, you should review the following steps:
   The numerator is 5,297 (adults and children only). Divide the numerator by the number of days (denominator) in May (31). Look at the number one place beyond the decimal and round appropriately (if the decimal is less than 0.5, drop it when rounding; if the decimal is 0.5 or larger, add 1 to the whole number). Remember, do not include newborn inpatient service days. Consider newborns separately. Watch the decimal point.

   b. 16

   There were 486 newborn inpatient service days for May. Divide the inpatient service days by the number of days in May (31). $\dfrac{486}{31} = 15.7 = 16$

2. **a.** 145

   There were 4,350 inpatient service days for June. Divide the inpatient service days by the number of days in June (30). The answer is a whole number, so no rounding is required.

   b. 12

   There were 360 newborn inpatient service days for June. Divide the inpatient service days by the number of days in June (30). The answer is a whole number, so rounding is not required.

3. Newborn: 11

   There were 298 newborn inpatient service days in February. Divide the newborn inpatient service days by the number of days in February (28) and round.

4. Every PCU creates a daily report of its census, admissions, discharges, and transfers as well as its patients-remaining census to the central collection area.

   The number of patients both admitted and discharged on that same day are added to the 11:59 p.m. census. This gives the inpatient service days for that particular PCU. Adding these over a period of time gives the total inpatient service days. This is not a new process but, rather, the same one followed for calculating total inpatient service days.

5. 12

   There were 358 inpatient service days in the Burn unit during December. Divide the inpatient service days by the number of days in December (31). $\dfrac{358}{31} = 11.5 = 12$

Chapter 4

Exercise 4.1

1. No.

   Beds set up for temporary and emergency use (for example, gurneys in the hall) are not included in the hospital's bed count because they are not continually staffed and available for use. Moreover, hospitals are licensed by the state for a certain number of beds, which does not include disaster needs, and so they cannot set up beds without proper licensure.

2. Bed count: The number of inpatient beds set up and staffed for use on a given day
   Bed capacity: The number of beds that a facility has been designed and constructed to house.
   Bed count must be less than or equal to the bed capacity.

Exercise 4.3

Children's Hospital June 20XX			
Unit	**Number of Beds**	**Inpatient Service Days**	**Percentage of Occupancy**
Pediatric Surgical	30	833	$\dfrac{833}{(30 \times 30)} = \dfrac{833}{900} = 0.9255$ Convert to a percent: $0.9255 \times 100 = 92.55\%$ Round to one decimal: 92.6%
Hematology Oncology	20	566	$\dfrac{566}{(20 \times 30)} = \dfrac{566}{600} = 0.9433$ Convert to a percent: $0.9433 \times 100 = 94.33\%$ Round to one decimal: 94.3%
Neurology/ Neurosurgical	30	756	$\dfrac{756}{(30 \times 30)} = \dfrac{756}{900} = 0.8400$ Convert to a percent: $0.8400 \times 100 = 84.00\%$ Round to one decimal: 84.0%
Renal/ Gastroenterology/ Endocrinology	20	555	$\dfrac{555}{(20 \times 30)} = \dfrac{555}{600} = 0.925$ Convert to a percent: $0.9250 \times 100 = 92.50\%$ Round to one decimal: 92.5%
Respiratory	30	897	$\dfrac{897}{(30 \times 30)} = \dfrac{897}{900} = 0.9966$ Convert to a percent: $0.9966 \times 100 = 99.66\%$ Round to one decimal: 99.7%
Cardiac Medicine/ Surgical	20	589	$\dfrac{589}{(20 \times 30)} = \dfrac{589}{600} = 0.9816$ Convert to a percent: $0.9816 \times 100 = 98.16\%$ Round to one decimal: 98.2%
Infant Care Unit	10	281	$\dfrac{281}{(10 \times 30)} = \dfrac{281}{300} = 0.9366$ Convert to a percent: $0.9366 \times 100 = 93.66\%$ Round to one decimal: 93.7%
Pediatric Intensive Care	20	540	$\dfrac{540}{(20 \times 30)} = \dfrac{540}{600} = 0.900$ Convert to a percent: $0.900 \times 100 = 90.0\%$ Round to one decimal: 90.0%
Total	180	5,017	$\dfrac{5,017}{(180 \times 30)} = \dfrac{5,017}{5,400} = 0.9290$ Convert to a percent: 0.9290×100 Round to one decimal: 92.9%

Example of unit totals:

For example, the pediatric surgical unit has 30 beds and 833 inpatient service days in the month of June (30 days). The percentage of occupancy is therefore the inpatient service days multiplied by 100 and divided by the product of the number of beds (30) and the number of days (30) to get 92.6%.

$$\frac{833}{(30 \times 30 \text{ days})} = \frac{833}{900} = 0.926 \text{ or } 92.6\%$$

To find the total, add the inpatient service days for each of the units to get 5,017. Multiply that by 100 and divide by the product of the total number of beds (180) and the number of days (30).

$$\frac{5,017}{(180 \times 30)} = \frac{5017}{5,400} = 0.929 \text{ or } 92.9\%$$

Excel formula version:

	A	B	C	D
1	Children's Hospital			
2	June 20XX			
3	Unit	Number of Beds	Inpatient Service Days	Percentage of Occupancy
4	Pediatrics Surgical	30	833	=C4/(B4*30)
5	Hematology Oncology	20	566	=C5/(B5*30)
6	Neurology/Neurosurgical	30	756	=C6/(B6*30)
7	Renal/ Gastroenterology/Endocrinology	20	555	=C7/(B7*30)
8	Respiratory	30	897	=C8/(B8*30)
9	Cardiac Medicine/Surgical	20	589	=C9/(B9*30)
10	Infant Care Unit	10	281	=C10/(B10*30)
11	Pediatric Intensive Care	20	540	=C11/(B11*30)
12	Total	=SUM(B4:B11)	=SUM(C4:C11)	=C12/(B12*30)

Excel calculated version:

	A	B	C	D
1	Children's Hospital			
2	June 20XX			
3	Unit	Number of Beds	Inpatient Service Days	Percentage of Occupancy
4	Pediatrics Surgical	30	833	92.6%
5	Hematology Oncology	20	566	94.3%
6	Neurology/Neurosurgical	30	756	84.0%
7	Renal/ Gastroenterology/Endocrinology	20	555	92.5%
8	Respiratory	30	897	99.7%
9	Cardiac Medicine/Surgical	20	589	98.2%
10	Infant Care Unit	10	281	93.7%
11	Pediatric Intensive Care	20	540	90.0%
12	Total	180	5017	92.9%

Exercise 4.5

Excel formula version:

	A	B	C	D
1	University Hospital			
2	January 20XX			
3	PCU	Inpatient Service Days	Bed Count	Percentage of Occupancy
4	Medicine	3752	130	=B4/(C4*31)
5	Rehabilitation/Neurology	600	35	=B5/(C5*31)
6	Orthopedics/Trauma	485	20	=B6/(C6*31)
7	Medicine/Surgical Oncology	1803	60	=B7/(C7*31)
8	Pediatrics	2142	80	=B6/(C6*31)
9	**Critical Care:**			
10	Medicine ICU	1603	55	=B10/(C10*31)
11	Surgical ICU (Adult)	1584	55	=B11/(C11*31)
12	Transplant	895	30	=B12/(C12*31)
13	Surgical ICU (Pediatrics)	923	40	=B13/(C13*31)
14	**Total**	=SUM(B4:B8) + SUM(B10:B13)	=SUM(C4:C8) + SUM(C10:C13)	=B14/(C14*31)

Excel calculated version:

	A	B	C	D
1	University Hospital			
2	January 20XX			
3	PCU	Inpatient Service Days	Bed Count	Percentage of Occupancy
4	Medicine	3,752	130	93.1%
5	Rehabilitation/Neurology	600	35	55.3%
6	Orthopedics/Trauma	485	20	78.2%
7	Medicine/Surgical Oncology	1,803	60	96.9%
8	Pediatrics	2,142	80	86.4%
9	**Critical Care:**			
10	Medicine ICU	1,603	55	94.0%
11	Surgical ICU (Adult)	1,584	55	92.9%
12	Transplant	895	30	96.2%
13	Surgical ICU (Pediatrics)	923	40	74.4%
14	**Total**	13,787	505	88.1%

Exercise 4.7

Patients discharged (includes deaths): 7,054
Average length of stay: 8.8 days
Bed occupancy rate: 85 percent

1. *To use the direct formula, divide patients discharged including deaths (7,054) by the number of beds (200) to get 35.3.*

$$\frac{7,054}{200} = 35.3$$

2. *To use the indirect formula, multiply the occupancy rate (85%) by the number of days in the year (365) and divide by the average length of stay (8.8 days) to get 35.3. Note: The indirect formula the bed occupancy percentage (85%) must be changed to a decimal (0.85). This example shows that during 20XX, each of the hospital's 200 beds changed occupants 35.3 times.*

$$\frac{(0.85 \times 365)}{8.8} = \frac{310.25}{8.8} = 35.3$$

Excel version:

⬒	A	B
1	**Direct Formula**	
2	Discharges (including deaths)	7054
3	Beds	200
4	Bed Turnover Rate - Direct	=B2/B3
5	Bed Turnover Rate - Direct Rounded	=B4
6		
7	**Indirect Formula**	
8	Occupancy Rate	0.85
9	Number of Days in Year	365
10	Average LOS	8.8
11	Bed Turnover Rate - Indirect	=(B8*B9/B10)
12	Bed Turnover Rate - Indirect Rounded	=B11
13		

⬒	A	B
1	**Direct Formula**	
2	Discharges (including deaths)	7054
3	Beds	200
4	Bed Turnover Rate - Direct	35.27
5	Bed Turnover Rate - Direct Rounded	35.3
6		
7	**Indirect Formula**	
8	Occupancy Rate	0.85
9	Number of Days in Year	365
10	Average LOS	8.8
11	Bed Turnover Rate - Indirect	35.25568
12	Bed Turnover Rate - Indirect Rounded	35.3
13		

Chapter 5

Exercise 5.1

Date Admitted	Date Discharged	Length of Stay
7/9	7/10	7/9 = 1 day
9/12	9/22	10 days (figure 5.1.1)
3/10	3/24	3/10, 3/11, 3/12, 3/13, 3/14, 3/15, 3/16, 3/17, 3/18, 3/19, 3/20, 3/21, 3/22, 3/23 14 days
6/17	7/18	6/17 to 6/30 = 30 − 17 = 13 days June to July transition = 1 day 7/1 to 7/18 = 18 − 1 = 17 days Total 13 + 1 + 17 = 31 days
10/20	11/25	Total 36 days (see figures 5.1.2 and 5.1.3)

Figure 5.1.1 – Method 2 for LOS from 9/12 to 9/22

2019 CALENDAR YEAR	SEPTEMBER CALENDAR MONTH		MONDAY FIRST DAY OF WEEK			
Monday	Tuesday	Wednesday	Thursday	Friday	Saturday	Sunday
26	27	28	29	30	31	01
02	03	04	05	06	07	08
09	10	11	Day 1 12 Admission	Day 2 13	Day 3 14	Day 4 15
Day 5 16	Day 6 17	Day 7 18	Day 8 19	Day 9 20	Day 10 21	Day 11 22 Discharge
23	24	25	26	27	28	29
30	01	02	03	04	05	06

Figure 5.1.2 LOS from 10/20 to 11/25

Excel – formula view

	A	B	C
1	Date Admitted	Date Discharged	LOS
2	20-Oct	25-Nov	=B2-A2
3			

Figure 5.1.3 LOS from 10/20 to 11/25

Excel – calculated view

	A	B	C
1	Date Admitted	Date Discharged	LOS
2	20-Oct	25-Nov	36
3			

Exercise 5.3

1. *Patient 1: Subtract 8:00 from 8:17 = 17-0 = 17 minutes wait time (Same hour)*
   Patient 2:
   LOS from 1:22 to 1:59 = 59 – 22 = 37 minutes
   LOS from 1:59 to 2:00 = 1 minute
   LOS from 2:00 to 2:05 = 5 – 0 = 5 minutes
   Total LOS = 37 + 1 + 5 = 43 minutes
   Patient 3:
   LOS from 10:30 to 10:59 = 59 – 30 = 29 minutes
   LOS from 10:59 to 11:00 = 1 minute
   LOS from 11:00 to 11:43 = 43 – 0 = 43 minutes
   Total LOS = 29 + 1 + 43 = 73 minutes or 1 hour 13 minute or 1:13
   Patient 4:
   LOS from 1:30 to 1:59 = 59 – 30 = 29 minutes
   LOS from 1:59 to 2:00 = 1 minute
   LOS from 2:00 to 2:59 = 59 – 0 = 59 minutes
   LOS from 2:59 to 3:00 = 1 minute
   Total LOS = 29 + 1 + 59 + 1 = 90 minutes or 1 hour 30 minute or 1:30
   Patient 5: Subtract 2:15 from 2:56 = 56 – 15 = 41 minutes wait time (Same hour)

2. a.

Excel – formula view

	A	B	C	D	
1	Patient	Time of Arrival	Time Patient was Triaged	Wait Time	
2	Patient A	8:00 AM	8:23 AM	=C2-B2	
3	Patient B	8:23 AM	8:56 AM	=C3-B3	
4	Patient C	8:56 AM	9:20 AM	=C4-B4	
5	Patient D	9:45 AM	10:46 AM	=C5-B5	
6	Patient E	10:20 AM	1:45 PM	=C6-B6	
7	Patient F	11:20 AM	1:50 PM	=C7-B7	
8	Patient G	12:15 PM	2:40 PM	=C8-B8	
9	Patient H	1:05 PM	2:56 PM	=C9-B9	
10	Patient I	3:27 PM	5:05 PM	=C10-B10	
11	Patient J	4:05 PM	4:56 PM	=C11-B11	
12					

Excel – Calculated view

	A	B	C	D	
1	Patient	Time of Arrival	Time Patient was Triaged	Wait Time	
2	Patient A	8:00 AM	8:23 AM	12:23:00 AM	
3	Patient B	8:23 AM	8:56 AM	12:33:00 AM	
4	Patient C	8:56 AM	9:20 AM	12:24:00 AM	
5	Patient D	9:45 AM	10:46 AM	1:01:00 AM	
6	Patient E	10:20 AM	1:45 PM	3:25:00 AM	
7	Patient F	11:20 AM	1:50 PM	2:30:00 AM	
8	Patient G	12:15 PM	2:40 PM	2:25:00 AM	
9	Patient H	1:05 PM	2:56 PM	1:51:00 AM	
10	Patient I	3:27 PM	5:05 PM	1:38:00 AM	
11	Patient J	4:05 PM	4:56 PM	12:51:00 AM	
12					

Column D must be formatted as time with no AM/PM designation. Right click on values in column D and select the time format highlighted in the figure below:

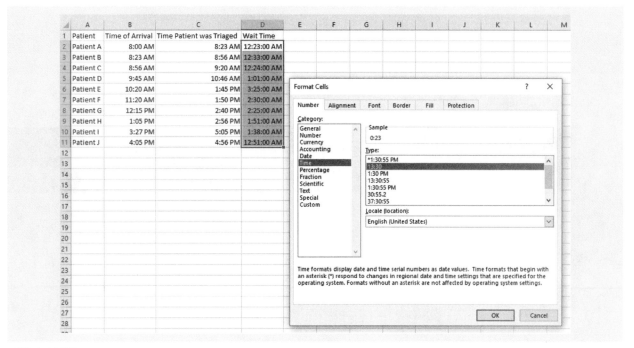

Click 'OK'

a. See Excel spreadsheet

b. Type the formula (without quotes) '=average (D2:D11)

answer is 1:30 (1 hour and 30 minutes)

c. No, the hospital ED is not in compliance

Exercise 5.5

1. Adults and Children: $\dfrac{923}{192} = 4.807$ days round to 4.8 days

2. a. $\dfrac{302}{15} = 20.1$ days

b. $\dfrac{203}{7} = 29.0$ days

c. $\dfrac{91}{4} = 22.75 = 22.8$ days

d. $\dfrac{8}{4} = 2$ days

e. $\dfrac{6}{3} = 2$ days

f. $\dfrac{89}{3} = 29.7$ days

g. $\dfrac{53}{3} = 17.7$ days

h. $\dfrac{44}{2} = 22$ days

i. $\dfrac{110}{4} = 27.5$ days

3.

University Medical Center January–June 20XX			
Clinical Units	**Discharges**	**Discharge Days**	**ALOS**
Medicine	12,280	61,400	$\dfrac{61,400}{12,280} = 5.0$
Surgery	10,320	51,762	$\dfrac{51,762}{10,320} = 5.0$
Neurology	12,464	68,320	$\dfrac{68,320}{12,464} = 5.5$
Oncology	6,228	61,280	$\dfrac{61,280}{6,228} = 9.8$
Orthopedics	4,906	20,624	$\dfrac{20,624}{4,906} = 4.2$
Rehabilitation	1,926	48,250	$\dfrac{48,250}{1,926} = 25.1$
Urology	678	2,698	$\dfrac{2,698}{678} = 4.0$
Psychiatry	936	22,400	$\dfrac{22,400}{936} = 23.9$
Ophthalmology	385	804	$\dfrac{804}{385} = 2.1$
Obstetrics/Gynecology	3,528	8,820	$\dfrac{8,820}{3,528} = 2.5$
Pediatrics	3,148	18,388	$\dfrac{18,388}{3,148} = 5.8$
Total	56,799	364,746	$\dfrac{364,746}{56,799} = 6.4$

Chapter 6

Exercise 6.1

1. $\dfrac{(4+1)}{(645+4+87+1)} = \dfrac{5}{737} = 0.00678$

   Convert to a percent: 0.00678 x 100 = 0.678%
   Round to two decimal places: 0.68%

2. $\dfrac{3}{58} = 0.0517.$

   Convert to percent and round: 5.17%

3. $\dfrac{3}{15} = 0.200$

   Convert to a percent: 0.200x100 = 20.00%

Exercise 6.3

$$Net\ Mortality\ Rate = \frac{5+1}{409+5+68\mp1} = \frac{6}{483} = 0.01242$$

Convert to a percent: $0.01242 \times 100 = 1.242\%$

Round to two decimal places: 1.24%

Note: Deaths within 48 hours of admission are removed from both the numerator and denominator of the net mortality rate.

Exercise 6.5

Excel – formula version

	A	B	C	D
1			Community Hospital	
2			July-December 20XX	
3			Number of Surgery Patients and Deaths, by Surgeon	
4	Physician Number	No. of Surgery Patients	No. of Deaths within 10 Days after Surgery	Postoperative Mortality rate
5	Dr. 102	298	6	=C5/B5
6	Dr. 237	247	4	=C6/B6
7	Dr. 391	110	2	=C7/B7
8	Dr. 518	144	2	=C8/B8
9	Dr. 637	206	8	=C9/B9
10	Dr. 802	82	3	=C10/B10
11	Dr. 900	120	3	=C11/B11
12	**Total**	=SUM(B5:B11)	=SUM(C5:C11)	=C12/B12
13				

Excel – calculated version

	A	B	C	D
1			Community Hospital	
2			July-December 20XX	
3			Number of Surgery Patients and Deaths, by Surgeon	
4	Physician Number	No. of Surgery Patients	No. of Deaths within 10 Days after Surgery	Postoperative Mortality rate
5	Dr. 102	298	6	2.0%
6	Dr. 237	247	4	1.6%
7	Dr. 391	110	2	1.8%
8	Dr. 518	144	2	1.4%
9	Dr. 637	206	8	3.9%
10	Dr. 802	82	3	3.7%
11	Dr. 900	120	3	2.5%
12	**Total**	1, 207	28	2.3%
13				

Exercise 6.7

Excel – formula version

	A	B	C	D	E
1		Community Hospital			
2		January–June20XX			
3		Selected MS-DRGs—Postoperative Deaths			
4		Number of Surgery Patients and Deaths			
5		Surgery Service			
6	MS-DRG	MS-DRG Title	No. of Surgery Patients	No. of Deaths within 10 Days after surgery	Postoperative Mortality rate
7	139	Salivary gland procedures	12	1	=D7/C7
8	217	Cardiac Valve & oth maj cardiothoracic proc w card w CC	427	5	=D8/C8
9	239	Amputation for circ sys disorders exc upper limb & toe w MCC	8	2	=D9/C9
10	327	Stomach, esophageal & duodenal proc w CC	84	3	=D10/C10
11	338	Appendectomy w complicated principal diag w MCC	6	1	=D11/C11
12	405	Pancreas, liver & shunt procedures w MCC	62	4	=D12/C12
13	469	Major joint replacement or reattachment of lower extremity w MCC	212	3	=D13/C13
14	625	Thyroid, parathyroid & thyroglossal procedures w MCC	207	1	=D14/C14
15	652	Kidney transplant	27	4	=D15/C15
16	736	Uterine & adnexa proc for ovarian or adnexal malignancy w MCC	143	4	=D16/C16
17	**Total**		=SUM(C7:C16)	=SUM(D7:D16)	=D17/C17
18					

Excel – calculated version

	A	B	C	D	E
1		Community Hospital			
2		Januar-June 20XX			
3		Selected MS-DRGs—Postoperative Deaths			
4		Number of Surgery Patients and Deaths			
5		Surgery Service			
6	MS-DRG	MS-DRG Title	No. of Surgery Patients	No. of Deaths within 10 Days after Surgery	Postoperative Mortality rate
7	139	Salivary gland procedures	12	1	8.33%
8	217	Cardiac valve & oth maj cardiothoracic proc w card cath w CC	427	5	1.17%
9	239	Amputation for circ sys disorders exc upper limb & toe w MCC	8	2	25.00%
10	327	Stomach, esophageal & duodenal proc w CC	84	3	3.57%
11	338	Appendectomy w complicated principal diag w MCC	6	1	16.67%
12	405	Pancreas, liver & shunt procedures w MCC	62	4	6.45%
13	469	Major joint replacement or reattachment of lower extremity w MCC	212	3	1.42%
14	625	Thyroid, parathyroid & thyroglossal procedures w MCC	207	1	0.48%
15	652	Kidney transplant	27	4	14.81%
16	736	Uterine & Adnexa proc for ovarian or adnexal malignancy w MCC	143	4	2.80%
17	Total		1,188	28	2.36%
18					

Exercise 6.9

Excel – formula version

	A	B
1	**University Hospital**	
2	**January–June 20XX**	
3	**Surgery Service**	
4	Discharges (Dose not include deaths)	2,642
5	Deaths	54
6	Within 10 days	12
7	After 10 days	42
8	Number of operations	2,645
9	Number of patients operated on	2,636
10	Number of anesthetics administered	2,636
11	General anesthesia	1,072
12	Regional anesthesia	1,017
13	Local anesthesia	547
14	Number of deaths due to anesthetic agents	7
15	General anesthesia	4
16	Regional anesthesia	2
17	Local anesthesia	1
18		
19	**Mortality Rates**	
20	General anesthesia	=B15/B11
21	Regional anesthesia	=B16/B12
22	Local anesthesia	=B17/B13

Excel – Calculated version:

	A	B
1	**University Hospital**	
2	**January–June 20XX**	
3	**Surgery Service**	
4	Discharges (does not include deaths)	2,642
5	Deaths	54
6	Within 10 days	12
7	After 10 days	42
8	Number of operations	2,645
9	Number of patients operated on	2,636
10	Number of anesthetics administered	2,636
11	General anesthesia	1,072
12	Regional anesthesia	1,017
13	Local anesthesia	547
14	Number of deaths due to anesthetic agents	7
15	General anesthesia	4
16	Regional anesthesia	2
17	Local anesthesia	1
18		
19	**Mortality Rates**	
20	General anesthesia	0.37%
21	Regional anesthesia	0.20%
22	Local anesthesia	0.18%

Exercise 6.11

The only cases that were direct obstetric deaths were the hemorrhage after C-section due to severed uterine artery and pre-eclampsia.

$$OB\ case\ fatality\ rate = \frac{2}{123} = 0.01626$$

Convert to a percent: $0.01626 \times 100 = 1.626\%$

Round to two decimal places: 1.63%

Exercise 6.13

$$\frac{1,231}{3,855,500} = 0.000319$$

Convert to per 100,000: $0.000319 \times 100,000 = 31.9$ per 100,000

Round to nearest whole number: 32 maternal deaths per 100,000 population.

Exercise 6.15

$$\frac{(4+3)}{(37+4+3)} = \frac{7}{44} = 0.15909$$

Convert to a percent: $0.15909 \times 100 = 15.909\%$
Round to two decimal places: 15.91%

Exercise 6.17

Excel formula version:

	A	B	C	D
1		Community Hospital		
2		Cancer Registry Annual Report		
3		Selected Cancers Reported		
4		20XX		
5	**Type of Cancer**	**No. of Discharges and Deaths**	**No. of Deaths**	**Cancer Mortality rate**
6	Breast	311	15	=C6/B6
7	Prostate	208	17	=C7/B7
8	Digestive System	102	13	=C8/B8
9	Lung and bronchus	162	12	=C9/B9
10	Urinary System	98	13	=C10/B10
11	Female Reproductive	48	3	=C11/B11
12	Melanoma of the skin	21	14	=C12/B12
13	All other sites	215	52	=C13/B13
14	**Total**	=SUM(B6:B13)	=SUM(C6:C13)	=C14/B14
15				

Excel calculated version

	A	B	C	D
1	Community Hospital			
2	Cancer Registry Annual Report			
3	Selected Cancers Reported			
4	20XX			
5	Type of Cancer	No. of Discharges and Deaths	No. of Deaths	Cancer Mortality rate
6	Breast	311	15	4.82%
7	Prostate	208	17	8.17%
8	Digestive System	102	13	12.75%
9	Lung and bronchus	162	12	7.41%
10	Urinary System	98	13	13.27%
11	Female Reproductive	48	3	6.25%
12	Melanoma of the skin	21	14	66.67%
13	All other sites	215	52	24.19%
14	Total	1,165	139	11.93%
15				

Exercise 6.19

Excel formula version:

	A	B	C	D
1	University Hospital			
2	Cancer Registry Annual Report			
3	Selected Cancers Reported			
4	20XX			
5	Type of Cancer	No. of Discharges and Deaths	No. of Deaths	Mortality rate
6	Oral Cavity and Pharynx	24	1	=C6/B6
7	Digestive System	198	5	=C7/B7
8	Respiratory System	242	16	=C8/B8
9	Bone and Joint	218	4	=C9/B9
10	Skin (excludes Basal Cell)	34	1	=C10/B10
11	Breast	190	12	=C11/B11
12	Female Genital System	47	8	=C12/B12
13	Male Genital System	228	25	=C13/B13
14	Urinary System	77	7	=C14/B14
15	Brain and Other Nervous System	42	19	=C15/B15
16	Endocrine System	28	1	=C16/B16
17	Lymphoma	47	6	=C17/B17
18	Myeloma	25	2	=C18/B18
19	Leukemia	15	4	=C19/B19
20	Total	=SUM(B6:B19)	=SUM(C6:C19)	=C20/B20

Excel calculated version

	A	B	C	D
1	University Hospital			
2	Cancer Registry Annual Report			
3	Selected Cancers Reported			
4	20XX			
5	**Type of Cancer**	**No. of Discharges and Deaths**	**No. of Deaths**	**Mortality rate**
6	Oral Cavity and Pharynx	24	1	4.17%
7	Digestive System	198	5	2.53%
8	Respiratory System	242	16	6.61%
9	Bone and Joint	218	4	1.83%
10	Skin (excludes Basal Cell)	34	1	2.94%
1	Breast	190	12	6.32%
12	Female Genital System	47	8	17.02%
13	Male Genital System	228	25	10.96%
14	Urinary System	77	7	9.09%
15	Brain and Other Nervous System	42	19	45.24%
16	Endocrine System	28	1	3.57%
17	Lymphoma	47	6	12.77%
18	Myeloma	25	2	8.00%
19	Leukemia	15	4	26.67%
20	**Total**	1,415	111	7.84%
21				

Chapter 7

Exercise 7.1

1. $\dfrac{6}{18} = 0.3333$

   Convert to a percent: $0.3333 \times 100 = 33.33\%$

   Round to nearest tenth of a percent: 33.3%

2. $\dfrac{2}{9} = 0.2222$

   Convert to a percent: $0.2222 \times 100 = 22.22\%$

   Round to nearest tenth of a percent: 22.2%

3. $\dfrac{15}{18} = 0.8333$

   Convert to a percent: $0.8333 \times 100 = 83.33\%$

   Round to nearest tenth of a percent: 83.3%

Exercise 7.3

Gross death rate: $\dfrac{267}{18,251} = 0.01462$

Convert to a percent: $0.01462 \times 100 = 1.462\%$

Round to two decimals: 1.46%

Gross autopsy rate: $\dfrac{170}{267} = 0.63670$

Convert to a percent: $0.63670 \times 100 = 63.670\%$

Round to two decimals: 63.67%

Net autopsy rate: $\dfrac{170}{(267-20)} = \dfrac{170}{247} = 0.68826$

Convert to a percent: $0.68826 \times 100 = 68.826\%$

Round to two decimals: 68.83%

Exercise 7.5

Excel formula version:

	A	B	C	D	E	F	G	H
2								
3								
4	Month	Discharges	Inpatient Deaths	Autopsies	Coroner's Cases	Gross Mortality Rate	Gross Autopsy Rate	Net Autopsy Rate
5	January	598	5	2	1	=C5/B5	=D5/D5	=D5/(C5-E5)
6	February	587	6	2	2	=C6/B6	=D6/D6	=D6/(C6-E6)
7	March	607	7	5	1	=C7/B7	=D7/D7	=D7/(C7-E7)
8	April	624	5	1	0	=C8/B8	=D8/D8	=D8/(C8-E8)
9	May	620	6	2	1	=C9/B9	=D9/D9	=D9/(C9-E9)
10	June	599	7	3	2	=C10/B10	=D10/D10	=D10/(C10-E10)
11	July	609	9	5	2	=C11/B11	=D11/D11	=D11/(C11-E11)
12	August	575	5	2	0	=C12/B12	=D12/D12	=D12/(C12-E12)
13	September	611	7	3	1	=C13/B13	=D13/D13	=D13/(C13-E13)
14	October	578	8	4	1	=C14/B14	=D14/D14	=D14/(C14-E14)
15	November	622	6	2	0	=C15/B15	=D15/D15	=D15/(C15-E15)
16	December	572	7	2	2	=C16/B16	=D16/D16	=D16/(C16-E16)
17	**Total**	=SUM(B5:B16)	=SUM(C5:C16)	=SUM(D5:D16)	=SUM(E5:E16)	=C17/B17	=D17/D17	=D17/(C17-E17)

Excel calculated version:

Month	Discharges	Inpatient Deaths	Autopsies	Coroner's Cases	Gross Mortality Rate	Gross Autopsy Rate	Net Autopsy Rate
			Annual Statistics				
			20XX				
January	598	5	2	1	0.84%	40.00%	50.00%
February	587	6	2	2	1.02%	33.33%	50.00%
March	607	7	5	1	1.15%	71.43%	83.33%
April	624	5	1	-	0.80%	20.00%	20.00%
May	620	6	2	1	0.97%	33.33%	40.00%
June	599	7	3	2	1.17%	42.86%	60.00%
July	609	9	5	2	1.48%	55.56%	71.43%
August	575	5	2	-	0.87%	40.00%	40.00%
September	611	7	3	1	1.15%	42.86%	50.00%
October	578	8	4	1	1.8%	50.00%	57.14%
November	622	6	2	-	0.96%	33.33%	33.33%
December	572	7	2	2	1.22%	28.57%	40.00%
Total	7,202	78	33	13	1.08%	42.31%	50.77%

Exercise 7.7

a, b, c, e, f (*d does not apply because the autopsy was done by the medical examiner, and g does not apply because fetal deaths and autopsies are calculated separately.*)

Exercise 7.9

Adjusted hospital autopsy rate:
Number of autopsies:
(3 IP autopsies + 2 ESD autopsies + 1 home health autopsy) = 6
Number of bodies available for autopsy:
[(12 IP deaths + 2 ESD deaths + 1 home health death) – 2 coroner's cases]
= 13

Adjusted autopsy rate $= \dfrac{6}{13} = 0.46154$

Convert to a percent: $0.46154 \times 100 = 46.154\%$
Round to two decimals: 46.15%

Exercise 7.11

Newborn autopsy rate $= \dfrac{1}{2} = 0.5000$

Convert to a percent: $0.5000 \times 100 = 50.00\%$

Round to two decimals: 50.0%

Exercise 7.13

Newborn death rate:

$$\frac{3}{686} = 0.004373$$

Convert to a percent: $0.004373 \times 100 = 0.4373\%$
Round to two decimals: 0.44%

Fetal death rate:

$$\frac{[(7 \text{ intermediate fetal deaths}+3 \text{ late fetal deaths})]}{(687 \text{ births}+7 \text{ intermediate}+3 \text{ late fetal deaths})} = \frac{10}{697} = 0.014347$$

Convert to a percent: $0.014347 \times 100 = 1.4347\%$
Round to two decimals: 1.43%

Newborn autopsy rate:

$$\frac{2}{3} = 0.66666$$

Convert to a percent: $0.66666 \times 100 = 66.666\%$
Round to two decimals: 66.67%

Fetal autopsy rate:

$$\frac{(1 \text{ intermediate autopsy}+2 \text{ late fetal autopsies})}{(7 \text{ intermediate fetal deaths}+3 \text{ late fetal deaths})} = \frac{3}{10} = 0.30000$$

Convert to a percent: $0.30000 \times 100 = 30.000\%$
Round to two decimals: 30.00%

Chapter 8

Exercise 8.1

Calculate the rates requested for Community Hospital.
Hospital-acquired infection rate for adults and children:

$$\frac{18}{2,190} = 0.008219$$

Convert to a percent: $0.008219 \times 100 = 0.8219\%$
Round to two decimal places: 0.82%

Hospital-acquired infection rate for newborns:

$$\frac{2}{127} = 0.01574$$

Convert to a percent: $0.01574 \times 100 = 1.574\%$
Round to two decimal places: 1.57%

Total Hospital-acquired infection rate for the hospital:

$$\frac{(18+2)}{(2,190+127)} = \frac{20}{2,317} = 0.008631$$

Convert to a percent: $0.008631 \times 100 = 0.8631\%$
Round to two decimal places: 0.86%

Gross mortality rate for this annual period:

$$\frac{(13+1)}{(2,190+127)} = \frac{14}{2,317} = 0.00604$$

Convert to a percent: $0.00604 \times 100 = 0.604\%$
Round to two decimal places: 0.60%

Exercise 8.3

Postoperative infection rate:

$$\frac{14}{2,176} = 0.00643$$

Convert to a percent: 0.643%
Round to two decimals: 0.64%

Postoperative morality rate:

$$\frac{8}{2,170} = 0.00368$$

Convert to a percent: 0.368%
Round to two decimals: 0.37%

Exercise 8.5

<table>
<tr><td colspan="3" style="text-align:center">Community Hospital
Infection Prevention Committee Report on Infections
January–March 20XX
389 discharges</td></tr>
<tr><th>Type of Infection</th><th>No. of Infections</th><th>Infection Rate</th></tr>
<tr><td>Central Line-associated bloodstream infections</td><td>8</td><td>$\frac{8}{389} = 0.02056$

Convert to a percent: $0.02056 \times 100 = 2.056\%$
Round to two decimals: 2.06%</td></tr>
<tr><td>Catheter-associated urinary tract infections</td><td>12</td><td>$\frac{12}{389} = 0.03084$

Convert to a percent: $0.03084 \times 100 = 3.084\%$
Round to two decimals: 3.08%</td></tr>
<tr><td>Ventilator-associated pneumonia</td><td>4</td><td>$\frac{4}{389} = 0.01028$

Convert to a percent: $0.01028 \times 100 = 1.028\%$
Round to two decimals: 1.03%</td></tr>
<tr><td>Surgical-site infections</td><td>6</td><td>$\frac{6}{389} = 0.01542$

Convert to a percent: $0.01542 \times 100 = 1.542\%$
Round to two decimals: 1.54%</td></tr>
<tr><td>Cardiovascular system infections</td><td>2</td><td>$\frac{2}{389} = 0.00514$

Convert to a percent: $0.00514 \times 100 = 0.514\%$
Round to two decimals: 0.51%</td></tr>
</table>

(continued on next page)

<table>
<tr><td colspan="3" align="center">**Community Hospital**
Infection Prevention Committee Report on Infections
January–March 20XX
389 discharges</td></tr>
<tr><td>**Type of Infection**</td><td>**No. of Infections**</td><td>**Infection Rate**</td></tr>
<tr><td>Gastrointestinal tract infections</td><td>3</td><td>$\dfrac{3}{389} = 0.00771$

Convert to a percent: $0.00771 \times 100 = 0.771\%$
Round to two decimals: 0.77%</td></tr>
<tr><td>Skin and soft-tissue infections</td><td>1</td><td>$\dfrac{1}{389} = 0.00257$

Convert to a percent: $0.00257 \times 100 = 0.257\%$
Round to two decimals: 0.26%</td></tr>
<tr><td>Ears, nose and throat infections</td><td>9</td><td>$\dfrac{9}{389} = 0.02313$

Convert to a percent: $0.02313 \times 100 = 2.313\%$
Round to two decimals: 2.31%</td></tr>
<tr><td>Central nervous system infections</td><td>7</td><td>$\dfrac{7}{389} = 0.01799$

Convert to a percent: $0.01799 \times 100 = 1.799\%$
Round to two decimals: 1.80%</td></tr>
<tr><td>Systemic infections</td><td>5</td><td>$\dfrac{5}{389} = 0.01285$

Convert to a percent: $0.01285 \times 100 = 1.285\%$
Round to two decimals: 1.29%</td></tr>
</table>

Exercise 8.7

Excel formula version:

	A	B	C	D
1		Community Hospital		
2		Complication Rate by Physician		
3		January-June 20XX		
4	Physician No.	No. Discharges and Deaths	No. Complications	Complication Rate
5	102	298	2	=C5/B5
6	237	247	4	=C6/B6
7	391	110	3	=C7/B7
8	518	144	2	=C8/B8
9	637	206	3	=C9/B9
10	802	82	1	=C10/B10
11	900	100	3	=C11/B11
12	**Total**	=SUM(B5:B11)	=SUM(C5:C11)	=C12/B12
13				

Excel calculated version:

	A	B	C	D
1	Community Hospital			
2	Complication Rate by Physician			
3	January–June 20XX			
4	Physician No.	No. Discharges and Deaths	No. Complications	Complication Rate
5	102	298	2	0.67%
6	237	247	4	1.62%
7	391	110	3	2.73%
8	518	144	2	1.39%
9	637	206	3	1.46%
10	802	82	1	1.22%
11	900	100	3	3.00%
12	Total	1,187	18	1.52%
13				

Exercise 8.9

Calculate the C-section rate, the newborn mortality rate, and the fetal mortality rate at University Hospital for the month of July.

C-section rate:

$$\frac{20}{130} = 0.15384$$

Convert to a percent: 0.15384 x 100 = 15.384%
Round to two decimals: 15.38%

Newborn mortality rate:

$$\frac{1}{130} = 0.00769$$

Convert to a percent: 0.00769 x 100 = 0.769%
Round to two decimals: 0.77%

Fetal mortality rate:

$$\frac{(2+2)}{(130+2+2)} = \frac{4}{134} = 0.02985$$

Convert to a percent: 0.02985 x 100 = 2.985%
Round to two decimals: 2.99%

Exercise 8.11

Excel formula version:

	A	B	C	D	E	F
1			Community Hospital			
2			Surgery Service			
3			Annual Statistics 20XX			
4	Month	Disch Including Deaths	Deaths	Consults	Consultation Rate	Gross Death Rate
5	January	602	18	119	=D5/B5	=C5/B5
6	February	675	12	107	=D6/B6	=C6/B6
7	March	598	11	92	=D7/B7	=C7/B7
8	April	555	14	74	=D8/B8	=C8/B8
9	May	630	10	105	=D9/B9	=C9/B9
10	June	592	6	96	=D10/B10	=C10/B10
11	July	581	9	85	=D11/B11	=C11/B11
12	August	593	7	72	=D12/B12	=C12/B12
13	September	621	5	89	=D13/B13	=C13/B13
14	October	610	12	56	=D14/B14	=C14/B14
15	November	601	10	95	=D15/B15	=C15/B15
16	December	581	14	82	=D16/B16	=C16/B16
17	**Total**	=SUM(B5:B16)	=SUM(C5:C16)	=SUM(D5:D16)	=D17/B17	=C17/B17
18						

Excel calculated version:

	A	B	C	D	E	F
1		Community Hospital				
2		Surgery Service				
3		Annual Statistics 20XX				
4	Month	Disch Including Deaths	Deaths	Consults	Consultation Rate	Gross Death Rate
5	January	602	18	119	19.77%	2.99%
6	February	675	12	107	15.85%	1.78%
7	March	598	11	92	15.38%	1.84%
8	April	555	14	74	13.33%	2.52%
9	May	630	10	105	16.67%	1.59%
10	June	592	6	96	16.22%	1.01%
11	July	581	9	85	14.63%	1.55%
12	August	593	7	72	12.14%	1.18%
13	September	621	5	89	14.33%	0.81%
14	October	610	12	56	9.18%	1.97%
15	November	601	10	95	15.81%	1.66%
16	December	581	14	82	14.11%	2.41%
18	**Total**	7,239	128	1,072	14.81%	1.77%
19						

Exercise 8.13

Excel formula version:

	A	B	C	D	E
1			Community Hospital		
2			Semiannual Statistics, 20XX		
3			Readmission by Selected MS-DRGs		
4	MS-DRG	Title	No. Live Disch	No. Readmissions within 30 days of Previous Discharge	Readmission Rate
5	190	COPD with MCC	12	2	=D5/C5
6	191	COPD with CC	14	5	=D6/C6
7	192	COPD without/MCC CC/MCC	42	11	=D7/C7
8	193	Simple pneumonia & pleurisy with MCC	8	1	=D8/C8
9	194	Simple pneumonia & pleurisy with CC	15	4	=D9/C9
10	195	Simple pneumonia & pleurisy without CC/MCC	97	8	=D10/C10
11	280	Acute myocardial infarction discharged alive, with MCC	10	3	=D11/C11
12	281	Acute myocardial infarction discharged alive, with CC	8	2	=D12/C12
13	282	Acute myocardial infarction discharged alive, without CC	180	10	=D13/C13
14	291	Heart failure & shock with MCC	3	1	=D14/C14
15	292	Heart failure & shock with CC	6	1	=D15/C15
16	293	Heart failure & shock without CC/MCC	63	2	=D16/C16
17	469	Major joint replacement or reattachment, lower extremity with MCC	15	2	=D17/C17
18	470	Major joint replacement or reattachment, lower extremity without MCC	49	4	=D18/C18

Excel calculated version:

	A	B	C	D	E
1		Community Hospital			
2		Semiannual Statistics, 20XX			
3		Readmission by Selected MS-DRGs			
4	MS-DRG	Title	No. Live Disch	No. Readmissions within 30 days of Previous Discharge	Readmission Rate
5	190	COPD with MCC	12	2	16.67%
6	191	COPD with CC	14	5	35.71%
7	192	COPD without CC/MCC	42	11	26.19%
8	193	Simple pneumonia & pleurisy with MCC	8	1	12.50%
9	194	Simple pneumonia & pleurisy with CC	15	4	26.67%
10	195	Simple pneumonia & pleurisy without CC/MCC	97	8	8.25%
11	280	Acute myocardial infarction discharged alive, with MCC	10	3	30.00%
12	281	Acute myocardial infarction discharged alive, with CC	8	2	25.00%
13	282	Acute myocardial infarction discharged alive, without CC/MCC	180	10	5.56%
14	291	Heart failure & shock with MCC	3	1	33.33%
15	292	Heart failure & shock with CC	6	1	16.67%
16	293	Heart failure & shock without CC/MCC	63	2	3.17%
17	469	Major joint replacement or reattachment, lower extremity with MCC	15	2	13.33%
18	470	Major joint replacement or reattachment, lower extremity without MCC	49	4	8.16%

Exercise 8.15

1. Percentage of total hospital patients in the medicine service:

$$\frac{5,967}{9,845} = 0.60609$$

Convert to a percent: 0.60609 x 100 = 60.609%
Round to two decimals: 60.61%

2. Complication rate for medicine service:

$$\frac{236}{5,967} = 0.03955$$

Convert to a percent: 0.03955 x 100 = 3.955%
Round to two decimals: 3.96%

3. Hospital-acquired infection rate for medicine service:

$$\frac{89}{5,967} = 0.01491$$

Convert to a percent: 0.01491 x 100 = 1.491%
Round to two decimals: 1.49%

4. Gross mortality rate for medicine service:

$$\frac{71}{5,967} = 0.01189$$

Convert to a percent: 0.01189 x 100 = 1.189%
Round to two decimals: 1.19%

Chapter 9

Exercise 9.1

1. $0.10 per line

$$\frac{\$31,200}{312,000} = \$0.10 \ per \ line$$

2. $0.12 per line

$$\frac{\$29,120}{234,000} = \$0.12 \ per \ line$$

3. Excel formula version:

	A	B	C	D	E	F
1	Transcriptionist	Hourly Rate	Daily Lines	Annual Salary	Annual Lines	Cost per Unit
2	1	14	1000	=B2*2080	=C2*260	=D2/E2
3	2	14.8	1000	=B3*2080	=C3*260	=D3/E3
4	3	14.8	1000	=B4*2080	=C4*260	=D4/C4
5	4	14.8	1000	=B5*2080	=C5*260	=D5/C5
6	5	16	1000	=B6*2080	=C6*260	=D6/E6
7	6	14.25	1100	=B7*2080	=C7*260	=D7/E7
8	7	17	1100	=B8*2080	=C8*260	=D8/E8
9	8	14	1200	=B9*2080	=C9*260	=D9/E9
10	Total			=SUM(D2:D9)	=SUM(E2:E9)	=D10/E10
11						

Excel calculated version:

	A	B	C	D	E	F
1	Transcriptionist	Hourly Rate	Daily Lines	Annual Salary	Annual Lines	Cost per Unit
2		$14.00	1000	$29,120	260,000	$ 0.11
3		$14.00	1000	$30,784	260,000	$ 0.12
4		$14.00	1000	$30,784	260,000	$ 0.12
5		$14.00	1000	$30,784	260,000	$ 0.12
6		$16.00	1000	$33,280	260,000	$ 0.13
7		$14.25	1100	$29,640	286,000	$ 0.10
8		$17.00	1100	$35,360	286,000	$ 0.12
9		$14.00	1200	$29,120	312,000	$ 0.09
10	Total			$248,872	2,184,000	$ 0.11
11						

a. The difference in cost per line is: $0.11 – $0.09 = $0.02

b. The employees make the same hourly rate, but one produces less than the other, resulting in a higher per line rate for the employee who produces 1,000 lines per day than the employee who produces 1,200 lines per day.

c. The difference in cost per line is: $0.13 – $0.10 = $0.03

d. 0.11 per line

4. a. Lead coder: *Salary = $20.35 × 2,080 = $42,328*

Productivity: 7.5 hours per day × 4 records per hour = 30 records per day

30 records × 5 days per week × 52 weeks per year = 7,800

$$\frac{\$42,328}{7,800} = \$5.43 \text{ per record}$$

New Graduate: *Salary = $15.50 × 2,080 = $32,240*

Productivity: 7.5 hours per day × 3 records per hour = 22.5 records per day

22.5 records × 5 days per week × 52 weeks per year = 5,850

$$\frac{\$32,240}{5,850} = \$5.51 \text{ per record}$$

Experienced coder: *Salary = $18.90 × 2,080 = $39,312*

Productivity: 7.5 hours per day × 6 records per hour = 45 records per day

45 records × 5 days per week × 52 weeks per year = 11,700

$$\frac{\$39,312}{11,700} = \$3.36 \text{ per record}$$

b. $$\frac{\$113,880}{25,350} = \$4.49 \text{ per record}$$

Salaries = Add all salaries together = $113,880

Productivity = Add all productivity together = 13 records per hour = 97.5 per day

97.5 × 5 days per week × 52 weeks per year = 25,350 records coded per year

$$\frac{\$113,880}{25,350} = \$4.49 \text{ per record}$$

5. Excel formula version:

	A	B	C	D	E	F
1	Coding Professional	Salary	Records coded per hour	Salary per year	Annual productivity	Unit Cost
2	A	15	4	31200	=C2*7.5*5*52	=D2/E2
3	B	15.45	5	32136	=C3*7.5*5*52	=D3/E3
4	C	15.1	4	31408	=C4*7.5*5*52	=D4/E4
5	D	16.70	6	34923	=C5*7.5*5*52	=D5/E5
6	E	18.22	6	37898	=C6*7.5*5*52	=D6/E6
7	F	22.65	6	47112	=C7*7.5*5*52	=D7/E7
8	G	16.03	6	33342	=C8*7.5*5*52	=D8/E8
9	H	16.85	6	35048	=C9*7.5*5*52	=D9/E9
10	I	21.76	8	45261	=C10*7.5*5*52	=D10/E10
11	J	17.34	6	36067	=C11*7.5*5*52	=D11/E11
12	**Total**			=SUM(D2:D11)	=SUM(E2:E11)	=D12/E12
13						

Excel calculated version

	A	B	C	D	E	F	G
1	Coding Professional	Salary	Records coded per hour	Salary per year	Annual productivity	Unit Cost	
2	A	$15.00	4	$31,200	7,800	$4.00	
3	B	$15.45	5	$32,136	9,750	$3.30	
4	C	$15.10	4	$31.408	7,800	$4.03	
5	D	$16.79	6	$34,923	11,700	$2.98	
6	E	$18.22	6	$37,898	11,700	$3.24	
7	F	$ 22.65	6	$47,112	11,700	$4.03	
8	G	$16.03	6	$33,342	11,700	$2.85	
9	H	$16.85	6	$35,048	11,700	$3.00	
10	I	$ 21.76	8	$45,261	15,600	$2.90	
11	J	$ 17.34	6	$36,067	11,700	$3.08	
12	**Total**			$364,395	111,150	$3.28	
13							

Exercise 9.3

1. Postage: $\dfrac{\$790}{550} = \$1.44$

Service contract: $\dfrac{\$265}{550} = \$0.48$

Equipment: $\dfrac{\$150}{550} = \$0.27$

Supplies: $\dfrac{\$95}{550} = \$0.17$

Wages: $\$13.00 \times 2{,}080 = \$27{,}040$

$\dfrac{\$27{,}040}{12 \text{ months}} = \$2{,}253$

$\dfrac{\$2{,}253}{550} = \$4.10$

2. $(\$1.44 + \$0.48 + \$0.27 + \$0.17 + \$4.10) = \$6.46$

   $\$6.46 \times 550 \text{ requests} = \$3{,}553$

3. $\$3{,}553 - \$1{,}800 = \$1{,}753$ per month in losses

4. Advantages: No financial loss to the facility; possible use of employee in other areas of department.

   Disadvantages: Possible loss of employee; not sure staff is qualified; loss of control of the ROI function.

5. a. $\dfrac{6{,}382}{100{,}000} = 0.6832$

   Convert to a percent: $0.6832 \times 100 = 6.382\%$

   Round to two decimals: 6.38%

   b. $\dfrac{3{,}375}{6{,}382} = 0.52883$

   Convert to a percent: $0.52883 \times 100 = 52.883\%$

   Round to two decimals: 52.88%

Exercise 9.5

1. Excel formula version:

	A	B	C
1		Community Hospital	
2		Electronic Signature System	
3		500 Physicians on staff; 489 Using the system	
4	Site	No. of Physicians Using the System at This Site	% of Physicians Using the System at This Site
5	Medicine, 2 West	54	=B5/489
6	Medicine, 2 East	62	=B6/489
7	Pediatrics, 3 West	42	=B7/489
8	Obstetrics, 1 West	12	=B8/489
9	Physician's lounge	87	=B9/489
10	HIM department	65	=B10/489
11	Personal mobile device	92	=B11/489
12	Physician home	75	=B12/489
13			

Excel calculated version:

	A	B	C	D
1	Community Hospital			
2	Electronic Signature System			
3	500 Physicians on staff; 489 Using the system			
4	Site	No. of Physicians Using the System at This Site	% of Physicians Using the System at This Site	
5	Medicine, 2 West	54	11.04%	
6	Medicine, 2 East	62	12.68%	
7	Pediatrics, 3 West	42	8.59%	
8	Obstetrics, 1 West	12	2.45%	
9	Physician's lounge	87	17.79%	
10	HIM department	65	13.29%	
11	Personal mobile device	92	18.81%	
12	Physician home	75	15.34%	
13				

2. $500 - 489 = 11$ not using the system

$$\frac{11}{500} = 0.0220$$

Convert to a percent: $0.0220 \times 100 = 2.20\%$

Round to one decimal: 2.2% are not using the system.

Exercise 9.7

1. $$\frac{9,000}{(100 \times 5)} = \frac{9,000}{500} = 18 \text{ FTEs}$$

The number of FTEs will be the total number of patients divided by the total number of records required per week (assume a 5-day work week).

2. $$\frac{65,104 \text{ records per year}}{52 \text{ weeks}} = 1,252 \text{ per week}$$

$$\frac{1,252}{5} \text{ days a week} = 250.4 \text{ more records per day}$$

$$\frac{250.4 \text{ records}}{100 \text{ records to be coded each day}} = 2.5 \text{ additional coders}$$

3. $$\frac{142,500}{20} = 7,125 \text{ lines per day}$$

$$\frac{7,125}{950} \text{ required lines} = 7.5 \text{ FTEs needed}$$

4. Excel formula version:

	A	B	C	D	E	F	G
1		Community Hospital					
2		Coding Productivity Report					
3		Coding Standard: 20 medical records per day					
4	Coding Professional	Week 1	Week 2	Week 3	Week 4	Total Records	Records per day
5	1	90	105	98	107	=SUM(B5:E5)	=F5/20
6	2	100	105	105	95	=SUM(B6:E6)	=F6/20
7	3	75	80	85	105	=SUM(B7:E7)	=F7/20
8	4	80	95	115	110	=SUM(B8:E8)	=F8/20
9							
10	Note: 4 weeks × 5 workdays per week = 20 days						
11							
12	Coder 3 is below the 20 records/day coding standard and may require assistance.						
13							

Excel calculated version:

	A	B	C	D	E	F	G	H	I	J
1		Community Hospital								
2		Coding Productivity Report								
3		Coding Standard: 20 medical records per day								
4	Coding Professional	Week 1	Week 2	Week 3	Week 4	Total Records	Records per day			
5	1	90	105	98	107	400	20			
6	2	100	105	105	95	405	20.25			
7	3	75	80	85	105	345	17.25			
8	4	80	95	115	110	400	20			
9										
10	Note: 4 weeks × 5 workdays per week = 20 days									
11										
12	Coder 3 is below the 20 records/day coding standard and may require assistance.									
13										

5. Excel formula version:

	A	B	C	D	E	F	G
1	Inpatient coding productivity calculation for September, 20XX						
2	Coding Professional	Work Output (All Records Coded)	Total Hours Worked	Average Work Output per Hour	Completed Work Percentage	Completed Work Output (Records Coded Accurately)	Completed Work per Hours Worked
3	1	400	150	2.67	0.9375	375	=F3/C3
4	2	405	150	2.7	0.9877	400	=F4/C4
5	3	345	140	1.75	0.9913	342	=F5/C5
6	4	400	140	2.86	0.95	380	=F6/C6
7							
8							

Excel calculated version:

	A	B	C	D	E	F	G
1	Inpatient coding productivity calculation for September, 20XX						
2	Coding Professional	Work Output (All Records Coded)	Total Hours Worked	Average Work Output per Hour	Completed Work Percentage	Completed Work Output (Records Coded Accurately)	Completed Work per Hours Worked
3	1	400	150	2.67	93.75%	375	2.50
4	2	405	150	2.7	98.77%	400	2.67
5	3	345	140	1.75	99.13%	342	2.44
6	4	400	140	2.86	95.00%	380	2.71
7							
8							

Exercise 9.9

1. 6.7 FTEs needed

20 minutes × 750 = 15,000 minutes

$$\frac{15,000\ minutes}{60\ minutes\ in\ an\ hour} = 250\ hours$$

$$\frac{250}{37.5}\ productive\ hours = 6.7\ FTEs\ needed$$

2. Excel formula version:

◢	A	B	C	D
1		**Community Physician's Clinic**		
2		**Coding Department**		
3		**Denials–October 20XX**		
4	**Payment source**	**Number of Claims Sent**	**Number of Denials**	**Percentage of Denials**
5	Medicare	460	43	=C5/C10
6	Medicaid	345	35	=C6/C10
7	Tricare/Military	182	14	=C7/C10
8	Commercial payers	1307	83	=C8/C10
9	Worker's Compensation	6	1	=C9/C10
10	**Total**	=SUM(B5:B9)	=SUM(C5:C9)	

Excel calculated version:

◢	A	B	C	D
1		**Community Physician's Clinic**		
2		**Coding Department**		
3		**Denials–October 20XX**		
4	**Payment Source**	**Number of Claims Sent**	**Number of Denials**	**Percentage of Denials**
5	Medicare	460	43	24.43%
6	Medicaid	345	35	19.89%
7	Tricare/Military	182	14	7.95%
8	Commercial payers	1,307	83	47.16%
9	Worker's Compensation	6	1	0.57%
10	**Total**	2,300	176	
11				

3. 264 hours

1.5 hours × 176 denials = 264 hours

4. 1.76 FTEs needed

20 work days × 7.5 hours = 150 hours available in the 20 work days

$$\frac{264 \text{ hours needed}}{150} = 1.76 \text{ FTEs needed}$$

5.

Charge-Lag Time Reason Attributed to:	Percentage of Non-Billed Claims
Physician	$\dfrac{120}{2,300} = 0.05217$ Convert to a percent: $0.05217 \times 100 = 5.217\%$ Round to two decimals: 5.22%
Coder	$\dfrac{18}{2,300} = 0.00782$ Convert to a percent: $0.00782 \times 100 = 0.782\%$ Round to two decimals: 0.78%
Business Office	$\dfrac{32}{2,300} = 0.01391$ Convert to a percent: $0.0139 \times 100 = 1.391\%$ Round to two decimals: 1.39%

Chapter 10

Exercise 10.1

1. True

2.

	A	B	C	D	E
1	Test Scores				
2	27				
3	35				
4	54				
5	56				
6	65				
7	74				
8	75				
9	76				
10	77				
11	84				
12	86				
13	88				
14	89				
15	91				
16	92				
17	93				
18	94				
19	95				
20	96				
21	97				
22	99				
23	100				
24					
25	Step 1: Sort scores in ascending order (smallest to largest).				
26	Step 2: Determine the number of scores: N = 22				
27	Step 3: Determine the rank of the score 86: 11th score				
28	Step 4: Percentile = 11/22 or 50th percentile				

3.

	A	B	C	D	E	F	G	H	I
1	Physician Number	Number of C-sections							
2	508	1							
3	710	2							
4	101	3							
5	911	4							
6	401	5							
7	202	7							
8	407	8							
9	629	9							
10	518	12							
11	944	15							
12	912	18							
13	975	20							
14	933	22							
15	303	27							
16	305	33							
17									
18	Step 1: Sort physicians by number of c-sections in ascending order (smallest to largest).								
19	Step 2: Determine the number of scores: N = 15								
20									
21	a. Which percentile is Dr. 975?								
22	Step 3: Determine the rank of Dr. 975: 12th score								
23	Step 4: Percentile = 12/15 or 80th percentile								
24									
25	b. Find the 60th percentile.								
26	Step 5: 60th percentile is the $0.60 \times 15 = 9$th observation.								
27	Step 6: The 9th observation is 12. The 60th percentile value is 12 c-sections.								

4.

	A	B	C	D	E	F	G	H	I	J	K
1	**Patient Number**	**Weight**									
2	232323	147									
3	980753	150									
4	764309	155									
5	745261	172									
6	142849	175	First quartile								
7	867342	180									
8	753254	185									
9	912356	186									
10	765497	189									
11	455656	192	Second quartile								
12	743952	195									
13	892345	196									
14	877654	207									
15	567815	209									
16	647382	222	Third quartile								
17	925627	232									
18	875408	242									
19	872345	245									
20	543465	307									
21											
22	Step 1: Sort scores in ascending order (smallest to largest).										
23	Step 2: Determine the number of scores: N = 19										
24	Step 3: Determine the second quartile or middle value.										
25	There are 19 values, so the 10th value will divide the set into two subsets of nine values each.										
26	Step 4: Determine the middle value of the top subset. There are 9 values, so the 5th value is the middle.										
27	Step 4: Determine the middle value of the bottom subset. There are 9 values, so the 5th value is the middle.										
28											

Exercise 10.3

1. The range for the data may be expressed as 18 (the difference) or as 1 to 19 (quoting the smallest and largest values); however, keep in mind that in mathematics, the range is usually expressed as one value.

2. **a.** 2 to 20 or 18

   a. 0 to 20 or 20

   b. 35 to 132 to 97

3. 2 + 20 = 22

4. 109 − 45 = 64

5. 245 − 125 = 120

Chapter 11

Exercise 11.1

1. This is an example of the nominal data or scale.

   In the nominal scale of measurement, you are only allowed to examine whether the data are equal to some particular value or to count the number of occurrences of each value. For example, gender is a nominal scale variable. You can examine whether the gender of a person is female or to count the number of males in a sample. The count of discharges is a ratio variable.

2. No.

   Temperature is an interval scale of measurement and the zero on the scale does not represent the absence of the thing being measured. Interval measurement ratios do not make sense: 80 degrees is not twice as hot as 40 degrees (although the attribute value is twice as large).

3. Yes.

   This is an example of ratio scale of measurement. There is a zero point; meaning, you can have zero patients.

4. This is an example of ordinal scale.

   Ordinal data are types of data where the values are in ordered categories. On the ordinal scale, the order of the labels is meaningful, not the label itself. This is because the intervals or distance between categories are not necessarily equal.

5. This is an example of an ordinal scale of measurement.

   Measurements with ordinal scales are ordered in the sense that higher numbers represent higher values. However, the intervals between the numbers are not necessarily equal. For example, on the five-point rating scale measuring correct information given by the clerk, the difference between a rating of 2 and a rating of 3 may not represent the same difference as the difference between a rating of 4 and a rating of 5.

Exercise 11.3

1. **a.** Table

   b. Graph

   c. Graph

   d. Table

2. Column A contains categories that are not mutually exclusive.

   For example, in which category would the data for a 30-year-old patient be grouped?

   Column B contains categories that are mutually exclusive and clearly defined.

   The categories are most suitable for continuous data when some values could include a decimal value, such as lab values or tumor size.

   Column C contains categories that are mutually exclusive and clearly defined. *However, the categories are appropriate for discrete data only (whole numbers).*

3.

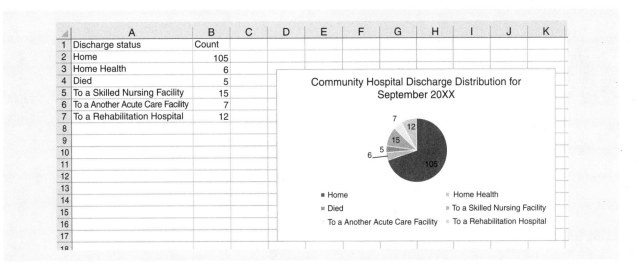

Note: use example 11.8 as a guide.

4.

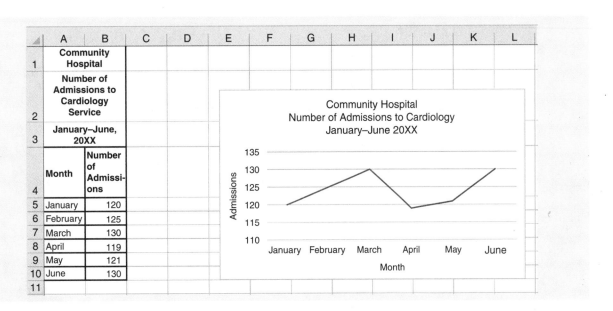

Chapter 12

Exercise 12.1

1. a

2. b

3. b

4. a

5. a

6. b

Exercise 12.3

1. g
2. f
3. d
4. c
5. b
6. a
7. e

Chapter 13

Exercise 13.1

68% C.I. = ___13.6 to 14.4___

95% C.I. = ___13.2 to 14.8___

99.7% C.I. = ___12.8 to 15.2___

To calculate these, take the mean (14) + and − the standard error of the mean for 68% C.I., and the standard error of the mean × 2 for the 95% C.I. and standard error of the mean × 3 for the 99.7% C.I.

For 68% confidence interval: 14 − 0.4 = 13.6 and 14 + 0.4 = 14.4

For 95% confidence interval: 14 − (0.4 × 2) = 14 − 0.8 = 13.2 and 14 + (0.4 × 2) = 14 + 0.8 = 14.8

For 99.7 % confidence interval: 14 − (0.4 × 3) = 14 − 1.2 = 12.8 and 14 + (0.4 × 3) = 14 + 1.2 = 15.2

Exercise 13.3

Fail to reject the null hypothesis

Index